Studies in Computational Intelligence

Volume 1124

The series "Studies in Computational Intelligence" (SCI) publishes new developments and advances in the various areas of computational intelligence—quickly and with a high quality. The intent is to cover the theory, applications, and design methods of computational intelligence, as embedded in the fields of engineering, computer science, physics and life sciences, as well as the methodologies behind them. The series contains monographs, lecture notes and edited volumes in computational intelligence spanning the areas of neural networks, connectionist systems, genetic algorithms, evolutionary computation, artificial intelligence, cellular automata, self-organizing systems, soft computing, fuzzy systems, and hybrid intelligent systems. Of particular value to both the contributors and the readership are the short publication timeframe and the world-wide distribution, which enable both wide and rapid dissemination of research output.

Indexed by SCOPUS, DBLP, WTI Frankfurt eG, zbMATH, SCImago.

All books published in the series are submitted for consideration in Web of Science.

Hazrat Ali · Mubashir Husain Rehmani ·
Zubair Shah
Editors

Advances in Deep Generative Models for Medical Artificial Intelligence

Springer

Editors
Hazrat Ali
College of Science and Engineering
Hamad Bin Khalifa University
Doha, Qatar

Mubashir Husain Rehmani
Department of Computer Science
Munster Technological University
Bishopstown, Cork, Ireland

Zubair Shah
College of Science and Engineering
Hamad Bin Khalifa University
Doha, Qatar

ISSN 1860-949X ISSN 1860-9503 (electronic)
Studies in Computational Intelligence
ISBN 978-3-031-46340-2 ISBN 978-3-031-46341-9 (eBook)
https://doi.org/10.1007/978-3-031-46341-9

This Springer imprint is published by the registered company Springer Nature Switzerland AG
The registered company address is: Gewerbestrasse 11, 6330 Cham, Switzerland

Paper in this product is recyclable.

Preface

The popularity of research on deep learning and artificial intelligence (AI) in computer-aided diagnosis and healthcare data is rising. Many new methods are being developed, and applications of existing models for many new tasks are being explored. For example, in the medical imaging, there has been rapid growth in deep learning methods for tumor detection, cancer diagnosis, pneumonia detection, COVID-19 detection, etc. Similarly, many studies are being published on deep learning for disease prognosis and precision medicine. However, deep learning methods for medical decision-making suffer poor generalization, particularly due to a lack of data on new tasks or due to a lack of diversity in the data. The latter phenomenon is also subjective to image acquisition as imaging standards may vary even for the same domain due to differences in equipment, manufacturers' specifications, geographical origin, etc.

Deep generative models such as generative adversarial networks (GANs), autoencoders, and neural diffusion models have the potential to learn the distribution of real data and augment the data by synthesis. While these models have been popular for generating synthetic medical image data, there has been an increasing interest in developing these models for other applications such as segmentation, diagnosis, and super-resolution. Besides, with the recent successful applications of diffusion models for the synthesis of art images (the now famous DALL-E 2 framework that uses diffusion models), it is expected to gain more insights into medical image data. Consequently, there is a rapid influx of new architectures for applications in medical imaging and healthcare data. Hence, there is a dire need to present the recent advancements and new generative AI methods for healthcare data.

This book highlights the recent advancements in generative artificial intelligence for medical and healthcare applications, using medical imaging and clinical and electronic health records data. The book presents the concepts and applications of deep learning-based AI methods such as GANs, convolutional neural networks (CNNs), and vision transformers (ViTs) in a comprehensive way.

Below, we present the summary and organization of the book.

Chapter "Deep Learning Techniques for 3D-Volumetric Segmentation of Biomedical Images" comprehensively reviews deep learning-based AI methods for 3D volumetric segmentation of medical images. It includes evaluating the performance of deep learning models based on their backbone network and task formulation. Various convolutional neural networks and GANs-based approaches reported in the scientific literature are discussed. Additionally, the techniques are categorized into semantic, instance, and panoptic tasks for volumetric medical image segmentation. The majority of AI methods employ CNN architectures as the backbone network for medical image segmentation models. However, there have been research efforts that explore GAN-based approaches in segmentation frameworks. For instance, GAN-based models have demonstrated superior performance in semantic segmentation tasks involving volumetric data from human brain MRI. Conversely, some studies have found that CNN-based methods like RDC-Net outperformed GAN-based approaches in the segmentation task of nuclei. Read the full chapter to find out the in-depth discussion of these advancements in generative AI models concerning medical image segmentation tasks.

Chapter "Analysis of GAN-Based Data Augmentation for GI-Tract Disease Classification" presents GANs-based approaches for the augmentation of image data of gastrointestinal (GI) disorders. GI disorders are a significant problem for the human digestive system. GI disorders are on the rise worldwide. Before the onset of symptoms, routine screening for patients at average risk can help with early identification and treatment. CNN models have been used by automated systems to help with GI disorder identification. A hurdle in the field of medical imaging is the requirement for a sizeable amount of annotated data to increase the results' quality. Furthermore, the class imbalance exacerbates the problem and adds bias toward classes with more images. In this connection, the study in this chapter makes use of GAN-based data augmentation and geometric transformation-based data augmentation for the classification of GI tract disorders. The results in the chapter suggest that GAN-based data augmentation prevents the classification model from being overly tailored to the dominant class. Additionally, training with this enriched data improves performance across classes by regularizing training.

Chapter "Deep Generative Adversarial Network-Based MRI Slices Reconstruction and Enhancement for Alzheimer's Stages Classification" presents a GAN-based approach for enhancing and reconstructing brain magnetic resonance imaging (MRI) that helps in Alzheimer's disease (AD) classification. AD is a neurodegenerative brain disorder that leads to a steady decline in brain function and the death of brain cells. AD condition causes dementia, which cannot be treated. Deep learning has quickly become an effective choice for analyzing MRI images in recent times. However, they often require a significant amount of training data, and medical data is frequently unavailable. In this connection, the study explores the use of GAN-based methods to enhance and reconstruct brain MRI data. The study presents an implementation of a Vanilla-GAN model for enhancing and reconstructing brain MRI. After generating the enhanced images, the study performs a classification task to identify the stages of Alzheimer's. Experiments are reported for the dataset collected by the Alzheimer's Disease Neuroimaging Initiative. Results reported in the study show that GAN frameworks can enhance both the performance of AD classification and the quality of images.

Chapter "Evaluating the Quality and Diversity of DCGAN-Based Generatively Synthesized Diabetic Retinopathy Imagery" presents a GAN-based approach for the synthesis of diabetic retinopathy (DR) images to address the problem of data imbalance for DR images. The publicly available datasets for DR are imbalanced that contain limited samples of images with DR. The data imbalance causes challenges to the training of a machine learning classifier and leads to model overfitting. The impact of this imbalance is exacerbated as the severity of the DR stage increases, affecting the classifiers' diagnostic capacity. The study explores addressing the data imbalance problem using GANs to augment the datasets with synthetic images. Generating synthetic images is advantageous if high-quality and diverse images are produced. To evaluate the quality and diversity of synthetic images, several evaluation metrics, such as Multi-Scale Structural Similarity Index (MS-SSIM), Cosine Distance (CD), and Fréchet Inception Distance (FID), are used. Understanding the effectiveness of each metric in evaluating the quality and diversity of synthetic images is critical to select images for augmentation. This chapter provides an empirical assessment of these evaluation metrics as applied to synthetic Proliferative DR imagery generated by a deep convolutional GAN (DCGAN). Furthermore, the metrics' capacity to indicate the quality and diversity of synthetic images and their correlation with classifier performance are also examined. This enables a quantitative selection of synthetic imagery and an informed augmentation strategy.

Chapter "Deep Learning Approaches for End-to-End Modeling of Medical Spatiotemporal Data" presents an overview of different medical applications of spatiotemporal DL for prognostic and diagnostic predictive tasks. For many medical applications, a single, stationary image may not be sufficient for detecting subtle pathology. Advancements in fields such as computer vision and deep learning have produced robust techniques able to learn complex interactions between space and time for prediction effectively. The chapter explores different deep learning approaches in computer vision that can be adapted to spatiotemporal medical data. While many techniques in the medical AI domain draw knowledge from previous work in other domains, adaptation to medical data brings unique challenges due to the complex nature of the data. Spatiotemporal deep learning provides unique opportunities to incorporate information about functional dynamics into prediction, which could be vital in many medical applications. Current medical applications of spatiotemporal deep learning have demonstrated the potential of these models, and recent advancements make this space poised to produce the state-of-the-art models for many medical applications.

Chapter "Skin Cancer Classification with Convolutional Deep Neural Networks and Vision Transformers Using Transfer Learning" presents a ViT-based method for skin cancer classification. The deadliest type of skin cancer is melanoma. Melanocytes are the cells where cancerous growths take place. The cells create melanin pigment, which gives skin its color. Sun exposure to bodily parts is the primary cause of cancer. The formation of a new pigment, changes to an existing mole, and unusual growth on the skin are all indicators of malignancy. Early detection and treatment of skin cancer helps in achieving better survival rates. A melanoma patient who has had malignant (cancerous) tissue removed can recover when the disease is still in its early stages. Malignant (non-cancerous) tumors frequently form in melanocytes. These benign tumors resemble melanoma in many ways and take the shape of moles (nevi). It might be challenging for doctors to distinguish benign tumors from melanoma. The study explores using CNNs and ViT to perform skin cancer classification tasks. It utilizes a pre-trained ViT model. The results show that EfficientNet-B3 performed best as compared to other CNN models and ViT with the same input image resolution of 224×224 and top layers configuration.

Chapter "A New CNN-Based Deep Learning Model Approach for Skin Cancer Detection and Classification" explores the use of CNNs for the diagnosis of basal cell carcinoma (BCC), a type of skin cancer caused by direct exposure to ultraviolet radiation. Depending on environmental or genetic factors, skin abrasions and tumors may occur. BCC and actinic keratosis (Akiec) are the most common of these tumors. BCC and Akiec species can be found anywhere on the skin, most commonly seen in the areas exposed to direct sunlight, such as the head and neck. Although the risk of metastasis in BCCs is low, if not diagnosed and treated, they can grow aggressively and even cause loss of tissue. When diagnosing BCCs, they can often be confused with a similar species, Akiecs. The study presents a deep learning pipeline using CNN to diagnose BCC. The pipeline is implemented in three steps. In the first step, the input images are evaluated in different color spaces in order to determine in which color space the lesion regions are more prominent. In the second step, Geodesic Active Contour (GAC), Chan and Vese (C-V), Selective Binary and Gaussian Filtering Regularized Level Set (SBGFRLS), and Online Region Active Contour (ORACM) methods are used to segment the ROI regions from the images. The best results in the first two steps are obtained with the C-V segmentation method in the HSV color space. In the last step, the obtained images are classified with the CNN-based MatConvNet-1.0-beta15 architecture. As a result of classification, accuracy and F1-score are reported.

Chapter "Machine Learning Based Miscellaneous Objects Detection with Application to Cancer Images" presents an adaptive boosting algorithm for the detection of objects of interest in medical images. With the technological developments in artificial intelligence, traditional machine learning methods and recently deep convolutional neural networks (DCNNs) have accomplished great success in several vision-related tasks. For example, object detection, object classification or recognition, and image segmentation are effectively achieved with the aid of the aforementioned technologies. Training an effective DCNN model needs a large amount of diverse and balanced data. However, the DCNNs are quite often constrained by several aspects, such as (i) data annotation cost, (ii) long-tailed dispersal of data or imbalanced data, and (iii) scarcity of relevant data. Moreover, these days generative adversarial networks (GANs) are widely used in image generation and synthesis-related tasks. Object detection, being an important but challenging problem in the field of image processing and computer vision, plays an important role in several applications. While different methods exist to detect objects that appear in an image, a detailed analysis regarding common object detection is still lacking. This chapter pertains to detecting objects that appear in an image with complex backgrounds using the adaptive boosting algorithm (ABA). Different from several previously published chapters or research articles that focus on the detection of six different objects, such as ships, vehicles, faces, or eyes on standard datasets, this chapter focuses on real-life objects, which include: (i) melanoma (actual malignant melanoma, nevus spilus, and blue nevus), (ii) license plates, (iii) vehicles, (iv) pedestrians, (v) players, and (vi) football. The ABA is applied on 8,525 test images, which include: 251 melanoma, 2512 license plates, 2400 vehicles, 2502 pedestrians, 590 players/sportsmen, and 270 football images. The chapter also analyzes the challenges of the current study while investigating several real-life objects' images and proposes a promising research direction, namely supervised learning cloud-based object detection.

Finally, Chapter "Advanced Deep Learning for Heart Sounds Classification" presents the applications of CNNs and ViTs to spectrogram data to help in the detection of abnormal patterns in heart sounds. Globally, cardiovascular diseases (CVDs) constitute the leading cause of death. A heart murmur is a frequently encountered anomaly that can be detected during the process of auscultation, which involves listening to the sounds produced by the heart. Recent research has focused on identifying representative features and patterns from heart signals to precisely detect abnormal heart sounds. Short-time Fourier transforms (STFT)-based spectrograms have gained attention as a means to learn characteristic patterns of normal and abnormal phonocardiogram (PCG) signals. In this study, authors investigated the use of advanced deep learning models, such as CNNs, convolutional autoencoders (CAEs), ViTs, and transfer learning techniques, for identifying abnormal patterns in spectrograms derived from PCGs. The PhysioNet/CinC and PASCAL challenges datasets were used for training and testing the deep learning models. Transfer learning was found to be a highly effective approach, achieving high accuracy and precision in all four approaches. ViTs and CAEs performed equally well. The bespoke CNN model employed in this study was less complex and lighter than previous competing research, yet it outperformed them with relatively excellent classification precision and accuracy, making it an appropriate tool for using PCG data to screen for abnormal heart sounds. By employing the transfer learning technique, spectrogram detection achieved noteworthy performance with respect to accuracy, F1-scores, sensitivity, specificity, and precision.

Primary audience: Computer science researchers and graduate students working in artificial intelligence and deep learning and interested in studying the potential of medical artificial intelligence. Basic knowledge of medical imaging and computer-aided diagnosis will be helpful for the readers to understand the applications and the challenges related to healthcare data (such as privacy, data scarcity, and complexity), as discussed in the book.

Secondary audience: Healthcare informatics and medical imaging researchers, as well as professionals interested in studying recent developments in the use of deep generative models to address challenges such as data scarcity, super-resolution, diagnosis, and prognosis using medical AI. Some prior knowledge of computer science algorithms and artificial intelligence will be helpful in understanding the concepts presented in the book.

Doha, Qatar Hazrat Ali
Bishopstown, Cork, Ireland Mubashir Husain Rehmani
Doha, Qatar Zubair Shah

Acknowledgements

We, the editors, thank all the chapter authors for their hard work in preparing their chapters. We are also thankful to the reviewers who helped us in reviewing the book chapters on time. Their feedback and comments have greatly improved the overall quality of the book.

We thank the leadership of the College of Science and Engineering, Hamad Bin Khalifa University, Qatar, for supporting us to work on this book.

Finally, we would like to thank our families for their unwavering patience and support throughout completing this book. Their encouragement provided the emotional strength to persevere through long hours preparing, reviewing, and editing this book.

Hazrat Ali
Mubashir Husain Rehmani
Zubair Shah

Contents

About the Editors

Hazrat Ali (SM'21, AFHEA) is a researcher at Hamad Bin Khalifa University, Qatar. His research interests lie in generative artificial intelligence, medical artificial intelligence, medical imaging, and speech and image processing. He is a senior member of IEEE and an associate editor at *IEEE Access* and *IET Signal Processing journals*. He has served as a reviewer at *Nature Scientific Reports*, *IEEE Transactions on Artificial Intelligence*, *IEEE Transactions on Neural Networks and Learning Systems*, *IEEE Transactions on Medical Imaging*, *Machine Learning for Health Symposium*, *IEEE IJCNN*, and many other reputed journals and conferences. He has published more than 70 peer-reviewed conference and journal papers. His research is featured in international media, including Quanta Magazine and the European Society of Radiology AI blog. He was selected as a young researcher at the 5th Heidelberg Laureate Forum, Heidelberg, Germany. He is the recipient of the 2021 best researcher award by COMSATS University, the HEC start-up research grant, the top 10 research pitch award by the University of Queensland, Australia, HEC, and the Erasmus Mundus STRoNGTiES research grant.

Mubashir Husain Rehmani (M'14-SM'15, SFHEA) received the B.Eng. degree in computer systems engineering from Mehran University of Engineering and Technology, Jamshoro, Pakistan, in 2004; the M.S. degree from the University of Paris XI, Paris, France, in 2008; and the Ph.D. degree from the University Pierre and Marie Curie, Paris, in 2011. He is currently working as a lecturer at the Department of Computer Science, Munster Technological University (MTU), Ireland. Prior to this, he worked as a postdoctoral researcher at the Telecommunications Software and Systems Group (TSSG), Waterford Institute of Technology (WIT), Waterford, Ireland. He also served for five years as an assistant professor at COMSATS Institute of Information Technology, Wah Cantt., Pakistan. He is serving as an editorial board member of *Nature Scientific Reports*. He is currently an area editor of the *IEEE Communications Surveys and Tutorials*. He served for three years (from 2015 to 2017) as an associate editor of the *IEEE Communications Surveys and Tutorials*. He served as a column editor for Book Reviews in *IEEE Communications Magazine*. He is appointed as an associate editor for *IEEE Transactions on Green*

Communication and Networking. Currently, he serves as an associate editor of *IEEE Communications Magazine*, Elsevier *Journal of Network and Computer Applications (JNCA)*, and the *Journal of Communications and Networks (JCN)*. He is also serving as a guest editor of Elsevier *Ad Hoc Networks journal*, Elsevier *Future Generation Computer Systems journal*, the *IEEE Transactions on Industrial Informatics*, and Elsevier *Pervasive and Mobile Computing journal*. He has authored/edited total eight books: two books with Springer, two books published by IGI Global, USA, three books published by CRC Press—Taylor and Francis Group, UK, and one book with Wiley, UK He received "Best Researcher of the Year 2015 of COMSATS Wah" award in 2015. He received the certificate of appreciation, "Exemplary Editor of the IEEE Communications Surveys and Tutorials for the year 2015" from the IEEE Communications Society. He received Best Paper Award from IEEE ComSoc Technical Committee on Communications Systems Integration and Modeling (CSIM), in IEEE ICC 2017. He consecutively received research productivity award in 2016–17 and also ranked # 1 in all engineering disciplines from Pakistan Council for Science and Technology (PCST), Government of Pakistan. He received Best Paper Award in 2017 from Higher Education Commission (HEC), Government of Pakistan. He is the recipient of Best Paper Award in 2018 from Elsevier *Journal of Network and Computer Applications*. He is the recipient of Highly Cited Researcher™ award thrice in 2020, 2021, and 2022 by Clarivate, USA. His performance in this context features in the top 1% by citations in the field of Computer Science and Crossfield in the Web of Science™ citation index. He is the only researcher from Ireland in the field of "Computer Science" who received this International prestigious award. In October 2022, he received Science Foundation Ireland's CONNECT Centre's Education and Public Engagement (EPE) Award 2022 for his research outreach work and being a spokesperson for achieving a work-life balance for a career in research.

Zubair Shah is an assistant professor at the Division of ICT, College of Science and Engineering, Hamad Bin Khalifa University, Qatar, where he leads the health informatics research group. Dr. Shah received an M.S. degree in Computer System Engineering from Politecnico di Milano, Italy, and a Ph.D. degree from the University of New South Wales, Australia. He was a research fellow from 2017 to 2019 at the Australian Institute of Health Innovation, Macquarie University, Australia. Dr. Shah's expertise is in the field of artificial intelligence and big data analytics and their application to health informatics. His research is focused on health informatics, particularly in relation to public health, using social media data (e.g., Twitter) and news sources to identify patterns indicative of population-level health. He has published his work in various A-tier international journals and conferences, including *Nature Scientific Reports*, *IEEE Transactions on Big Data*, and *Journal of Medical Informatics*.

Deep Learning Techniques for 3D-Volumetric Segmentation of Biomedical Images

Sikandar Afridi, Muhammad Irfan Khattak, Muhammad Abeer Irfan, Atif Jan, and Muhammad Asif

Abstract A thorough review of deep learning (DL) methods for the 3D-Volumetric segmentation of biomedical images is presented in this chapter. The performance of these deep learning methods for 3D-Volumetric segmentation of biomedical images has been assessed by the classification of these methods into tasks. We have devised two main categories, i.e., the backbone network and the task formulation. We have categorized various methods based on the backbone network into a convolutional neural network (CNN)-based and generative adversarial network (GAN)-based. These techniques are further divided into the semantic, instance, and panoptic tasks for the 3D-Volumetric segmentation of biomedical images based on the task formulation. The majority of the most prominent deep learning architectures used to segment biomedical images employ CNNs as their standard backbone network. In this field, 3D networks and architectures have been developed and put into use to fully take advantage of the contextual information in the spatial dimension of 3D biomedical images. Because of the advancements in deep generative models, various GAN-based models have been designed and implemented by the research community to address the challenging task of biomedical image segmentation. The challenges are addressed, and recommendations are provided for future studies in the domain of DL methods for 3D-Volumetric segmentation of biomedical images at the conclusion of

S. Afridi (✉) · M. I. Khattak · A. Jan
Department of Electrical Engineering, University of Engineering and Technology, Peshawar, Pakistan
e-mail: 13mseesafridi@seecs.edu.pk

M. I. Khattak
e-mail: m.i.khattak@uetpeshawar.edu.pk

A. Jan
e-mail: atifjan@uetpeshawar.edu.pk

M. A. Irfan
Department of Computer Systems Engineering, University of Engineering and Technology, Peshawar, Pakistan
e-mail: abeer.irfan@uetpeshawar.edu.pk

M. Asif
Department of Electrical Engineering, University of Science and Technology, Bannu, Pakistan
e-mail: masifeed@ustb.edu.pk

H. Ali et al. (eds.), *Advances in Deep Generative Models for Medical Artificial Intelligence*, Studies in Computational Intelligence 1124,
https://doi.org/10.1007/978-3-031-46341-9_1

the study. The non-local U-Net based on CNN outperforms the GAN-based FM-GAN with a Dice Similarity Coefficient (DSC) of 89% for 3D-Volumetric semantic segmentation of 6-month infant Magnetic Resonance Imaging (MRI) on the iSeg dataset. The GAN-based model MM-GAN performs better than the best CNN-based model 3D FCN with multiscale for the 3D-Volumetric semantic segmentation of the human brain, obtaining a DSC of 89.90% and 86.00% for the whole tumor (WT), respectively on the BRATS 17 dataset. For 3D-Volumetric segmentation of nuclei, RDC-Net outperforms the best GAN-based model SpCycleGAN with average precision (AP) values of 99.40% and 93.47%, respectively.

1 Introduction

To perform non-invasive diagnostic procedures, medical imaging is one of the most vital and significant components of healthcare systems nowadays [1]. Medical imaging represents visually and functionally the interior and different human organs to be analyzed for clinical purposes. Medical images have different types, such as MRI, Ultrasound Imaging (US), Computed Tomography (CT), X-ray imaging, Optical Coherence Tomography (OCT), and Microscopic Images. Besides these imaging techniques, the use of medical images has increased to diagnose various conditions or diseases [2], such as skin diseases, heart diseases, different kinds of tumors, brain tumors, etc.

Medical imaging and its analysis have been playing a vital role in basic medical studies and different clinical treatments such as data management for medical records [3], biomedical medical robotics, image-based applications [4], and computer-aided diagnosis (CADx) [5]. It guides medical professionals to analyze and understand various diseases and clinical issues with better accuracy to enhance healthcare systems. As a result, there have been significant developments in the designing of models and algorithms for biomedical image processing; hence, automated image analysis and different evaluation algorithms used for the extraction of useful information have been developed. Segmentation is the basic step for automated image analysis. It divides the image into distinct regions depending on its visual appearance, such that each region has a semantic meaning for the given task [6]. Clear segmentation of images with distinguishable regions is very important for biomedical image analysis, which may include learning the similarity levels of texture or thickness of the layers [7]. In order to be understood and analyzed with ease, 3D biomedical images are segmented to change and simplify their representation.

Semantic segmentation, instance segmentation, and panoptic segmentation are the three main types of image segmentation tasks. The focus of instance segmentation is on individual differences, whereas the focus of semantic segmentation is on differences between categories. For instance, the semantic segmentation task only separates the categories, i.e., teeth, jaws, and background, in the CT image and does not distinguish the individuals in each of the categories, as shown in Fig. 1. However, instance segmentation distinguishes the individuals in each category of teeth or jaw by

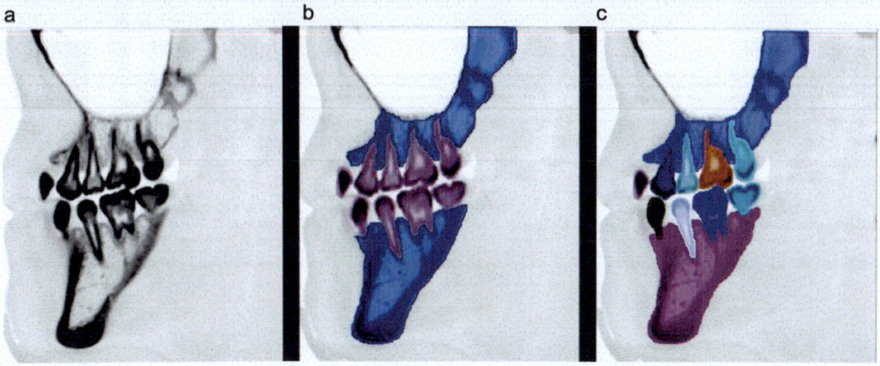

Fig. 1 Teeth segmentation (**a**) The actual image. **b** Semantic segmentation segments actual image into different categories (teeth, jaws, and background) by assigning labels to each category only. **c** Instance segmentation assigns labels to different categories as well as to each instance in the same class

assigning labels to the category as well as the instance of the class. When performing an image segmentation task, panoptic segmentation combines the predictions from the instance and semantic segmentation into a broad, unified output [1].

Due to limitations, such as manually designing the features, the traditional image segmentation algorithms are very challenging to apply directly to complex scenes directly [8]. Being among the most promising branches of machine learning (ML), DL has the capability to process raw data. Hence, the need to design features manually is eliminated [6]. The segmentation of medical images is now more effective and efficient because of advancements in DL in the past few years [9]. Because of developments in the learning algorithms and the availability of faster CPUs and GPUs, the training time and execution time have been largely reduced, and larger datasets can be accessed with ease [10]. Hence, DL methods have been effectively applied to segment biomedical images.

In recent years, convolutional neural networks (CNNs) have been among the most promising DL approaches in various areas of research, such as computer vision [11–14] and medical image computing [15–18], for the task of image recognition and classification. Due to their outstanding practical and theoretical segmentation capabilities, CNNs have already established themselves as a standard for image segmentation problems and can be very useful tools to segment biomedical images [19]. In addition to CNNs, GANs have been a significant breakthrough in deep learning networks and have been proven to be applicable for the 3D-Volumetric segmentation of biomedical images [20–22]. GANs are a different kind of neural network than traditional neural networks, where two different networks, i.e., generators and discriminators, are concurrently trained [23]. The generator tends to predict a perfect feature map of the original image to deceive the discriminator. Meanwhile, the discriminator tends to differentiate between actual and fake images. These two models work in a game-theoretic manner [24].

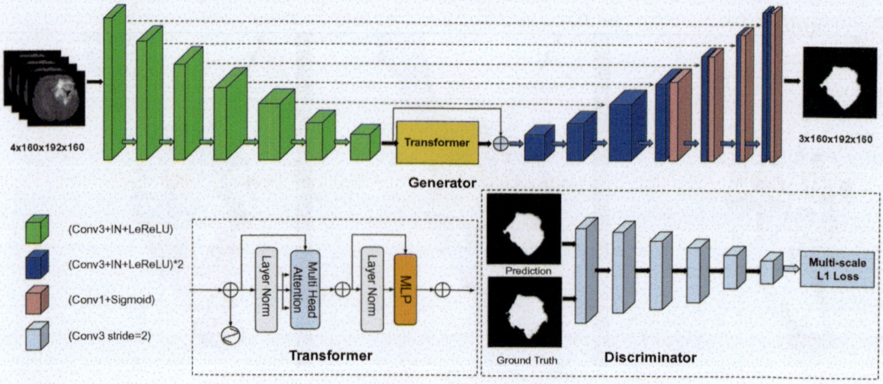

Fig. 2 GAN-based 3D-volumetric segmentation model

An architectural overview of the GAN-based 3D volumetric segmentation model is presented in Fig. 2. The GAN-based framework consists of two modules: a generator module and a discriminator module, both trained in a game-theoretic max-min game process for 3D-Volumetric Brian tumor segmentation using multi-modalities MRI [25]. Figure 2 depicts the generator's U-shaped transformer-based architecture with an encoder-decoder. In order to produce high-dimensional semantic features, a down-sampling encoder based on 3D CNN is used with a contracting path having seven spatial layers. Brain tumor images are cropped to form random patches in four channels with a patch size of $160 \times 192 \times 160$ voxels. These patches are then followed by the ($3\times3\times3$) down-sampling 3D convolution layers and a stride set to 2. Every convolution operation is followed by instance normalization (IN) and a leakyReLU activation operation. Normalization, activation layers, and dropout layers follow the two unbiased layers of convolution with a size of ($3\times3\times3$). A ResNet-based transformer module is used at the bottom of the encoder to estimate the global long-distance dependencies and ensure the flow of the semantic information [26]. Each layer of the transformer is composed of a Multi-Head Attention (MHA) block, a layer normalization (LN), and a feed-forward network (FFN). Spatial relations at each stage in long-range and short-range, which the encoder extracts, can flow blue to the decoder via the skip connections.

The decoder performs 3D transpose convolution of the size $2 \times 2 \times 2$, unlike the encoder for up-sampling. As shown in Fig. 2, skip connections are followed by a couple of 3D convolution layers of size ($3 \times 3 \times 3$). Interpolation is performed at the first up-sampling layer, while deconvolution is performed at the remaining up-sampling layers with a stride set to 2. Deep supervision is used to ensure improved gradient flow and improved supervision performance [27], which calculates the loss function with the help of the last three levels of decoders. The ground truth is down-sampled to the same resolution as the outputs to calculate an aggregated sum of the loss function at individual levels. The discriminator has an architecture similar to the encoder of the generator, which extracts feature maps hierarchically independent of the ground truth and the prediction in order to calculate the L1 loss with multi-scale. Six similar blocks compose the discriminator, each consisting of convolution layers of size (3×3×3) voxels and a stride of 2, a batch normalization, and an activation layer composed of leakyReLU. In order to find the difference between the prediction and the ground truth, the discriminator uses their L1 norm distance.

Despite extensive research being done to develop DL algorithms for 3D-Volumetric segmentation of biological images, no evidence of a survey in this area has been found [4, 5, 28]. This chapter provides a survey of 3D-Volumetric biomedical image segmentation architectures to assist the research community in selecting an appropriate DL-based segmentation technique and architecture based on the following criteria: (1) To use either a 2D-DL with multiple slices-based approaches or a 3D-DL end-to-end volumetric approach for the selected architecture to perform the desired 3D-Volumetric biomedical image segmentation task. (2) To use either semantic, instance, or panoptic segmentation after choosing one of the approaches in the above two considerations. (3) To segment 3D-Volumetric biomedical images using either the CNN-based or GAN-based DL approach.

2 Deep Learning for 3D-Volumetric Segmentation of Biomedical Images

In medical image computing, a major portion of medical imaging modalities, i.e., CT, MRI, etc., comprise volumetric data. DL architectures have been initially designed for operations with 2D data or images as an input, hence 2D data such as the segmentation of a 3D CT image as a 2D sectional image, i.e., a slice at once. Furthermore, data analysis is usually needed, even in a higher dimension from a temporal series, for volumetric diagnosis. To provide aid and quantitative measurements to surgical procedures, the segmentation of volumetric images has a very important role in CADx in clinical practices.

For instance, to identify and analyze the complete context of an anatomical structure accurately, all the views of the CT volumes need to be studied. Anatomical borders are usually discernible by very fine changes in shape or texture; however, they are not easily visible in the case of two consecutive 2D slices [29]. Addressing these limitations, different approaches have been proposed to design architecture in a 2.5D style [30] or with multiple 2D patches around the segmentation target that analyze at the same time all three views of 3D biomedical images [31]. Studies on 3D biomedical image segmentation have exploded most recently, driven by the need for 3D-Volumetric biomedical image segmentation, the ease with which neural network architectures adjust to variations in the dimensions, and the increased processing capacity of GPUs. Due to the huge memory footprints of 3D biomedical images, such as CT volumes, attempts to leverage the full resolution are still challenging and cause bottlenecks such as high dimensionality, high model complexity, a large number of parameters, issues with overfitting, and long training times for volumetric

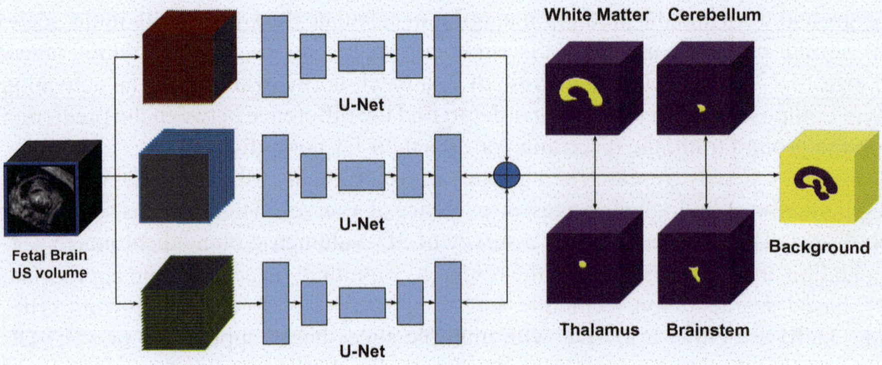

Fig. 3 U-net based 2D CNN for 3D-volumetric segmentation for fetal brain ultrasound

image segmentation. Despite these challenges, the 3D context in biomedical images can be accessed by processing the raw image volumes in a slab-wise or block-wise fashion [32]. Also, the approaches widely used for segmentation and instance detection of 2D biomedical images [33, 34] have powerful architectures and therefore can be translated with ease to 3D by designing the region proposal layer, but this is a memory-intensive approach, and the training time can be challenging.

CNNs developed for the segmentation of volumetric data can be categorized as follows: the first category includes an improved 2D CNN model that uses orthogonal planes (i.e., sagittal, axial, and coronal) or aggregated neighboring slices as inputs to obtain complementary spatial information [35]. However, these approaches fall short in their ability to fully exploit the contextual data, making them unable to carry out precise volumetric segmentation. The second category of CNNs, known as 3D CNNs, has been developed with an impressive performance in order to extract sufficient contextual information from volumetric data for volumetric segmentation [36]. End-to-end volumetric segmentation is performed by 3D CNNs that utilize the entire volume as an input rather than adjacent slices. However, these approaches have their own drawbacks, such as the limited representation capabilities achieved by using shallow depth or issues of optimization degradation caused if the network depth is increased [36].

A performance comparison of 2D U-Net architecture and its 3D version V-Net is carried out by [37]. 2D slices of 3D fetal brain ultrasound are fed to the 2D U-Net and, at the output, give the segmentation map of every slice, which is then stacked to perform the full 3D segmentation as shown in Fig. 3. The volume is sliced in three different ways so that contextual information from other views can also be incorporated [38]. A soft segmentation mask is predicted at the output of each 2D network, with a value for every voxel between 0 and 1 in every structure that corresponds to the network's confidence. In the final step, the output is aggregated from every network to exploit the information to segment in 3D. Being a 3D variant, V-Net replaces all 2D operations of 2D U-Net with 3D operations and segments the 3D fetal brain ultrasound volume as illustrated in Fig. 4.

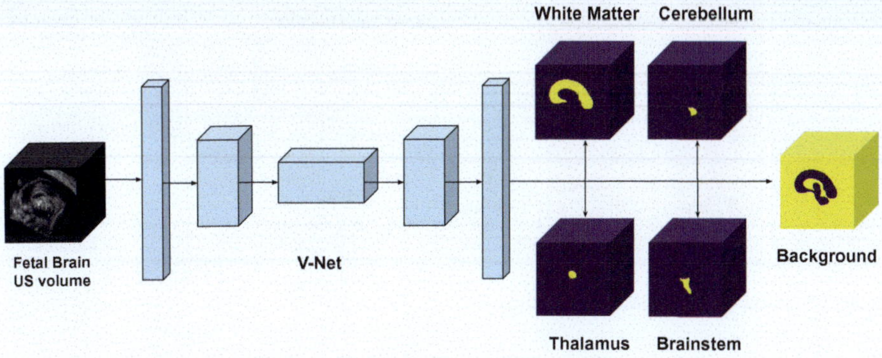

Fig. 4 V-net based 3D CNN for 3D-volumetric segmentation for fetal brain ultrasound

According to the quantitative results, V-Net outperforms the 2D U-Net architecture for 3D fetal brain ultrasound by more than a 22% increase in the DSC for every brain structure using the INTERGROWTH-21 study dataset for ultrasounds. This performance increase is because the segmented brain structures share anatomical boundaries as they are spatially close to each other. It means that they share common features that can be used to segment them. To compare the 2D U-Net in terms of complexity with the 3D U-Net, the GPU's performance was tested using a dataset of 80 3D CT images for organ segmentation in an independent study by [39]. The GPU savings of 2D U-Net are more than sixfold in the training and more than fivefold in the model application. The 2D U-Net is exactly 40 s, or 7% faster on average.

3 CNN-Based Algorithms for 3D-Volumetric Segmentation of Biomedical Images

CNN-based algorithms can be divided into semantic, instance, and panoptic tasks for the 3D-Volumetric segmentation of biomedical images based on the task formulation. An overview of CNN-based algorithms for 3D-Volumetric segmentation of biomedical images is presented in Fig. 5.

3.1 Algorithms for 3D-Volumetric Semantic Segmentation of Biomedical Images

In recent years, **3D fully convoluted network (FCN)** has emerged as one of the most feasible methods to make voxel-wise predictions using dense network architecture for volumetric images. 2D FCN is not always optimal to localize and segment the

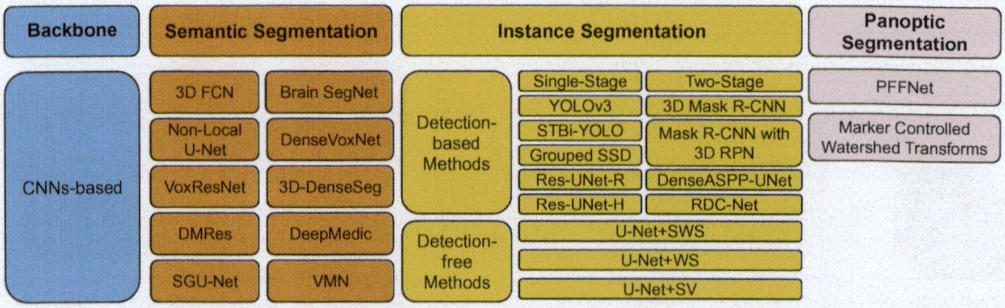

Fig. 5 Overview of CNN-based algorithms

most common type of volumetric data in medical image computing because of the consideration of limited spatial information [13]. In order to segment intervertebral discs (IVDs) using volumetric data, i.e., 3D MRI, an extended 3D variant of 2D FCN is implemented to generate voxel-wise predictions with end-to-end learning and interference and evaluated on the 3D MRI data of the MICCAI 2015 Challenge on Automatic Intervertebral Disc Localization and Segmentation. The main architectural advancement consists of replacing the 2D convolution, max-pooling, and up-sampling layers with their 3D versions. Results show that 3D FCN achieves increased localization and segmentation accuracy compared to 2D FCN. 3D FCN achieves a 94.3% success rate for detection with a 2.9% improvement 88.4% DSC for segmentation with a 5.2% improvement over 2D FCN. It shows the importance of volumetric information to carry out 3D localization and segmentation [40].

An earlier version of 3D FCN, a multiscale loss function-based 3D FCN, combined higher resolution features with initial lower resolution features to perform the task of segmentation [41]. The following main challenges exist to segment the brain tumor: context modelling for both the image and the label domains, the problem of MRI being qualitative in nature, and the issue of the class imbalance that persists in the analysis of biomedical images. Appreciated results were obtained during testing with the Brain Tumor Segmentation (BraTS) 2017 challenge, with DSC of 71%, 86%, and 78.3% for the enhanced tumor (ET), WT, and core tumor (CT), respectively [41].

Another variant of 3D FCN is used for CT-based 3D segmentation of liver tumors with a novel level-set method (LSM) [42, 43]. In order to refine the liver segmentation and tumor localization, the 3D FCN is used. To improve the previously implemented 3D FCN-based tumor segmentation, a novel LSM using the probabilistic distribution of fuzzy c-means clustering for liver tumors and an enhanced object indication function is used. The proposed 3D FCN with LSM outperforms the conventional 3D FCN by 5.69% improvement in the average DSC and 12.19% improvement in the minimum DSC for the liver CT image segmentation challenge in the 2019 international symposium on Image Computing and Digital Medicine [44].

A **cascaded 3D FCN** architecture is applied to resolve the issue of multi-organ and blood vessel segmentation [45]. To overcome segmentation inaccuracies around the boundaries, a coarse-to-fine approach is used, where a two-stage cascaded 3D FCN reduces the voxels to 40% by generating a mask of the patient's body in the first stage, and then the voxel quantity is reduced further to 10% in the second stage. Using this method, the FCN search space is narrowed down to determine if a voxel belongs in the background or in the foreground [46]. The results predict 7.5% improvements in DSC score per organ. Small and tiny organs, especially arteries, benefit from the cascaded approach, with an improvement in DSC scores from 54.8 to 63.1% and 59% to 79.6% for the pancreas and arteries, respectively. Improvement for large organs is less significant.

The skip connections between the encoder and the decoder in **U-Net** result in better segmentation performance [16]. A 3D variant of 2D U-Net that has the ability to extract both local and global information for image segmentation tasks is introduced to segment 3D volumetric medical images [47–49]. 3D U-Net learns spatial and temporal features hierarchically when trained, which improves segmentation performance.

An earlier version of the **3D U-Net** is implemented and tested on 3D-Volumetric segmentation of the sparsely annotated 3D-Volumetric images of the Xenopus kidney [47]. The main architectural advancement consists of replacing the 2D convolution, max-pooling, and up-convolution layers with their 3D versions. Moreover, the batch normalization approach is used to avoid bottlenecks such as high training time [50, 51]. The 3D model is compared with its 2D version to find the gain achieved by using the 3D context using intersection over union (IoU) as an accuracy measure. Results show an IoU of 86% for the 3D architecture, with an improvement of 7% compared to 2D U-Net the semi-autonomous mode, while the fully autonomous mode of the 3D architecture shows a performance gain equivalent to the 2D implementation.

DCE MRIs are 3D volumetric images that need accurate and robust 3D image segmentation techniques in order to accelerate the translation of the GRF technique into clinical practices and reduce the burden on radiologists [52, 53]. Applying 3D U-Net to the renal segmentation task is divided into two steps that can be performed more efficiently in terms of memory and time. In the first stage, low-resolution and augmented data are taken, and a modified 3D U-Net is used to localize the left and right kidneys. During the second stage, U-Net is applied to segment all the kidney regions extracted in the previous stage [54]. For the segmentation of normal and abnormal kidneys, the 3D U-Net achieves 91.4% and 83.6% DSC, respectively (Table 1).

Existing DL models based on U-Net for various biomedical image segmentations rely primarily on the encoder-decoder architecture along with stacked local operators for the gradual aggregation of long-range information. But using only local operators limits its efficiency and effectiveness. The latest variant of 3D U-Net with flexible global aggregation is known as the **non-local U-Net** [55], where these blocks are inserted into the model as size-preserving processes, down-sampling, and up-sampling layers. 3D MRIs of the infant's brain were used in experiments to check the model. It shows a DSC of 92.2% with the iSeg dataset.

In **Segmentation Networks (SegNet)**, the pooling indices are utilized to capture the missing information in the spatial domain using an up-sampling process, which speeds up model convergence [61, 62]. SegNet based on a 3D framework with residual connections for automatic voxel-wise segmentation and has the ability to predict

Table 1 CNN-based algorithms for 3D-volumetric semantic segmentation for biomedical images

Model	Dataset	Features	Evaluation metric (DSC)
3D FCN [44]	Liver CT image segmentation challenge (2019) international symposium on Image Computing and Digital Medicine with 24 training and 36 testing images	A novel LSM is presented along with enhanced object detection It refines the liver segmentation and localizes the tumor	91.03%
Non-local U-Net [55]	iSeg 2017 dataset with 10 T1 training MRIs and 13 testing MRIs	It is a 3D U-Net with flexible global aggregation The aggregation blocks are inserted into the model as a process to preserve size, down-sampling layers, and up-sampling layers	92.00%
Brain SegNet [56]	BRATS 2015 with a test set of 110 MRIs and ISLES 2017 with a test set of 32 MRIs	SegNet is based upon 3D residual framework for automatic voxel-wise segmentation Brain SegNet introduces a 3D refinement module to achieve voxel-level segmentation A new training strategy is introduced based on curriculum and focal loss, allows more effective learning, and effectively handles the problem of dense training and class imbalance	86.00%
DeepMedic [49]	ISLES 2015 with total 64 MRIs and BRATS 2015 with a test set of 110 MRIs	DeepMedic is 3D CNN based 11-Layers deep neural network with multi-scale A hybrid training scheme is applied using dense training It utilizes small-sized kernels, which enables training deeper networks Parallel convolutional pathways for multi-scale processing are performed to improve the segmentation results	89.80% Brain Tumor 66% Ischemic stike lesion
DMRes [32]	BRATS 2015 with 220 MRIs and BRATS 2016 with 191 MRIs	Residual connections are added to DeepMedic in order to improve DSC for CT and ET classes It is evaluated for robustness with less training data or fewer filters on BRATS 2015 It is also benchmarked on the BRATS 2016	89.80%
DenseVoxNet [57]	HVSMR 2016 challenge dataset with 10 3D cardiac MRIs in each training and testing set	A layer is directly connected to all the following layers, which makes the network easier to be trained It has fewer parameters compared to other 3D CNNs because it avoids learning redundant feature maps Auxiliary side paths in the network enable it to improve the gradient flow and stabilize the learning process	82.1±4% Myocardium 93±1% Blood pool

(continued)

Table 1 (continued)

Model	Dataset	Features	Evaluation metric (DSC)
3D-DenseSeg [58]	iSeg 2017 dataset with 10 T1 training MRIs and 13 testing MRIs	To preserve the spatial information, 3D-DenseSeg replaces the pooling layer with a convolution layer BC is used at each dense block and reduces the number of feature maps as a result the number of learned parameters is reduced Hence the computational efficiency is improved than the existing models	92.50%
VoxResNet [36]	MICCAI MRBrainS challenge data with 20 3T MRI scans (10 male and 10 female)	Based on its 2D version VoxResNet is designed for the task of volumetric brain segmentation The image features with low-level, information with an implicit shape and context with high-level is integrated into an auto-context version of the VoxResNet	86.62%
SGU-Net [59]	CHAOS dataset with 40 CT scans and 40 MRIs	It simultaneously implies double separable convolutions known as the ultralight convolution	94.68%
	LiTS dataset with 131 labeled 3D CT scans, 90, 10, and 30 scans to train, validate, and test	An additional shape-guided strategy is introduced to make the network learn the shape of the target	95.90%
VMN [60]	MSD Dataset with lung subset containing 64 training and 32 testing and colon subset containing 126 training and 64 testing 3D CT volumes	VMN acts as a memory-augmented network, encodes previous segmentation information, and retrieves for segmentation future slices	82±8.8% Lung cancer 80.4±11.2% Colon cancer
	KiTS19 dataset with 210 3D volumetric images, 162 training, and 48 testing 3D CT volumes	A quality assurance module is incorporated for segmentation by suggesting the next slice to interact with based on the quality of segmentation of each slice generated in the previous loop	97.0±1.7% Kidney organ 89.1 ± 7.4% kidney tumor

dense voxel segmentation directly. One such SegNet is presented for voxel-wise segmentation of brain tumors and the ischemic stroke region using 3D brain MRIs, known as **Brain SegNet** by [56]. 3D brain SegNet is inspired by the 3D convolutional architecture, which uses multi-scale MRIs in combination with a Conditional Random Field (CRF) [49, 63]. In order to achieve accurate voxel-level segmentation, Brain SegNet introduces a 3D refinement module that has the capability to aggregate 3D deep features with a rich and fine-scale from multi-modal brain MRIs and helps to capture the local detailed features as well as the high-level contextual information in the 3D domain. A new training strategy is introduced in the architecture that is based on curriculum and focal loss, allows for more effective learning, and effectively handles the problems of dense training and class imbalance. Due to these technical improvements, the model directly predicts dense voxel-wise segmentation in one pass. The BRATS 2015 [64] and Ischemic Stroke Lesion Segmentation (ISLES) 2017 [65] databases were used to evaluate Brain SegNet. Improved results are reported with 86% DSC for brain tumor segmentation.

DeepMedic is a 3D CNN-based 11-layer deep neural network with multi-scale devised to overcome the limitations of current networks, with the following main features [49]: A hybrid training scheme is applied using dense training [13] on image segments, which is also analyzed for its adaptation capabilities for the problem of segmentation class imbalance. A very deep 3D CNN has been developed and has been analyzed to be more discriminative but computationally more efficient. Using a design-level approach to utilize small-sized kernels, initially found effective in 2D networks [12] has an even more prominent impact on 3D CNNs, enabling the training of deeper networks. Furthermore, to include local as well as contextual information, multi-scale processing is performed in a parallel manner using the convolutional pathways to improve the segmentation results [57]. A 3D fully connected CRF is used to effectively remove false positives. DeepMedic outperforms many latest models, with top rankings in two MICCAI challenges, ISLES 2015 and BRATS 2015, achieving a DSC of 89.8% and 66% for the challenging tasks of brain tumor and ischemic stroke lesion segmentation, respectively, which shows the generalization capabilities of the model. DeepMedic was further improved by adding residual connections known as **DMRes** in terms of DSC for CT and ET classes [32]. Its robustness was further evaluated for less training data or fewer filters using BRATS 2015 and was also benchmarked on the BRATS 2016 challenge, with high performance despite the simplicity.

In order to get full leverage of the contextual representations of the volumetric data for the task of recognition, a deep voxel-wise residual network known as **VoxResNet** is proposed [36]. Based on its 2D version, VoxResNet is applied to the task of volumetric brain segmentation. To further improve the performance of volumetric segmentation, image features with low-level, information with an implicit shape, and context with a high level are integrated together in the VoxResNet with the feature of auto-context [36]. Deep residual learning with a network deep enough addresses the problem of optimization degradation with the objective of the residual function instead of stacking the layers only [26]. The architecture is composed of the VoxRes Modules, i.e., a stacked residual module with 25 convolutional layers and 4 deconvolutional layers for volumetric segmentation, one of the deepest proposed 3D convolutional architectures. Furthermore, multi-modal images are used as volumetric information for segmentation in order to acquire complementary information and provide robust diagnostic results. It concatenates the multi-modal data and fuses the complementary information while training the network implicitly, hence showing a performance improvement over the single modality. The VoxResNet is validated on the MICCAI MRBrainS challenge data and has outperformed state-of-the-art methods such as 3D U-net [47], MDGRU, and PyraMiD-LSTM [66] in terms of DSC, the 95th percentile of the Hausdorff distance (HD), and the absolute volume difference (AVD). Results show that the DCS can be further improved by incorporating auto-contextual information. Out of thirty-seven competing teams, VoxResNet has secured the top spot in the challenge with the highest DSC of 86.62%, HD of 1.86 mm, and AVD of 6.566%.

Recent studies suggest that if CNNs have shorter connections between the layers closer to the input layer and those closer to the output layer, it makes the network potentially more deeper, more efficient, and more accurate to train. **Dense convolution Networks (DenseNet)** were designed with all the layers connected to every other layer in the network in a feed-forward manner, which increases the number of connections from L to L(L+1)/2 in DenseNet compared to the traditional CNNs to maximize the flow of information between the layers [67]. For all the layers, the feature maps of every preceding layer act as the inputs, and their own feature maps act as the inputs to every layer to follow. DenseNet has several significant advantages, such as reducing the issue of vanishing gradients, enhancing the propagation and reuse of features, and reducing the number of parameters.

To ease the training of CNNs, an extended DenseNet for volumetric cardiac segmentation known as **DenseVoxNet** is presented for segmentation of the cardiac and vascular structures using 3D cardiac MRIs [57]. It adopts the architecture of 3D FCN for volume-to-volume segmentation and incorporates the concept of dense connectivity; therefore, it has the three compelling advantages of DenseNet from the perspective of learning [57]. 1) It connects each layer directly to all the other layers, providing additional supervision due to the shorter connection. It makes the training of the network easier. 2) It has fewer parameters as compared to the rest of the 3D CNNs because the layers have the ability to access the feature from the preceding layers; therefore, it is possible to avoid learning the redundant feature maps. It is very essential for the training of CNNs with a limited number of images in order to have a lower chance of overfitting problems. 3) Auxiliary side paths enable the network to improve the gradient flow and stabilize the learning process. DenseVoxNet is evaluated with the dataset of the MICCAI Workshop on Whole-Heart and Great Vessel Segmentation from 3D Cardiovascular MRI in Congenital Heart Disease (HVSMR). It achieves the best DSC of 82.1±4.1% and outperforms the method, which ranked second by around 2% in the challenge and 93±1% for 3D-Volumetric segmentation of myocardium and blood pool, respectively.

3D-DenseSeg with very deep architecture and a dense connection between the layers is proposed based on DenseNet for volumetric brain segmentation [58]. It captures multi-scale contextual information by combining local and global predictions and concatenating fine and coarse dense block feature maps. In the traditional DenseNet architecture [68], reduced feature resolution is used in the pooling layer, and it may have to lose the spatial information to increase the abstract representation of features. The spatial information is maintained by 3D-DenseSeg by incorporating a convolutional layer and a stride set to 2 instead of the pooling layer, which improves the segmentation performance significantly by increasing the number of parameters in a very small proportion. Also, a bottleneck with compression (BC) module is used at each dense block to decrease the number of feature maps, thereby decreasing the number of learned parameters. As a result, better computational efficiency is achieved than the existing model [47, 57]. The experimental results show that 3D-DenseSeg is better in terms of accuracy and efficiency in terms of the number of parameters for segmentation in the MICCAI grand challenge on the 6-month infant brain MRI segmentation iSeg dataset. The state-of-the-art DenseVoxNet [57] has 32 layers with 4.34 million learned parameters and a DSC of 89.23%, as compared to 18 layers with 19 million learned parameters in the 3D U-Net with a DSC of 91.58% [47]. The 3D-DenseSeg architecture has a deeper network with 47 layers, but it has just 1.55 million learned parameters due to the use of the BC model with a higher DSC of 92.50%.

To address the issue of a larger number of parameters resulting in difficulties in deploying CNNs on hardware with limited resources, such as mobile devices and embedded systems. A **Shape-Guided Ultralight Network (SGU-Net)** is presented in [59]. It offers extremely low computational complexity without any loss in segmentation accuracy. SGU-Net has two main features: first, it has the ability to simultaneously execute convolutions in a double-separable manner, i.e., asymmetrically as well as depthwise, known as the ultralight convolution. Secondly, an additional adversarial shape constraint is introduced to make the network learn the shape of the target, known as a shape-guided strategy.

For further improvement of the segmentation performance for the abdominal medical images, a shape adversarial autoencoder (SAAE) is introduced as a self-supervision by enabling the network to predict the target in a low-dimensional manifold [69]. SGU-Net achieves a DSC of 94.68±1.64% with 4.99 million parameters, compared to U-Net, which achieves a DSC of 94.02±2.32% with 34.53 million parameters on the Combined (CT-MR) healthy abdominal organ segmentation (CHAOS) dataset [70] for liver volumetric segmentation. The network is also evaluated with the Liver Tumor Segmentation Challenge (LiTS) dataset [71], which achieved a DSC of 95.90±1.08% for liver volumetric segmentation.

Fully automated results still cannot meet the required clinical accuracy and need further refinement, despite the enormous development in automatic medical image segmentation methods. A state-of-the-art **Volumetric Memory Network (VMN)** performs the segmentation of a 3D medical image in an interactive manner for the improvement of segmentation accuracy [60]. In the first stage, a 2D network is used in an interactive manner to perform 2D segmentation on a chosen slice by providing hints to the network. In the second stage, the segmentation mask obtained in the first stage is propagated by the VMN to all the slices of the whole volume in a bidirectional manner. The proposed VMN acts as a memory-augmented network [72] and has the ability to easily encode the information from previous segmentation and retrieve it for the segmentation of upcoming slices in the future. Similarly, the refinement induced by the user interaction can be incorporated into other slices. Also, in order to assist the segmentation in a human-in-the-loop manner, a quality assurance unit is incorporated for segmentation by suggesting the coming slice interact based upon the segmentation quality of all the slices generated in the previous loop. Thus, direct estimation of the quality of prediction for each segmentation can be easily carried out to build an active learning paradigm for multi-round refinement. VMN has been evaluated with the Medical Segmentation Decathlon (MSD) dataset [73], achieving a DSC of 82±8.8% and 80.4±11.2% for 3D-Volumetric segmentation of lung tumor and colon cancer with extreme clicking, respectively. The network also achieves a DSC of 97.0±1.7% and 89.1 ± 7.4% on the 2019 Kidney and Kidney Tumor Segmentation Challenge (KiTS19) dataset [74] for volumetric segmentation of kidney organs and kidney tumor volumetric segmentation with extreme clicking, respectively.

3.2 Algorithms for 3D-Volumetric Instance Segmentation of Biomedical Images

CNN-based 3D-Volumetric Instance segmentation can be classified into two categories based on the algorithms: detection-based methods and detection-free methods.

3.2.1 Detection Based Methods

Detection-based methods obtain the bounding boxes. Segmentation is performed inside these bounding boxes. These bounding boxes are obtained by using object detection methods. These methods are viewed as an extension of object detection and are further divided into single-stage and two-stage methods. 3D-Volumetric instance segmentation follows the principle of detecting first and then segmenting with these methods. The segmentation performance of these methods depends on the performance of the object detector. A common example of a single-stage CNN-based method, for instance, segmentation is the YOLO [75], which performs instance segmentation by generating masks [76].

Single-Stage Methods

A novel approach was presented to locate, detect, and segment volumes containing cells fast and accurately in [77]. A recently modified CNN-based network known as 2D **YOLOv2** is used in combination with a tuned 3D U-Net in this method. New image processing and fusion algorithms are incorporated. The volumes of microscopy are converted to slices, stacked over one another, and fed to YOLOv2. It estimates the 2D bounding boxes of the objects. These 2D bounding boxes are combined by the fusion algorithm, and the relevant bounding cubes are extracted for each object. A fast 3D segmentation using 3D U-Net has performed more accurately only in the regions containing bounding cubes, which have knowledge of localized cells. Segments from the cells were detected in the post-processing step by using the interface detection in the 3D U-Net using the information obtained from the fusion algorithm about the bounding cubes. This method touching cells as an instance task with multiple synthetic volumes [77]. The mean average precision (mAP) for the three approaches of 3D watershed (WS) segmentation on the original synthetic data without any noise (3DWS-GT), 3D WS segmentation, for instance, segmentation of the cells with total variation (3DWS-TV), 3D U-Net network to perform segmentation (3D U-Net-GT), and the proposed method are 87%, 72%, 85%, and 76% respectively. The proposed method outperforms 3DWS-TV without using the ground truth while showing results comparable to 3DWS-GT and 3D U-Net-GT that use the ground truth.

Another YOLO-based method, along with the content-sensitive-based technique for superpixels, a deep CNN known as ResCNN with residual connections, and particle spam optimization (PSO), is proposed to perform prostate instance segmentation on 3D MRI scans [78]. It uses **YOLOv3** CNN for the important step of prostate detection to limit the use of MRIs to the target region only and separate the unwanted details of other organs from the image. YOLO can be preferred over other object detection methods because it is extremely fast for detection, predicts the bounding box using the information from the entire image, and has the capability to be generalized [34]. In the segmentation step, the content-sensitive technique is applied slice by slice to group the pixels, and using the Intrinsic Manifold Simple Linear Iterative Clustering (IMSLIC) algorithm, the superpixels are formed [79]. The ResCNN is used to classify the superpixels into prostate tissues and non-prostate tissues. The method is tested for performance using two databases, i.e., the Prostate 3T database and the PROMISE12 database. It shows a DSC of 86.68%, a Jaccard-index (JI) of 76.58%, a volumetric similarity of 96.69%, and a relative volume difference of 3.92%. It also achieves 93.43% specificity, 91.97% accuracy, 90.90% area under the ROC curve, and 88.36% sensitivity (Table 2).

Stochastic-pooling-based spatial pyramid pooling network and bidirectional feature pyramid network (STBi-YOLO) originated from YOLO-v5 and is proposed for lung node recognition with performance improvements over YOLO [80]. The basic network structure is first modified using spatial pyramid pooling, a stochastic pooling-based method [90]. In order to achieve multi-scale feature fusion, a bidirectional feature pyramid network (BiFPN) is applied [91], and finally, the loss of the YOLO-v5 is improved using the EIoU, which in turn optimizes the training model. STBi-YOLO is evaluated with the Lung Nodule Analysis (LUNA) 16 experimental dataset. According to the results, STBi-YOLO has a 95.9% mAP and a 93.3% recall rate for lung nodules detection. STBi-YOLO has 2FPS slower detection speed but has improved mAP and recall rate by 5.1% and 5.6%, respectively, compared to YOLO-v5 [80].

A single-stage model such as the Single Shot MultiBox Detector (SSD) detects the category of the objects and the bounding box from the feature maps directly compared to the two-stage model, which completes the same task in two stages [76]. The goal of single-stage models is to perform faster training and better inference, resulting in a speed-accuracy trade-off in order to have a performance similar to the two-stage models [92]. SSD, along with grouped convolutions, is used to detect liver lesions from multi-phase CT volumes known as **Grouped SSD (GSSD)** [81]. The grouped convolution utilizes the information in the form of multi-phase data to perform object detection and mitigates the generalization gap issue in SSD. The input to the model is created by stacking three slices consecutively from all the phases to make the model recognize the z-axis information. The model is evaluated with a CT database of 64 subjects containing four phases of CT for liver lesion detection, with

Table 2 CNN-based algorithms for 3D-volumetric instance segmentation of biomedical images

Model	Dataset	Features	Evaluation metric
YOLOv3 [77]	Prostate 3T and PROMISE12 with 30 and 50 MRI scans including the ground truth, respectively	It uses YOLOv3 CNN for detection in order to limit the span of MRIs only to the target region Content-sensitive superpixels technique, deep ResCNN and the PSO are used in combination to perform segmentation	76.58% JI 91.97% Accuracy
STBi-YOLO [80]	LUNA16 Dataset containing 888 3D lung CT scans with 70%, 15%, and 15% used to train, test and validate, respectively	YOLO-v5 is modified using spatial pyramid pooling and applying BiFPN to achieve a multi-scale feature fusion In order to optimize the training, the loss function is improved using EIoU function for YOLO-v5	96.10% Accuracy
Grouped SSD [81]	In-house CT database of 64 subjects containing four phases with a total of 613 data points	SSD along with grouped convolutions is used to detect liver lesions from multi-phase CT volumes The model is created by stacking three consecutive slices from each phase	53.30% AP
Res-UNet-R [82]	MitoEM Dataset contains $(30um)^3$ two EM images from a rat tissue and a human tissue, respectively	Network performance is boosted with the deployment of the multi-scale training strategy	91.70% AP@75
Res-UNet-H [82]		A denoising pre-processing is added to generalize the trained model on the test set	82.80% AP@75
3D Mask R-CNN [83]	In-house dataset of DSCE MRI perfusion images with 1260 3D MRI volumes	Mask R-CNN for brain tumor segmentation using DSCE MRI perfusion image volumes It localizes and segments the tumor from extracted regions of the kidney, simultaneously	91±4% Precision
Mask R-CNN [84]	LUNA16 and Ali TianChi challenge datasets with 888 and 800 3D lung CT scan, respectively	Pulmonary nodules detection and segmentation is performed using 3D CT scans. Ray-casting volume rendering algorithm is used to generate the 3D models	88.20% AP@50
Mask R-CNN with 3D RPN [85]	In-house dataset of 20 3D CT	The mask R-CNN is extended to its 3D version by introducing 3D RPN NMS is used to remove duplicate region proposals	91.98% DSC
DenseASPP U-Net [86]	In-house dataset of 20 3D CBCT head scans	The center-sensitive mechanism ensures accurate center of the tooth A label optimization method and a boundary-aware dice loss are used	96.2% DSC

(continued)

Table 2 (continued)

Model	Dataset	Features	Evaluation metric
RDC-Net [87]	3D-ORG nuclei dataset with 49 3D images	A minimalist RNN with an SDC layer refines the output and interpretable intermediate predictions The network has few hyperparameters and light weights	99.40% Instance Precision @50
U-Net+SWS [88]	Manually annotated dataset of 124 3D confocal images using SEGMENT3D [89]	U-net is combined with the watershed strategies for 3D segmentation of microscopic images	87% JI
U-Net+WS [88]		The network performs well in the limitations of seeding and boundary constraints	84.30% JI
U-Net+SV [88]		Auxiliary side paths in the network enable it to improve the gradient flow and stabilize the learning process	84.30% JI

the approval of the international review board of Seoul National University Hospital. GSSD achieves a 53.3% AP score with a speed of three seconds per volume.

Instance segmentation of the mitochondria using electron microscope images has witnessed significant progress with the introduction of DL methods. Inspired by 3D U-Net, two advanced DL networks are proposed for 3D instance segmentation of mitochondria of human and rat samples, known as **Res-UNet-H** and **Res-UNet-R**, respectively [82]. Network performance is boosted using the deployment of the multi-scale training strategy and anisotropic convolution block, which are simple and effective. To generalize the trained model to the test data, a denoising pre-processing step is also included [93]. These networks are evaluated using the MitoEM dataset with an AP@75 of 82.8% Res-UNet-H. Res-UNet-R achieves an AP@75 of 91.7%, JI of 89.5%, and a DSC of 94.5%.

Two-Stage Methods

Mask R-CNN with RoIAlign for feature extraction and a branch of an object mask to a faster R-CNN for prediction is one of the two-stage methods [33]. An automatic 3D instance segmentation-based method is proposed to segment brain tumors in dynamic susceptibility contrast-enhanced (DSCE) MRI perfusion images known as **3D Mask R-CNN** [83]. It localizes and segments the tumor simultaneously. It contains both ROI localization as well as voxel-wise segmentation with regression. The proposed network evaluated the perfusion images of 21 patients with 50 and 70 time point volumes, and 1260 3D volumes in total. It has an average DSC, precision, and recall of 90±4%, 91±4%, and 90±6%.

In the field of surgical research and application, 3D visualization diagnosis has become a very promising area for the detection and segmentation of pulmonary nodules. A **Mask R-CNN-based** based method to detect and segment 3D CT scans for pulmonary nodules is proposed with a ray-casting volume rendering algorithm in order to assist the radiologists in diagnosing the pulmonary nodule more accurately [84]. Resnet50 is used as a backbone in the Mask R-CNN; furthermore, the multi-scale feature maps are fully explored by using the Feature Pyramid Network (FPN) [94]. For the proposal of the candidate boxes, a Region Proposal Network (RPN) is introduced. The sequence of predicted pulmonary nodules is obtained by multiplying of the mask values with the sequences of the medical images. Finally, 3D models of pulmonary nodules are generated with the ray-casting volume rendering algorithm. The method is evaluated with the LUNA16 dataset and the Ali TianChi challenge dataset. Using Mask R-CNN, the model achieves 88.2% AP@50 with the weighted loss on the labelme_LUNA15 dataset with 88.1% and 88.7% of sensitivity, at 1 and 4 false positives per scan, respectively.

The Mask R-CNN is extended to its 3D version by creating a **3D region proposal network (RPN)** for key point tracking [95]. Motivated by the performance of the 3D version of Mask R-CNN in [95], a two-stage deep CNN is formulated to perform accurate voxel-wise automatic instance tooth recognition and segmentation from cone beam CT (CBCT) [85]. The network extracts an edge map in the first stage for the enhancement of the contrast along the boundaries of the shapes in the input CBCT volume. The learned edge map features are concatenated with image features at the input and fed into the second stage of the network built upon the 3D RPN. A group of region proposals is generated by the 3D RPN module. Using non-maximum suppression (NMS), the duplicate region proposals are removed before being sent to the 3D RoIAlign module. The network is evaluated with a dataset of 20 3D CTs from some patients before and after orthodontics. It achieves a DSC of 91.98%, detection accuracy (DA) of 97.75%, and identification accuracy (FA) of 92.79%.

The tooth instance segmentation is extremely useful for computer-aided orthodontic treatment [96]. To achieve 3D tooth instance segmentation, a two-level hierarchical deep network is proposed, known as **DenseASPP-UNet** [86]. In the first stage, the accurate center of the tooth is ensured, and the localization of the tooth instances is guided using the center-sensitive mechanism. The individual tooth is then segmented and classified by DenseASPP-UNet. A label optimization method and a boundary-aware dice loss are used in order to refine the boundary in cases where teeth overlap and improve the accuracy of segmentation at the boundaries. The model is evaluated with a dataset of 20 CBCT head scans approved by the institutional review board, with a DSC of 96.2% and an average symmetric surface distance (ASD) of 12.2%.

Instance segmentation can be performed using two slightly different methods. One method is based on the proposal, where the segmentation stage is followed by detection. The other method segments first and then detects. One of the most common neural networks based on this method, the Recurrent Neural Network (RNN), uses instance embedding, which predicts similar pixel embedding within the same instance and dissimilar pixel embedding across the different instances [97, 98]. A minimalist RNN with a shared stacked convolution (sSDC) layer is proposed and known as the **Recurrent Dilated Convolution Network (RDC-Net)** [87]. The network is evaluated on a 3D dataset of nuclei called 3D-ORG. It refines the output, and interpretable intermediate predictions are generated in an iterative manner. The network has a few hyperparameters and light weights depending on physical parameters, i.e., the sizes or densities of the objects. It achieves 99.4% instance precision at 50% IoU and 92.4% aggregated JI.

3.2.2 Detection Free Methods

Detection-free methods predict the embedded vectors, and then, by means of clustering, the corresponding pixels are grouped together [19]. The discriminative power of CNNs to pre-process data and watershed-based post-processing strategies are combined to segment 3D microscopy images. Three distinct watershed strategies, namely seeded watershed (SWS), native watershed (WS), and superpixel approach (SV), were merged with the U-Net to build three distinct networks: **U-Net + SWS, U-Net + WS, and U-Net + SV** [88]. These networks were able to segment the shapes of the objects, even with limitations such as rough seeding and boundary constraints. All three networks are evaluated with manually annotated 3D confocal microscopy images [89]. The highest JI of 87% and DSC of 93.1% are achieved by U-Net + SWS.

3.3 Algorithms for 3D-Volumetric Panoptic Segmentation of Biomedical Images

Both the proposal-based and the proposal-free methods suffer from a loss of information because they cannot target both the global levels and the local levels simultaneously. In order to counter this shortcoming, panoptic segmentation combines the semantic and instance features [99]. One of such methods is **Panoptic Feature Net (PFFNet)**, which contains a feature fusion mechanism based on residual attention in order to embed the prediction from the instance segmentation stage with the extracted features by the semantic segmentation [100]. Also, to set the confidence score for every object with the quality of mask prediction, a sub-branch is designed for mask quality. A regularization mechanism is used to maintain consistency between the semantic branch and the instance branch. The network is evaluated with the Cancer Genome Atlas (TCGA)- KUMAR, Triple Negative Breast Cancer (TNBC), BBBC039V1 for fluorescence microscopy images, and Computer Vision Problem in Plant Phenotyping (CVPPP) datasets. On the TNBC dataset, it attains a JI of 63.13%, a DSC of 80.37%, and a panoptic quality (PQ) of 62.98% (Table 3).

Among the most prominent methods for nuclei panoptic segmentation is the **marker-controlled watershed transforms** enhanced by DL [102]. In this method, CNNs are used to create the masks of the nuclei along with the markers, and for instance, in the segmentation task, the watershed strategy is applied [101]. An edge-emphasizing CNN, i.e., U-Net, was introduced along with the optimized H-minima

Table 3 CNN-based algorithms for 3D-volumetric panoptic segmentation of biomedical images

Model	Dataset	Features	PQ (%)	Evaluation matrix (JI) (%)
	TCGA KUMAR Dataset consists of 30 histopathology images	A residual attention feature fusion mechanism is integrated	58.71	61.07
PFFNet [100]	TNBC Dataset consists of 30 histopathology images	To ensure mask segmentation quality sub-branch of mask quality is added	62.98	63.13
	BBBC039V1 Dataset consists of 200 fluorescence images	A semantic task consistency mechanism is introduced to regularize the training of the semantic segmentation task	83.31	84.77
Marker controlled watershed transform [101]	3D twelve HepG2 spheroids dataset consists of twelve 3D HepG2 nuclei spheroid images	Edge emphasizing U-Net is used along with the optimized H-minima transform to perform the segmentation of densely cultivated 3D nuclei The masks and markers are generated by the U-Net and the H-minima transform respectively	76.00	77.00

transform [103] to improve the performance of 3D nuclei segmentation with dense cultivation. The CNN generates the mask, and the transform generates the marker [28]. The 3D images of twelve HepG2 spheroids were used for training and evaluating the method.

An edge emphasizing CNN with 3D architecture and the H-minima transform method with optimization scores of 76% PQ and 77% aggregated JI compared to the baseline DL-enhanced marker-controlled watershed with 69% PQ and 66% aggregated JI. Results indicate that this method can improve segmentation using the U-Nets architecture with edge-emphasizing and H-minima transforms with optimization in the case of densely cultivated 3D nuclei.

4 GAN-Based Algorithms for 3D-Volumetric Segmentation of Biomedical Images

Similar to the CNN-based algorithms, the GAN-based algorithms can also be divided into semantic, instance, and panoptic tasks for the 3D-Volumetric segmentation of biomedical images based on the task formulation as shown in Fig. 6.

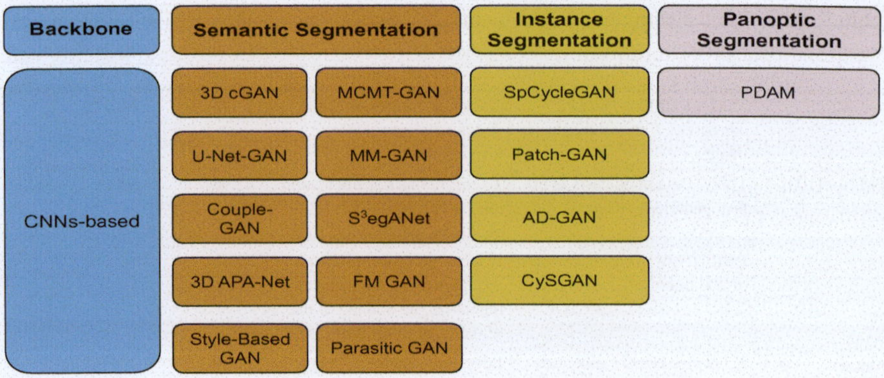

Fig. 6 Overview of GAN-based algorithms

4.1 Algorithms for 3D-Volumetric Semantic Segmentation of Biomedical Images

With their powerful capabilities in image synthesis, GANs have demonstrated themselves to be among the most effective methods used for the improvement of image segmentation. GANs consist of a generator module that tends to learn the mapping of real images and a discriminator module that distinguishes the real images from the synthesized image. Recently, the **conditional Generative Adversarial Network (cGAN)** has achieved better performance on biomedical image synthesis, which trains the two modules to beat each other [104–106]. 3D cGANs are proposed to prevent the information loss taking place in the 2D segmentation and learn contextual information among the voxels for accurate 3D-Volumetric segmentation of biomedical images [107]. A **3D cGAN** is proposed for FLAIR image synthesis, which can be utilized to train a 3D CNN to improve segmentation of brain tumor [108]. The proposed 3D cGAN addresses the issue of discontinuous estimation due to the 2D cGANs across the slices. A 3D cGAN model can improve the synthesis of FLAIR images by considering contextual information. It considers the larger image patches and hierarchical features as compared to the 2D cGANs. A method of locally adaptive synthesis is introduced to improve the synthesized flair, which in turn improves the segmentation performance. 3D cGAN is evaluated on BRATS 2015 for 3D biomedical image segmentation and achieves a DSC of 68.23% and 72.28% for the WT and the CT, respectively.

The ability to segment organs-at-risk (OARs) accurately and on time is critical for efficient radiation therapy planning [109]. A GAN-based 3D network is designed for 3D semantic segmentation and is used for multiple organs in thoracic CT volumes; it is known as the **U-Net-Generative Adversarial Network (U-Net-GAN)** [110]. Together, it trains the generator, consisting of a group of U-Nets, and the discriminator, consisting of a group of FCNs. By learning end-to-end maps from the CT images to the multiorgan-segmented OARs, the U-Net-based generators are responsible for producing an image map to segment multiple organs. The FCN-based discriminator is responsible for differentiating ground truth from segmented OARs. An optimal segmentation map for multiple organs is generated as a result of the contest between the generator and the discriminator against each other. The 2017 AAPM thoracic auto-segmentation challenge dataset with thoracic CT volumes of 35 subjects is used for the evaluation of U-Net-GAN [111]. The DSC for the 3D semantic segmentation is 97% for the left lung and 97% for the right lung, 90% for the spinal cord, 75% for the esophagus, and 87% for the heart. A mean surface distance (MSD) of 0.4–1.5 mm is achieved among all the subjects for the above-mentioned five OARs.

An efficient novel method for 3D left ventricle segmentation using 3D echocardiography is proposed in combination with a GAN network known as the **Couple Generator Adversarial Network (Couple-GAN)** [23]. An information consistency constraint is used to overcome the challenges of the high dimensionality of data, complex anatomical structures, and limited data annotation. The proposed model is merged with the novel framework to make it model capable of learning global semantic information. The framework achieves 1.52 mm, 5.6 mm, and 97% MSD, HD, and DSC, respectively, on the 3D echocardiography dataset consisting of 25 subjects to train, 10 subjects to validate, and 35 subjects to test.

3D-Volumetric segmentation using MRIs of the prostate with high accuracy and reliability is crucial to diagnosing and treating prostate diseases. Many DL methods have been presented for the automatic segmentation of the prostate gland; still, there is room for improvement in the segmentation performance due to the variations, interference, and anisotropic spatial resolution in the images [112]. A 3D GAN known as the **3D adversarial pyramid anisotropic convolutional network (3D APA-Net)** is modeled to improve the performance of prostate segmentation using MRIs [20]. 3D PA-Net acting as a generator consists of an encoder-decoder with a 3D ResNet encoder, an anisotropic convolution (AS-Conv), and multi-level pyramid convolutional (Py-Conv) skip connections to produce image segmentation results. The discriminator consists of a seven-layer 3D adversarial Deep Convolutional Neural Network (DCNN) that differentiates the segmentation result from the ground truth. The model is evaluated with PROMISE12 [113], ASAP13, and a hybrid dataset consisting of 110 T2-weighted prostate MRIs. It achieves a DSC of 90.6%, an HD of 4.128, and an average boundary distance (ABD) of 1.454 mm for PROMISE12. For ASAP13, the model achieves a DSC of 89.3±2.5% and an ABD of 1.167±0.285. The network is compared with the V-Net, 3D U-Net, and 3D Global Convolutional Network (3D GCN) using the hybrid dataset and achieves the best DSC of 90.1±3.3% and ABD of 0.944±0.364 among all the models in comparison.

A **Style-Based GAN** is modeled for the semantic segmentation of pulmonary nodules using 3D CT images. The network first augments the training data to address the issues of data scarcity and imbalance in labeled data faced by the nodule segmentation [21]. In the first step, the GAN is trained, and the generator, as well as the style encoder, are optimized and given the task of using the semantic labels and the style matrix to reconstruct the real image. In the second step, the augmented image is generated using the style encoder by extracting the style bank from every training sample, which randomly provides the style matrix. A region-aware network architecture is used for fine control of the style in a specific region, such as lung nodules, pleural surfaces, and vascular structures. Finally, a 3D U-Net model is used for 3D-Volumetric segmentation. The model is evaluated with the lung image database consortium and image database resource initiative (LIDC-IDRI) dataset [114]. Style-based GAN gives a DSC of 83.68%, a sensitivity score of 84.31%, and a positive predictive value (PPV) of 85.50% without GAN augmentation. It gives a DSC of 85.21%, a sensitivity of 86.22%, and a PPV of 86.68% with GAN augmentation.

The synthesis of multi-modal data is highly desirable for the 3D segmentation of biomedical images [115], because it provides diverse and complementary information useful for segmentation. However, collecting multi-modal images is limited due to a variety of factors, including their high cost, inconvenience to patients, and scarcity. A **multi-task coherent modality transferable GAN (MCMT-GAN)** is proposed to synthesize 3D brain MRI used for 3D segmentation [116]. The network is more robust for the synthesis of multi-modal brain images and segments by merging the bidirectional adversarial loss, cycle-consistency loss, domain-adapted losses, and manifold regularization in a volumetric space. The generator and discriminator work collaboratively to ensure the usefulness of the synthesizer for segmentation. The model is evaluated with the IXI dataset for synthesizing different cross-modalities, such as proton density-weighted as a T2-weighted MRI (PD-w $\rightarrow$ T2-w) with a DSC of 89.82% and a T2-weighted MRI as a proton density-weighted (T2-w $\rightarrow$ PD-w) with a DSC of 86.09%.

A cGAN architecture known as **MM-GAN** is proposed for MRI augmentation and segmentation [117]. It translates the labeled maps to a 3D MRI without affecting the pathological characteristics. The 3D U-Net is used as a generator in this end-to-end architecture to synthesize the 3D MRIs for 3D-Volumetric segmentation of biomedical images [47]. The discriminator of SimGAN is modified for 3D images in MM-GAN, which is a reliable and effective method to simulate the local features in 2D images [118]. A series of tests are performed for the evaluation of MM-GAN for tumor segmentation on the BRATS 2017 dataset. It achieves a performance close to that of the models trained with real data when trained with pure fake data, using only 29 samples to fine-tune the model. A DSC of 89.90% is achieved for the WT with 500% fake and 100% real data for training.

3D-Volumetric segmentation is very crucial for the spinal structures in order to save time and perform quantitative analysis for diagnosis, surgical procedures, and disease treatments. A complete voxel-wise solution with a multi-stage adversarial learning strategy (MSAL) is presented to semantically segment in a 3D fashion the multiple spinal structures, simultaneously known as **S^{3}egANet** [119]. To address the issue of very high diversity and variations in the complex 3D spinal structures, a multi-modality auto-encoder (MMAE) with the capability to extract fine structural information was introduced [120]. To improve the performance of segmentation, a cross-modality voxel fusion strategy (CMVF) is incorporated to gain detailed spatial information using multi-modal MRIs [121]. The adversarial learning strategy achieves high reliability and accuracy for simultaneous 3D segmentation of multiple spinal structures. S^{3}egANet achieves a sensitivity of 91.45% and a DSC of 88.3% after evaluation of a dataset of 90 sets of clinical patients' lumber scans (Table 4).

Table 4 GAN-based algorithms for 3D-volumetric semantic segmentation of biomedical images

Model	Dataset	Features	Evaluation metrics (DSC)
3D cGAN [108]	BRATS 2015 with 230 MRIs as a training set and 44 MRIs as a testing set	3D cGAN addresses the issue of discontinuous estimation caused by the 2D cGANs across the slices 3D cGAN improves the synthesis of FLAIR images by considering contextual information	68.23% WT 72.28% CT
U-Net-GAN [110]	2017 AAPM Thoracic Auto-segmentation challenge Dataset with 34 sets of CT images for training and validation and 1 for testing	A series of U-Nets and FCNs are trained together as generators and discriminators respectively An optimal segmentation map for multiple organs is generated as a result of the contest between the generator and the discriminator against each other	97% Left Lungs 97% Right Lungs 90% Spinal Cord 75% Esophagus
Couple-GAN [23]	In-house dataset of 3D echocardiography with 25 subjects to train, 10 to validate, and 35 to test	To overcome the challenges of high dimensional data, complex anatomical environments, and limited annotation data, an information consistency constraint is used The global semantic information of the proposed couple-GAN is combined with the novel framework	97%
3D APA-Net [20]	PROMISE12 with 50 MRIs for training and 30 for testing	3D PA-Net acting as a generator consists of an encoder-decoder with a 3D ResNet encoder, AS-	90.60%
	ASAP 13 with 60 MRIs for training and 10 for testing	conv, and multi-level Py-Conv to perform image segmentation for the prostate	89.3±2.5%
	Hybrid dataset with 110 MRIs	The discriminator consists of a seven-layer 3D adversarial DCNN	90.1±3.3%
Style-based GAN [21]	LIDC-IDRI dataset containing 1010 CT scans	Styles and semantic labels are first extracted from the whole dataset The augmented CT images are synthesized for each semantic label and used for the segmentation of the pulmonary nodules	85.21%
MCMT-GAN [116]	IXI Dataset with 578 brain MRIs of normal and healthy subjects	MCMT-GAN combines the bidirectional adversarial loss, cycle-consistency loss, domain-adapted losses, and manifold regularization in a volumetric space The generator and discriminator work collaboratively to ensure the usefulness of the synthesizer for the segmentation	89.82%
MM-GAN [117]	BRATS 2017 consisting of 210 HGG and 75 LGG brain MRI scans for training	The 3D U-Net is used as a generator in this end-to-end framework for brain tumor segmentation The 2D discriminator of SimGAN is modified into a 3D discriminator	89.90%

(continued)

Table 4 (continued)

Model	Dataset	Features	Evaluation metrics (DSC)
S^3egANet [119]	In-house dataset of 90 sets of clinical patients' lumber scans	MMAE is used to address the issue of very high diversity and variations of complex 3D spinal structures CMVF is used to gain detailed spatial information to improve the segmentation performance	91.45%
FM GAN [122]	iSeg 2017 dataset with 10 T1 training and 13 testing brain MRIs	FM GAN reducing the problem of over-fitting It outperforms 3D U-Net when trained with few samples	89% WT
Parasitic GAN [123]	BRATS 2017 with 285 brain MRIs as the training images and 46 as validation images	3D U-Net serves as a segmentor for 3D-volumetric segmentation A modified 3D GAN generator and an extended 3D version of the patch GAN discriminator are used as a generator and discriminator, respectively	77.7% WT

To address the issue of 3D semantic segmentation of multi-modal biomedical images with very few labeled training examples, a GAN-based novel semi-supervised method is introduced to train a 3D segmentation model known as **feature mapping (FM) GAN** [122]. FM GAN discriminates between true and fake patches with the generator and discriminator models, reducing the problem of over-fitting. It outperforms many of the modern-day networks, such as 3D U-Net, when trained with very few samples. The proposed model is evaluated with the iSeg 2017 dataset and achieves a DSC of 89% and an ASD of 27% for Cerebrospinal Fluid (CSF) with one training image. It achieves a DSC of 88% and an ASD of 25% for CSF with two training images.

To address the issue of a shortage of annotated data for 3D semantic segmentation, especially for biomedical images, a GAN-based model known as **Parasitic GAN** is introduced [123]. Parasitic GAN has the ability to exploit unlabeled data more efficiently for 3D segmentation of brain tumor. It consists of a segmentation module, a generator, and a discriminator. 3D U-Net is used as a segmentor for 3D-Volumetric segmentation. VoxResNet [36] and V-Net [48] can also be used for volumetric segmentation. The generator of parasitic GAN is a modified version of the 3D GAN generator accompanied by the leaky ReLu and the original activation function, and the normalization method is replaced with the instance normalization [124]. An extended 3D version of the Patch GAN discriminator is used in the parasitic GAN [125]. The segmentor and GAN are associated in a parasitic manner to limit the overfitting issue and enhance network generalization. On the BRAT 2017 dataset, it achieves a DSC of 73.3%, 75.1, and 77.7% for WT, 63.8%, 71.1%, and 74.9% for CT, and 57.3%, 64.9%, and 67.3% ET for 30, 50, and 80% labeled data.

4.2 *Algorithms for 3D-Volumetric Instance Segmentation of Biomedical Images*

3D-Volumetric segmentation of nuclei is a very crucial and important factor in the analysis of subcellular structures in tissues. Based upon the well-known **spatially constrained cycle-consistent adversarial network (SpCycleGAN)** [126], a two-stage instance segmentation method is introduced for 3D nuclei fluorescence microscopy volumes [127]. It tends to solve the problem of limited ground truth for 3D images. First, realistic synthetic 3D volumes are generated using the SpCycleGAN without using actual volumes to train the CNN [128]. An architecture similar to U-Net, with 3D batch normalization and ReLu as an activation function, serves as the CNN. The central area of the nuclei is extracted to avoid overlapping the surfaces of the nuclei. Another CNN is used for nuclei instance segmentation, which is segmentation with distinct labels for the individual detected nuclei. The method is evaluated on three rat kidney datasets and achieves a precision of 93.47%, a recall of 96.80%, and an F1 score of 95.10%.

Another cGAN-based approach is presented to generate 3D fluorescence microscopy to address the limited ground truth availability issue for 3D-Volumetric segmentation of cellular structures [129]. A patch-wise strategy is followed by a full-size resembled method for the generation of images of different sizes and organisms. The combination of mask simulation approaches yields a 3D, fully annotated microscopy dataset. The data for different quality levels and position-dependent intensity characteristics are generated using a positional conditioning strategy. The dataset is publicly available and can be used for the purpose of training and benchmarking instance segmentation networks. Two different datasets were used to evaluate this method. The first dataset consists of 125 3D image stacks of Arabidopsis thaliana [89], and the second dataset contains 394 3D image stacks of Danio rerio [130]. It gives a structural similarity index measure (SSIM) of 70.6%.

Existing methods, such as CycleGAN, have produced significant results for unsupervised cell nuclei 3D instance segmentation using unmatched image-to-image mapping among the cell nuclei volumes and randomly synthesized masks [131]. First, the CycleGAN is trained in order to generate data using the synthetic masks, and the process of learning is performed using a segmentation model [126]. Also, a SpCycleGAN is developed to address the issue of spatial offset occurring in 3D volumes. It uses a synthetic paired dataset on a 3D model developed to segment [132]. But these methods have a two-stage channel and are unable to perform end-to-end learning in 3D images of cell nuclei. As a result, the "lossy transformation" becomes more severe because of the increase in content inconsistency between the actual image and the related output of the segmentation [133]. A "text-based framework", known as **Aligned Disentangling Generative Adversarial Network (AD-GAN)**, is a novel unsupervised framework proposed to address these issues [134]. It performs end-to-end learning. AD-GAN incorporates a novel strategy called disentanglement in order to split the content and the style representation from each other, preserve the spatial structure, and reduce the lossy transformation. The generator consists of an encoder and a decoder with domain labels and is different from multimodal unsupervised image-to-image translation (MUNIT), which extracts the style code with the help of a style encoder. Hence, a multi-layer perceptron learns a representation with a single style for each domain. The encoder as well as the decoder are incorporated with a layer of Adaptive Instance Normalization (AdaIN) for style representation. Finally, a unified framework is developed to learn style representations in both domains. In this framework, a novel algorithm is introduced for training that aligns the disentangled content in order to decrease the lossy transformation. AD-GAN performs better than many of the latest unsupervised frameworks, with an average improvement of 16.1% in DSC on a dataset of four cell nuclei, and offers a performance close to that of the supervised models. **BBBC024** [135] and **Scaffold-A549** are 3D fluorescence microscopy datasets utilized to evaluate AD-GAN for the 3D-Volumetric instance segmentation of cell nuclei. AD-GAN achieves 93.1% precision, 91.5% recall, and 92.6% DSC for the BBBC024 dataset and 89% precision, 78.2% recall, and 83.3% DSC for the Scaffold-A549 dataset (Table 5).

Collecting annotated data with the help of experts is time-consuming as well as expensive; thus, segmentation of unlabeled image modality is a challenging yet necessary task. Current methods for 3D-Volumetric segmentation of new modalities involve either a pre-trained model optimization on a training set with diverse data or performing domain translation and segmentation as two separate steps [137, 138]. A novel **Cyclic Segmentation Generative Adversarial Network (CySGAN)** is proposed, which performs the task of image instance segmentation and translation for 3D neuronal nuclei simultaneously using a unified framework [134]. An additional self-supervised and segmentation-based adversarial objective is introduced to improve the performance of the model using the unlabeled target domain images. CySGAN is evaluated with the NpenucEXM dataset [139], containing expansion microscopy (ExM) volumes of cell nuclei and achieves an AP of 93.1%.

4.3 Algorithms for 3D-Volumetric Panoptic Segmentation of Biomedical Images

One of the GAN-based methods for panoptic segmentation of 3D-Volumetric biomedical images based on an unsupervised domain adoption (UDA) [140, 141] method is known as **Panoptic Domain Adaptive Mask R-CNN (PDAM)**, which is proposed to segment 3D microscopic images [142]. A baseline Domain Adaptive Mask (DAM) R-CNN is designed first, with features for cross-domain alignment on the instance and image levels. There is also the possibility of the existence of domain bias in the contextual information at the semantic level. Therefore, there is a need to design a domain discriminator at the semantic level in order to fill the gap between the domains. At the panoptic level, the cross-domain features are aligned by the integration of semantic and instance-level feature adaptations. The trade-off weights of the semantic and instance loss functions are assigned using a task re-

Table 5 GAN-based algorithms for 3D-volumetric instance segmentation of biomedical images

Model	Dataset	Features	Evaluation metrics
SpCycleGAN [127]	In-house rat kidney dataset consisting of three sets of 512, 415, and 45 images	3D volumes are generated using the SpCycleGAN without using actual ground truth for the training of CNN A U-NET-like architecture with 3D batch normalization and ReLu as activation is used as the CNN The central area of the nuclei is extracted to avoid overlapping among the surfaces of nuclei	93.45% Precision
Patch-GAN [129]	Arabidopsis thaliana dataset with 125 3D images of cell membranes and Danio rerio dataset with 394 3D images of cell membranes and nuclei	A patch-wise working principle is combined with a full-size resembled strategy for the generation of images of different sizes and organisms The data of different quality levels and position-dependent intensity characteristics are generated using a positional conditioning strategy	70.6% SSIM
AD-GAN [134]	BBBC024 Dataset 80 HL60 cell nuclei simulated images	It separates the content representation from the style representation, preserves the spatial structure, and reduces the lossy transformation	92.6% DSC
	Scaffold-A549 dataset with 20 3D fluorescent images for training and 1 annotated image	A novel algorithm is used to train the framework, which aligns the disentangled content in order to reduce the lossy transformation	83.3% DSC
CySGAN [136]	NucExM dataset with 2 Zebrafish brain ExM volumes	It performs the task of image instance segmentation and translation for 3D neuronal nuclei simultaneously A self-supervised segmentation-based adversarial objective is introduced for the improvement of the model performance using the unlabeled target domain images	93.1% AP

weighting strategy to solve the domain bias issue. In order to enhance instance-level feature adaptation, a feature similarity mechanism is designed. CycleGAN is used to generate images like the target images using the images provided by the source domain. It is trained by using synthesized images for the source domain and real images for the target domain. The network achieve an aggregated JI of 59.74% and a PQ of 48.08% on the EPLF, consisting of 132 images to train and 33 images to validate to VNC dataset consisting of 13 images to train and 7 images to test.

5 Challenges

The majority of the issues with 2D image segmentation are more severe with 3D image segmentation. The following section discusses some of the main challenges faced by 3D-Volumetric segmentation for biomedical images.

5.1 Limited Data Annotation

To train a model for improved segmentation performance, DL networks need a lot of annotated samples. Acquiring a dataset of annotated images is typically very difficult and expensive in the field of medical image processing. With 3D-Volumetric segmentation, which requires voxel-wise labeling of a volume rather than pixel-wise labeling of an image, the issue is made more challenging. Transfer learning, which transfers the annotations or information from a properly constructed model to another model in the same or even a different region, is one approach to resolving this problem. Because of this, the problem of inadequate data annotation for 3D-Volumetric segmentation has enormous potential to be solved via transfer learning. Splitting the image or volume into several random patches is another tactic to address this problem, particularly in 3D-Volumetric segmentation [143]. Although they converge more quickly and have a higher variance, these random patches have a problem with class imbalance [144]. The model learns from labeled voxels in sparsely annotated data, and the weights of unlabeled data are adjusted to zero in the sparse annotation technique. Because of the rarity of properly labeled data, this method is frequently employed for 3D-Volumetric segmentation [47].

5.2 High Computational Complexity

The computational complexity of 3D-Volumetric segmentation is one of the most significant challenges. The inherited high dimensionality of the 3D volumes makes the problem of computational complexity more essential. High-performance computational equipment, such as GPUs, must be used for it. In order to shorten the inference time, a dense inference is applied, which is one way to lower the computational complexity of inference for 3D-Volumetric segmentation. According to [145], their technique reduces the inference time for a single brain scan by about a minute. Another method eliminates the patches by making them less likely to contain the target organs using a rule-out strategy. This method speeds up inference since it narrows the search space.

5.3 *Overfitting*

In contrast to the unprocessed instances in the problem, over-fitting occurs when the model captures patterns and regularities with extremely high accuracy during training. One of the main causes of over fitting during training for 3D-Volumetric segmentation is using datasets with smaller sizes. One method to address the issue of over fitting is to use dropouts in the training phase in order to drop the output of random sets of neurons in fully connected layers in each iteration.

5.4 *Training Time*

For 3D-Volumetric segmentation, deep learning models need a lot of training time. The goal of many studies has been to speed up network convergence and decrease training time. Among the most prominent solutions to the problem is using the pooling layers to lowers the dimensionality of the parameters [146]. One of the most recent pooling-based techniques that lower the network parameters is convolution with strides [12]. Compared to pooling, batch normalization is a more effective method for enhancing network convergence since it prevents the loss of useful information [147].

The aforementioned difficulties indicate that there are still many opportunities to study the deep learning algorithms for 3D-Volumetric segmentation of biomedical images.

6 Conclusion

One of the most crucial and difficult processes in biomedical imaging for diagnostic procedures and clinical therapies has been 3D-Volumetric segmentation, which is the focus of a current study. As a result, no single DL-based standard method can be claimed to perform equally well on all tasks. When attempting to address a 3D-Volumetric segmentation problem for biomedical imaging, it is essential to investigate various models and techniques that are now accessible. The degree of accuracy required and the complexity of the problem determine whether to use a 2D-DL with numerous slice-based techniques or a 3D-DL end-to-end volumetric approach for segmentation. Because medical applications of segmentation are particularly sensitive to accuracy and learning spatial contextual information is critical for effective 3D-Volumetric segmentation, a 3D-DL end-to-end volumetric approach is preferred at the expense of computing complexity. This article aids researchers in selecting a 3D-Volumetric segmentation method for a particular biomedical image that is either CNN-based or GAN-based, semantic, instance, or panoptic task.

Different 3D-DL approaches are compared for the same segmentation problems and evaluated with the same datasets based on the models provided and the quantitative analysis in the form of evaluation matrices in this work. First, models for both the CNN-based and the GAN-based approaches for 3D-Volumetric segmentation of biomedical images are compared in each task-based subdivision, i.e., semantic, instance, and panoptic. On BRATS 2015, the CNN-based models **DeepMedic** and **DMRes** provided the best DSC of 89.8% for 3D-Volumetric semantic segmentation of the human brain. With a 96.1% AP on the LUNA16 dataset, the **STBi-YOLO** model can be regarded as the most efficient CNN-based volumetric instance segmentation model for segmenting lung nodes. Among the GAN-based models for volumetric semantic segmentation of the human brain, **MM-GAN** achieves the highest DSC of 89.90% with BRATS 2017. For 3D instance segmentation of nuclei, the GAN-based models **SpCycleGAN** and **CySGAN** reach the best AP of 93.47% and 93.1%, respectively.

Due to the lack of a shared segmentation task and dataset for both the CNN-based and GAN-based models, these models are compared independently for semantic and instance tasks. For 3D-Volumetric semantic segmentation of 6-month infant MRI on the iSeg dataset, CNN-based **Non-local U-Net** performs better than GAN-based **FM-GAN** with a DSC of 89%. However, when trained on a small sample size, FM-GAN outperforms **3D U-Net**, making it a good choice for segmentation problems with insufficient labeled data. Given that U-Net performs better in 3D-Volumetric semantic segmentation, it is frequently utilized as a segmentor in the generators of GAN-based models for this task. For the 3D-Volumetric semantic segmentation of the human brain, the GAN-based model **MM-GAN** performs better, achieving a DSC of 89.9% for WT than the best CNN-based model, **3D FCN** with multiscale achieving a DSC of 86% for WT on the BRATS 17 dataset. To compare the CNN-based models with the GAN-based models for 3D-Volumetric instance segmentation, **RDC-Net** outperforms the best GAN-based model **SpCycleGAN**, with an AP of 99.4% and 93.47% for nuclei segmentation, respectively. As the panoptic models are very few and are not evaluated with the same dateset to perform the same 3D-Volumetric segmentation task for biomedical images, therefore there is no proper comparison possible.

References

1. Intisar Rizwan I Haque and Jeremiah Neubert. Deep learning approaches to biomedical image segmentation. *Informatics in Medicine Unlocked*, 18:100297, 2020.
2. Anabik Pal, Akshay Chaturvedi, Utpal Garain, Aditi Chandra, and Raghunath Chatterjee. Severity grading of psoriatic plaques using deep cnn based multi-task learning. In *2016 23rd International Conference on Pattern Recognition (ICPR)*, pages 1478–1483. IEEE, 2016.
3. Ge Wang. A perspective on deep imaging. *IEEE access*, 4:8914–8924, 2016.
4. Zhihua Liu, Lei Tong, Long Chen, Zheheng Jiang, Feixiang Zhou, Qianni Zhang, Xiangrong Zhang, Yaochu Jin, and Huiyu Zhou. Deep learning based brain tumor segmentation: a survey. *Complex & Intelligent Systems*, pages 1–26, 2022.

5. Kunio Doi. Computer-aided diagnosis in medical imaging: historical review, current status and future potential. *Computerized medical imaging and graphics*, 31(4-5):198–211, 2007.
6. Flávio Henrique Schuindt da Silva. *Deep learning for corpus callosum segmentation in brain magnetic resonance images*. PhD thesis, Universidade Federal do Rio de Janeiro, 2018.
7. Tobias Volkenandt, Stefanie Freitag, and Michael Rauscher. Machine learning powered image segmentation. *Microscopy and Microanalysis*, 24(S1):520–521, 2018.
8. Mutasem K Alsmadi. A hybrid fuzzy c-means and neutrosophic for jaw lesions segmentation. *Ain Shams Engineering Journal*, 9(4):697–706, 2018.
9. Xiangrong Zhou, Kazuma Yamada, Takuya Kojima, Ryosuke Takayama, Song Wang, Xinxin Zhou, Takeshi Hara, and Hiroshi Fujita. Performance evaluation of 2d and 3d deep learning approaches for automatic segmentation of multiple organs on ct images. In *Medical Imaging 2018: Computer-Aided Diagnosis*, volume 10575, pages 520–525. Spie, 2018.
10. Dinggang Shen, Guorong Wu, and Heung-Il Suk. Deep learning in medical image analysis. *Annual review of biomedical engineering*, 19:221, 2017.
11. Alex Krizhevsky, Ilya Sutskever, and Geoffrey E Hinton. Imagenet classification with deep convolutional neural networks. *Communications of the ACM*, 60(6):84–90, 2017.
12. Karen Simonyan and Andrew Zisserman. Very deep convolutional networks for large-scale image recognition. *arXiv preprint* arXiv:1409.1556, 2014.
13. Jonathan Long, Evan Shelhamer, and Trevor Darrell. Fully convolutional networks for semantic segmentation. In *Proceedings of the IEEE conference on computer vision and pattern recognition*, pages 3431–3440, 2015.
14. C Szegedy, W Liu, Y Jia, et al. Going deeper with convolutions 2015 ieee conference on computer vision and pattern recognition (cvpr) june 2015boston. *MA, USA1–9*, 10.
15. Adhish Prasoon, Kersten Petersen, Christian Igel, François Lauze, Erik Dam, and Mads Nielsen. Deep feature learning for knee cartilage segmentation using a triplanar convolutional neural network. In *International conference on medical image computing and computer-assisted intervention*, pages 246–253. Springer, 2013.
16. Olaf Ronneberger, Philipp Fischer, and Thomas Brox. U-net: Convolutional networks for biomedical image segmentation. In *International Conference on Medical image computing and computer-assisted intervention*, pages 234–241. Springer, 2015.
17. Hao Chen, Dong Ni, Jing Qin, Shengli Li, Xin Yang, Tianfu Wang, and Pheng Ann Heng. Standard plane localization in fetal ultrasound via domain transferred deep neural networks. *IEEE journal of biomedical and health informatics*, 19(5):1627–1636, 2015.
18. Hoo-Chang Shin, Holger R Roth, Mingchen Gao, Le Lu, Ziyue Xu, Isabella Nogues, Jianhua Yao, Daniel Mollura, and Ronald M Summers. Deep convolutional neural networks for computer-aided detection: Cnn architectures, dataset characteristics and transfer learning. *IEEE transactions on medical imaging*, 35(5):1285–1298, 2016.
19. Dan Luo, Wei Zeng, Jinlong Chen, and Wei Tang. Deep learning for automatic image segmentation in stomatology and its clinical application. *Frontiers in Medical Technology*, page 68, 2021.
20. Haozhe Jia, Yong Xia, Yang Song, Donghao Zhang, Heng Huang, Yanning Zhang, and Weidong Cai. 3d apa-net: 3d adversarial pyramid anisotropic convolutional network for prostate segmentation in mr images. *IEEE transactions on medical imaging*, 39(2):447–457, 2019.
21. Haoqi Shi, Junguo Lu, and Qianjun Zhou. A novel data augmentation method using style-based gan for robust pulmonary nodule segmentation. In *2020 Chinese Control and Decision Conference (CCDC)*, pages 2486–2491. IEEE, 2020.
22. Sibaji Gaj, Mingrui Yang, Kunio Nakamura, and Xiaojuan Li. Automated cartilage and meniscus segmentation of knee mri with conditional generative adversarial networks. *Magnetic resonance in medicine*, 84(1):437–449, 2020.
23. Suyu Dong, Gongning Luo, Clara Tam, Wei Wang, Kuanquan Wang, Shaodong Cao, Bo Chen, Henggui Zhang, and Shuo Li. Deep atlas network for efficient 3d left ventricle segmentation on echocardiography. *Medical image analysis*, 61:101638, 2020.
24. Ahmed Iqbal, Muhammad Sharif, Mussarat Yasmin, Mudassar Raza, and Shabib Aftab. Generative adversarial networks and its applications in the biomedical image segmentation: a

comprehensive survey. *International Journal of Multimedia Information Retrieval*, pages 1–36, 2022.
25. Liqun Huang, Long Chen, Baihai Zhang, and Senchun Chai. A transformer-based generative adversarial network for brain tumor segmentation. *arXiv preprint* arXiv:2207.14134, 2022.
26. Kaiming He, Xiangyu Zhang, Shaoqing Ren, and Jian Sun. Deep residual learning for image recognition. In *Proceedings of the IEEE conference on computer vision and pattern recognition*, pages 770–778, 2016.
27. Qikui Zhu, Bo Du, Baris Turkbey, Peter L Choyke, and Pingkun Yan. Deeply-supervised cnn for prostate segmentation. In *2017 international joint conference on neural networks (IJCNN)*, pages 178–184. IEEE, 2017.
28. Abdul Mueed Hafiz and Ghulam Mohiuddin Bhat. A survey on instance segmentation: state of the art. *International journal of multimedia information retrieval*, 9(3):171–189, 2020.
29. David Bouget, André Pedersen, Johanna Vanel, Haakon O Leira, and Thomas Langø. Mediastinal lymph nodes segmentation using 3d convolutional neural network ensembles and anatomical priors guiding. *Computer Methods in Biomechanics and Biomedical Engineering: Imaging & Visualization*, pages 1–15, 2022.
30. Xiahai Zhuang and Juan Shen. Multi-scale patch and multi-modality atlases for whole heart segmentation of mri. *Medical image analysis*, 31:77–87, 2016.
31. Arnaud Arindra Adiyoso Setio, Francesco Ciompi, Geert Litjens, Paul Gerke, Colin Jacobs, Sarah J Van Riel, Mathilde Marie Winkler Wille, Matiullah Naqibullah, Clara I Sánchez, and Bram Van Ginneken. Pulmonary nodule detection in ct images: false positive reduction using multi-view convolutional networks. *IEEE transactions on medical imaging*, 35(5):1160–1169, 2016.
32. Konstantinos Kamnitsas, Enzo Ferrante, Sarah Parisot, Christian Ledig, Aditya V Nori, Antonio Criminisi, Daniel Rueckert, and Ben Glocker. Deepmedic for brain tumor segmentation. In *International workshop on Brainlesion: Glioma, multiple sclerosis, stroke and traumatic brain injuries*, pages 138–149. Springer, 2016.
33. Kaiming He, Georgia Gkioxari, Piotr Dollár, and Ross Girshick. Mask r-cnn. In *Proceedings of the IEEE international conference on computer vision*, pages 2961–2969, 2017.
34. Joseph Redmon and Ali Farhadi. Yolov3: An incremental improvement. *arXiv preprint* arXiv:1804.02767, 2018.
35. Hao Chen, Lequan Yu, Qi Dou, Lin Shi, Vincent CT Mok, and Pheng Ann Heng. Automatic detection of cerebral microbleeds via deep learning based 3d feature representation. In *2015 IEEE 12th international symposium on biomedical imaging (ISBI)*, pages 764–767. IEEE, 2015.
36. Hao Chen, Qi Dou, Lequan Yu, and Pheng-Ann Heng. Voxresnet: Deep voxelwise residual networks for volumetric brain segmentation. *arXiv preprint* arXiv:1608.05895, 2016.
37. Lorenzo Venturini, Aris T Papageorghiou, J Alison Noble, and Ana IL Namburete. Multi-task cnn for structural semantic segmentation in 3d fetal brain ultrasound. In *Annual Conference on Medical Image Understanding and Analysis*, pages 164–173. Springer, 2020.
38. Abhijit Guha Roy, Sailesh Conjeti, Nassir Navab, Christian Wachinger, Alzheimer's Disease Neuroimaging Initiative, et al. Quicknat: A fully convolutional network for quick and accurate segmentation of neuroanatomy. *NeuroImage*, 186:713–727, 2019.
39. Nico Zettler and Andre Mastmeyer. Comparison of 2d vs. 3d u-net organ segmentation in abdominal 3d ct images. *arXiv preprint* arXiv:2107.04062, 2021.
40. Hao Chen, Qi Dou, Xi Wang, Jing Qin, Jack CY Cheng, and Pheng-Ann Heng. 3d fully convolutional networks for intervertebral disc localization and segmentation. In *International Conference on Medical Imaging and Augmented Reality*, pages 375–382. Springer, 2016.
41. Andrew Jesson and Tal Arbel. Brain tumor segmentation using a 3d fcn with multi-scale loss. In *International MICCAI Brainlesion Workshop*, pages 392–402. Springer, 2017.
42. Yue Zhang, Jiong Wu, Wanli Chen, Yifan Chen, and Xiaoying Tang. Prostate segmentation using z-net. In *2019 IEEE 16th International Symposium on Biomedical Imaging (ISBI 2019)*, pages 11–14. IEEE, 2019.

43. Jiong Wu, Yue Zhang, and Xiaoying Tang. A multi-atlas guided 3d fully convolutional network for mri-based subcortical segmentation. In *2019 IEEE 16th International Symposium on Biomedical Imaging (ISBI 2019)*, pages 705–708. IEEE, 2019.
44. Yue Zhang, Jiong Wu, Benxiang Jiang, Dongcen Ji, Yifan Chen, Ed X Wu, and Xiaoying Tang. Deep learning and unsupervised fuzzy c-means based level-set segmentation for liver tumor. In *2020 IEEE 17th International Symposium on Biomedical Imaging (ISBI)*, pages 1193–1196. IEEE, 2020.
45. Holger R Roth, Hirohisa Oda, Xiangrong Zhou, Natsuki Shimizu, Ying Yang, Yuichiro Hayashi, Masahiro Oda, Michitaka Fujiwara, Kazunari Misawa, and Kensaku Mori. An application of cascaded 3d fully convolutional networks for medical image segmentation. *Computerized Medical Imaging and Graphics*, 66:90–99, 2018.
46. P Viola and MJ Jones. Robust real-time face detection (2004). *Computational Vision. Disponível em:*< http://www.vision.caltech.edu/html-files/EE148-2005-Spring/pprs/viola04ijcv.pdf>. *Acesso em*, 19, 2018.
47. Özgün Çiçek, Ahmed Abdulkadir, Soeren S Lienkamp, Thomas Brox, and Olaf Ronneberger. 3d u-net: learning dense volumetric segmentation from sparse annotation. In *International conference on medical image computing and computer-assisted intervention*, pages 424–432. Springer, 2016.
48. Fausto Milletari, Nassir Navab, and Seyed-Ahmad Ahmadi. V-net: Fully convolutional neural networks for volumetric medical image segmentation. In *2016 fourth international conference on 3D vision (3DV)*, pages 565–571. IEEE, 2016.
49. Konstantinos Kamnitsas, Christian Ledig, Virginia FJ Newcombe, Joanna P Simpson, Andrew D Kane, David K Menon, Daniel Rueckert, and Ben Glocker. Efficient multi-scale 3d cnn with fully connected crf for accurate brain lesion segmentation. *Medical image analysis*, 36:61–78, 2017.
50. Christian Szegedy, Vincent Vanhoucke, Sergey Ioffe, Jon Shlens, and Zbigniew Wojna. Rethinking the inception architecture for computer vision. In *Proceedings of the IEEE conference on computer vision and pattern recognition*, pages 2818–2826, 2016.
51. Sergey Ioffe and Christian Szegedy. Batch normalization: Accelerating deep network training by reducing internal covariate shift. In *International conference on machine learning*, pages 448–456. PMLR, 2015.
52. Frank G Zöllner, Rosario Sance, Peter Rogelj, María J Ledesma-Carbayo, Jarle Rørvik, Andrés Santos, and Arvid Lundervold. Assessment of 3d dce-mri of the kidneys using non-rigid image registration and segmentation of voxel time courses. *Computerized Medical Imaging and Graphics*, 33(3):171–181, 2009.
53. Béatrice Chevaillier, Yannick Ponvianne, Jean-Luc Collette, Damien Mandry, Michel Claudon, and Olivier Pietquin. Functional semi-automated segmentation of renal dce-mri sequences. In *2008 IEEE International Conference on Acoustics, Speech and Signal Processing*, pages 525–528. IEEE, 2008.
54. Marzieh Haghighi, Simon K Warfield, and Sila Kurugol. Automatic renal segmentation in dce-mri using convolutional neural networks. In *2018 IEEE 15th International Symposium on Biomedical Imaging (ISBI 2018)*, pages 1534–1537. IEEE, 2018.
55. Zhengyang Wang, Na Zou, Dinggang Shen, and Shuiwang Ji. Non-local u-nets for biomedical image segmentation. In *Proceedings of the AAAI conference on artificial intelligence*, volume 34, pages 6315–6322, 2020.
56. Xiaojun Hu, Weijian Luo, Jiliang Hu, Sheng Guo, Weilin Huang, Matthew R Scott, Roland Wiest, Michael Dahlweid, and Mauricio Reyes. Brain segnet: 3d local refinement network for brain lesion segmentation. *BMC medical imaging*, 20(1):1–10, 2020.
57. Lequan Yu, Jie-Zhi Cheng, Qi Dou, Xin Yang, Hao Chen, Jing Qin, and Pheng-Ann Heng. Automatic 3d cardiovascular mr segmentation with densely-connected volumetric convnets. In *International conference on medical image computing and computer-assisted intervention*, pages 287–295. Springer, 2017.
58. Toan Duc Bui, Jitae Shin, and Taesup Moon. 3d densely convolutional networks for volumetric segmentation. *arXiv preprint* arXiv:1709.03199, 2017.

59. Tao Lei, Rui Sun, Xiaogang Du, Huazhu Fu, Changqing Zhang, and Asoke K Nandi. Sgu-net: Shape-guided ultralight network for abdominal image segmentation. *IEEE Journal of Biomedical and Health Informatics*, 2023.
60. Tianfei Zhou, Liulei Li, Gustav Bredell, Jianwu Li, Jan Unkelbach, and Ender Konukoglu. Volumetric memory network for interactive medical image segmentation. *Medical Image Analysis*, 83:102599, 2023.
61. Chaitra Dayananda, Jae-Young Choi, and Bumshik Lee. Multi-scale squeeze u-segnet with multi global attention for brain mri segmentation. *Sensors*, 21(10):3363, 2021.
62. Vijay Badrinarayanan, Alex Kendall, and Roberto Cipolla. Segnet: A deep convolutional encoder-decoder architecture for image segmentation. *IEEE transactions on pattern analysis and machine intelligence*, 39(12):2481–2495, 2017.
63. Philipp Krähenbühl and Vladlen Koltun. Efficient inference in fully connected crfs with gaussian edge potentials. *Advances in neural information processing systems*, 24, 2011.
64. Bjoern H Menze, Andras Jakab, Stefan Bauer, Jayashree Kalpathy-Cramer, Keyvan Farahani, Justin Kirby, Yuliya Burren, Nicole Porz, Johannes Slotboom, Roland Wiest, et al. The multimodal brain tumor image segmentation benchmark (brats). *IEEE transactions on medical imaging*, 34(10):1993–2024, 2014.
65. Oskar Maier, Bjoern H Menze, Janina von der Gablentz, Levin Häni, Mattias P Heinrich, Matthias Liebrand, Stefan Winzeck, Abdul Basit, Paul Bentley, Liang Chen, et al. Isles 2015-a public evaluation benchmark for ischemic stroke lesion segmentation from multispectral mri. *Medical image analysis*, 35:250–269, 2017.
66. Marijn F Stollenga, Wonmin Byeon, Marcus Liwicki, and Juergen Schmidhuber. Parallel multi-dimensional lstm, with application to fast biomedical volumetric image segmentation. *Advances in neural information processing systems*, 28, 2015.
67. Gao Huang, Zhuang Liu, Laurens Van Der Maaten, and Kilian Q Weinberger. Densely connected convolutional networks. In *Proceedings of the IEEE conference on computer vision and pattern recognition*, pages 4700–4708, 2017.
68. A Vedaldi, Y Jia, E Shelhamer, J Donahue, S Karayev, J Long, and T Darrell. Convolutional architecture for fast feature embedding. *Cornell University*, 2014.
69. Nathan Painchaud, Youssef Skandarani, Thierry Judge, Olivier Bernard, Alain Lalande, and Pierre-Marc Jodoin. Cardiac segmentation with strong anatomical guarantees. *IEEE transactions on medical imaging*, 39(11):3703–3713, 2020.
70. A Emre Kavur, N Sinem Gezer, Mustafa Barış, Sinem Aslan, Pierre-Henri Conze, Vladimir Groza, Duc Duy Pham, Soumick Chatterjee, Philipp Ernst, Savaş Özkan, et al. Chaos challenge-combined (ct-mr) healthy abdominal organ segmentation. *Medical Image Analysis*, 69:101950, 2021.
71. Patrick Bilic, Patrick Christ, Hongwei Bran Li, Eugene Vorontsov, Avi Ben-Cohen, Georgios Kaissis, Adi Szeskin, Colin Jacobs, Gabriel Efrain Humpire Mamani, Gabriel Chartrand, et al. The liver tumor segmentation benchmark (lits). *Medical Image Analysis*, 84:102680, 2023.
72. Sainbayar Sukhbaatar, Jason Weston, Rob Fergus, et al. End-to-end memory networks. *Advances in neural information processing systems*, 28, 2015.
73. Amber L Simpson, Michela Antonelli, Spyridon Bakas, Michel Bilello, Keyvan Farahani, Bram Van Ginneken, Annette Kopp-Schneider, Bennett A Landman, Geert Litjens, Bjoern Menze, et al. A large annotated medical image dataset for the development and evaluation of segmentation algorithms. *arXiv preprint* arXiv:1902.09063, 2019.
74. Nicholas Heller, Niranjan Sathianathen, Arveen Kalapara, Edward Walczak, Keenan Moore, Heather Kaluzniak, Joel Rosenberg, Paul Blake, Zachary Rengel, Makinna Oestreich, et al. The kits19 challenge data: 300 kidney tumor cases with clinical context, ct semantic segmentations, and surgical outcomes. *arXiv preprint* arXiv:1904.00445, 2019.
75. Daniel Bolya, Chong Zhou, Fanyi Xiao, and Yong Jae Lee. Yolact: Real-time instance segmentation. In *Proceedings of the IEEE/CVF international conference on computer vision*, pages 9157–9166, 2019.
76. Joseph Redmon, Santosh Divvala, Ross Girshick, and Ali Farhadi. You only look once: Unified, real-time object detection. In *Proceedings of the IEEE conference on computer vision and pattern recognition*, pages 779–788, 2016.

77. Amirkoushyar Ziabari, Abbas Shirinifard, Matthew R Eicholtz, David J Solecki, and Derek C Rose. A two-tier convolutional neural network for combined detection and segmentation in biological imagery. In *2019 IEEE Global Conference on Signal and Information Processing (GlobalSIP)*, pages 1–5. IEEE, 2019.
78. Giovanni Lucca França da Silva, João Vitor Ferreira França, Petterson Sousa Diniz, Aristófanes Corrêa Silva, Anselmo Cardoso de Paiva, and Elton Anderson Araújo de Cavalcanti. Automatic prostate segmentation on 3d mri scans using convolutional neural networks with residual connections and superpixels. In *2020 International Conference on Systems, Signals and Image Processing (IWSSIP)*, pages 51–56. IEEE, 2020.
79. Yong-Jin Liu, Minjing Yu, Bing-Jun Li, and Ying He. Intrinsic manifold slic: A simple and efficient method for computing content-sensitive superpixels. *IEEE transactions on pattern analysis and machine intelligence*, 40(3):653–666, 2017.
80. Kehong Liu. Stbi-yolo: A real-time object detection method for lung nodule recognition. *IEEE Access*, 10:75385–75394, 2022.
81. Sang-gil Lee, Jae Seok Bae, Hyunjae Kim, Jung Hoon Kim, and Sungroh Yoon. Liver lesion detection from weakly-labeled multi-phase ct volumes with a grouped single shot multibox detector. In *International Conference on Medical Image Computing and Computer-Assisted Intervention*, pages 693–701. Springer, 2018.
82. Mingxing Li, Chang Chen, Xiaoyu Liu, Wei Huang, Yueyi Zhang, and Zhiwei Xiong. Advanced deep networks for 3d mitochondria instance segmentation. In *2022 IEEE 19th International Symposium on Biomedical Imaging (ISBI)*, pages 1–5. IEEE, 2022.
83. Jiwoong Jeong, Yang Lei, Shannon Kahn, Tian Liu, Walter J Curran, Hui-Kuo Shu, Hui Mao, and Xiaofeng Yang. Brain tumor segmentation using 3d mask r-cnn for dynamic susceptibility contrast enhanced perfusion imaging. *Physics in Medicine & Biology*, 65(18):185009, 2020.
84. Linqin Cai, Tao Long, Yuhan Dai, and Yuting Huang. Mask r-cnn-based detection and segmentation for pulmonary nodule 3d visualization diagnosis. *Ieee Access*, 8:44400–44409, 2020.
85. Zhiming Cui, Changjian Li, and Wenping Wang. Toothnet: automatic tooth instance segmentation and identification from cone beam ct images. In *Proceedings of the IEEE/CVF Conference on Computer Vision and Pattern Recognition*, pages 6368–6377, 2019.
86. Xiyi Wu, Huai Chen, Yijie Huang, Huayan Guo, Tiantian Qiu, and Lisheng Wang. Center-sensitive and boundary-aware tooth instance segmentation and classification from cone-beam ct. In *2020 IEEE 17th International Symposium on Biomedical Imaging (ISBI)*, pages 939–942. IEEE, 2020.
87. Raphael Ortiz, Gustavo de Medeiros, Antoine HFM Peters, Prisca Liberali, and Markus Rempfler. Rdcnet: Instance segmentation with a minimalist recurrent residual network. In *International Workshop on Machine Learning in Medical Imaging*, pages 434–443. Springer, 2020.
88. Dennis Eschweiler, Thiago V Spina, Rohan C Choudhury, Elliot Meyerowitz, Alexandre Cunha, and Johannes Stegmaier. Cnn-based preprocessing to optimize watershed-based cell segmentation in 3d confocal microscopy images. In *2019 IEEE 16th International Symposium on Biomedical Imaging (ISBI 2019)*, pages 223–227. IEEE, 2019.
89. Lisa Willis, Yassin Refahi, Raymond Wightman, Benoit Landrein, José Teles, Kerwyn Casey Huang, Elliot M Meyerowitz, and Henrik Jönsson. Cell size and growth regulation in the arabidopsis thaliana apical stem cell niche. *Proceedings of the National Academy of Sciences*, 113(51):E8238–E8246, 2016.
90. Yi-Fan Zhang, Weiqiang Ren, Zhang Zhang, Zhen Jia, Liang Wang, and Tieniu Tan. Focal and efficient iou loss for accurate bounding box regression. *Neurocomputing*, 506:146–157, 2022.
91. Tianyi Zhao, Dashan Gao, Jiao Wang, and Zhaozheng Yin. Lung segmentation in ct images using a fully convolutional neural network with multi-instance and conditional adversary loss. In *2018 IEEE 15th International Symposium on Biomedical Imaging (ISBI 2018)*, pages 505–509. IEEE, 2018.

92. Jonathan Huang, Vivek Rathod, Chen Sun, Menglong Zhu, Anoop Korattikara, Alireza Fathi, Ian Fischer, Zbigniew Wojna, Yang Song, Sergio Guadarrama, et al. Speed/accuracy trade-offs for modern convolutional object detectors. In *Proceedings of the IEEE conference on computer vision and pattern recognition*, pages 7310–7311, 2017.
93. Donglai Wei, Zudi Lin, Daniel Franco-Barranco, Nils Wendt, Xingyu Liu, Wenjie Yin, Xin Huang, Aarush Gupta, Won-Dong Jang, Xueying Wang, et al. Mitoem dataset: large-scale 3d mitochondria instance segmentation from em images. In *International Conference on Medical Image Computing and Computer-Assisted Intervention*, pages 66–76. Springer, 2020.
94. Tsung-Yi Lin, Piotr Dollár, Ross Girshick, Kaiming He, Bharath Hariharan, and Serge Belongie. Feature pyramid networks for object detection. In *Proceedings of the IEEE conference on computer vision and pattern recognition*, pages 2117–2125, 2017.
95. Rohit Girdhar, Georgia Gkioxari, Lorenzo Torresani, Manohar Paluri, and Du Tran. Detect-and-track: Efficient pose estimation in videos. In *Proceedings of the IEEE Conference on Computer Vision and Pattern Recognition*, pages 350–359, 2018.
96. Matvey Ezhov, Adel Zakirov, and Maxim Gusarev. Coarse-to-fine volumetric segmentation of teeth in cone-beam ct. In *2019 IEEE 16th International Symposium on Biomedical Imaging (ISBI 2019)*, pages 52–56. IEEE, 2019.
97. Long Chen, Martin Strauch, and Dorit Merhof. Instance segmentation of biomedical images with an object-aware embedding learned with local constraints. In *International Conference on Medical Image Computing and Computer-Assisted Intervention*, pages 451–459. Springer, 2019.
98. Davy Neven, Bert De Brabandere, Marc Proesmans, and Luc Van Gool. Instance segmentation by jointly optimizing spatial embeddings and clustering bandwidth. In *Proceedings of the IEEE/CVF Conference on Computer Vision and Pattern Recognition*, pages 8837–8845, 2019.
99. Alexander Kirillov, Kaiming He, Ross Girshick, Carsten Rother, and Piotr Dollár. Panoptic segmentation. In *Proceedings of the IEEE/CVF Conference on Computer Vision and Pattern Recognition*, pages 9404–9413, 2019.
100. Dongnan Liu, Donghao Zhang, Yang Song, Heng Huang, and Weidong Cai. Panoptic feature fusion net: a novel instance segmentation paradigm for biomedical and biological images. *IEEE Transactions on Image Processing*, 30:2045–2059, 2021.
101. Tuomas Kaseva, Bahareh Omidali, Eero Hippeläinen, Teemu Mäkelä, Ulla Wilppu, Alexey Sofiev, Arto Merivaara, Marjo Yliperttula, Sauli Savolainen, and Eero Salli. Marker-controlled watershed with deep edge emphasis and optimized h-minima transform for automatic segmentation of densely cultivated 3d cell nuclei. *BMC bioinformatics*, 23(1):1–19, 2022.
102. Jierong Cheng, Jagath C Rajapakse, et al. Segmentation of clustered nuclei with shape markers and marking function. *IEEE Transactions on Biomedical Engineering*, 56(3):741–748, 2008.
103. Chanho Jung and Changick Kim. Segmenting clustered nuclei using h-minima transform-based marker extraction and contour parameterization. *IEEE transactions on biomedical engineering*, 57(10):2600–2604, 2010.
104. Mehdi Mirza and Simon Osindero. Conditional generative adversarial nets. *arXiv preprint* arXiv:1411.1784, 2014.
105. Avi Ben-Cohen, Eyal Klang, Stephen P Raskin, Michal Marianne Amitai, and Hayit Greenspan. Virtual pet images from ct data using deep convolutional networks: initial results. In *International workshop on simulation and synthesis in medical imaging*, pages 49–57. Springer, 2017.
106. Xin Yi and Paul Babyn. Sharpness-aware low-dose ct denoising using conditional generative adversarial network. *Journal of digital imaging*, 31(5):655–669, 2018.
107. Dong Nie, Roger Trullo, Jun Lian, Caroline Petitjean, Su Ruan, Qian Wang, and Dinggang Shen. Medical image synthesis with context-aware generative adversarial networks. In *International conference on medical image computing and computer-assisted intervention*, pages 417–425. Springer, 2017.
108. Biting Yu, Luping Zhou, Lei Wang, Jurgen Fripp, and Pierrick Bourgeat. 3d cgan based cross-modality mr image synthesis for brain tumor segmentation. In *2018 IEEE 15th international symposium on biomedical imaging (ISBI 2018)*, pages 626–630. IEEE, 2018.

109. Shalini K Vinod, Michael G Jameson, Myo Min, and Lois C Holloway. Uncertainties in volume delineation in radiation oncology: a systematic review and recommendations for future studies. *Radiotherapy and Oncology*, 121(2):169–179, 2016.
110. Xue Dong, Yang Lei, Tonghe Wang, Matthew Thomas, Leonardo Tang, Walter J Curran, Tian Liu, and Xiaofeng Yang. Automatic multiorgan segmentation in thorax ct images using u-net-gan. *Medical physics*, 46(5):2157–2168, 2019.
111. Jinzhong Yang, Harini Veeraraghavan, Samuel G Armato III, Keyvan Farahani, Justin S Kirby, Jayashree Kalpathy-Kramer, Wouter van Elmpt, Andre Dekker, Xiao Han, Xue Feng, et al. Autosegmentation for thoracic radiation treatment planning: a grand challenge at aapm 2017. *Medical physics*, 45(10):4568–4581, 2018.
112. Haozhe Jia, Yong Xia, Yang Song, Weidong Cai, Michael Fulham, and David Dagan Feng. Atlas registration and ensemble deep convolutional neural network-based prostate segmentation using magnetic resonance imaging. *Neurocomputing*, 275:1358–1369, 2018.
113. Geert Litjens, Robert Toth, Wendy van de Ven, Caroline Hoeks, Sjoerd Kerkstra, Bram van Ginneken, Graham Vincent, Gwenael Guillard, Neil Birbeck, Jindang Zhang, et al. Evaluation of prostate segmentation algorithms for mri: the promise12 challenge. *Medical image analysis*, 18(2):359–373, 2014.
114. Samuel G Armato III, Geoffrey McLennan, Luc Bidaut, Michael F McNitt-Gray, Charles R Meyer, Anthony P Reeves, Binsheng Zhao, Denise R Aberle, Claudia I Henschke, Eric A Hoffman, et al. The lung image database consortium (lidc) and image database resource initiative (idri): a completed reference database of lung nodules on ct scans. *Medical physics*, 38(2):915–931, 2011.
115. Mohammad Havaei, Nicolas Guizard, Nicolas Chapados, and Yoshua Bengio. Hemis: Hetero-modal image segmentation. In *International Conference on Medical Image Computing and Computer-Assisted Intervention*, pages 469–477. Springer, 2016.
116. Yawen Huang, Feng Zheng, Runmin Cong, Weilin Huang, Matthew R Scott, and Ling Shao. Mcmt-gan: multi-task coherent modality transferable gan for 3d brain image synthesis. *IEEE Transactions on Image Processing*, 29:8187–8198, 2020.
117. Yi Sun, Peisen Yuan, and Yuming Sun. Mm-gan: 3d mri data augmentation for medical image segmentation via generative adversarial networks. In *2020 IEEE International conference on knowledge graph (ICKG)*, pages 227–234. IEEE, 2020.
118. Ashish Shrivastava, Tomas Pfister, Oncel Tuzel, Joshua Susskind, Wenda Wang, and Russell Webb. Learning from simulated and unsupervised images through adversarial training. In *Proceedings of the IEEE conference on computer vision and pattern recognition*, pages 2107–2116, 2017.
119. Tianyang Li, Benzheng Wei, Jinyu Cong, Xuzhou Li, and Shuo Li. S 3 eganet: 3d spinal structures segmentation via adversarial nets. *IEEE Access*, 8:1892–1901, 2019.
120. Jonathan Masci, Ueli Meier, Dan Cireşan, and Jürgen Schmidhuber. Stacked convolutional auto-encoders for hierarchical feature extraction. In *International conference on artificial neural networks*, pages 52–59. Springer, 2011.
121. Kuan-Lun Tseng, Yen-Liang Lin, Winston Hsu, and Chung-Yang Huang. Joint sequence learning and cross-modality convolution for 3d biomedical segmentation. In *Proceedings of the IEEE conference on Computer Vision and Pattern Recognition*, pages 6393–6400, 2017.
122. Arnab Kumar Mondal, Jose Dolz, and Christian Desrosiers. Few-shot 3d multi-modal medical image segmentation using generative adversarial learning. *arXiv preprint* arXiv:1810.12241, 2018.
123. Yi Sun, Chengfeng Zhou, Yanwei Fu, and Xiangyang Xue. Parasitic gan for semi-supervised brain tumor segmentation. In *2019 IEEE international conference on image processing (ICIP)*, pages 1535–1539. IEEE, 2019.
124. Jiajun Wu, Chengkai Zhang, Tianfan Xue, Bill Freeman, and Josh Tenenbaum. Learning a probabilistic latent space of object shapes via 3d generative-adversarial modeling. *Advances in neural information processing systems*, 29, 2016.
125. Phillip Isola, Jun-Yan Zhu, Tinghui Zhou, and Alexei A Efros. Image-to-image translation with conditional adversarial networks. In *Proceedings of the IEEE conference on computer vision and pattern recognition*, pages 1125–1134, 2017.

126. Chichen Fu, Soonam Lee, David Joon Ho, Shuo Han, Paul Salama, Kenneth W Dunn, and Edward J Delp. Three dimensional fluorescence microscopy image synthesis and segmentation. In *Proceedings of the IEEE conference on computer vision and pattern recognition workshops*, pages 2221–2229, 2018.
127. David Joon Ho, Shuo Han, Chichen Fu, Paul Salama, Kenneth W Dunn, and Edward J Delp. Center-extraction-based three dimensional nuclei instance segmentation of fluorescence microscopy images. In *2019 IEEE EMBS International Conference on Biomedical & Health Informatics (BHI)*, pages 1–4. IEEE, 2019.
128. Jun-Yan Zhu, Taesung Park, Phillip Isola, and Alexei A Efros. Unpaired image-to-image translation using cycle-consistent adversarial networks. In *Proceedings of the IEEE international conference on computer vision*, pages 2223–2232, 2017.
129. Dennis Eschweiler, Malte Rethwisch, Mareike Jarchow, Simon Koppers, and Johannes Stegmaier. 3d fluorescence microscopy data synthesis for segmentation and benchmarking. *Plos one*, 16(12):e0260509, 2021.
130. Emmanuel Faure, Thierry Savy, Barbara Rizzi, Camilo Melani, Olga Stašová, Dimitri Fabrèges, Róbert Špir, Mark Hammons, Róbert Čúnderlík, Gaëlle Recher, et al. A workflow to process 3d+ time microscopy images of developing organisms and reconstruct their cell lineage. *Nature communications*, 7(1):1–10, 2016.
131. Moritz Böhland, Tim Scherr, Andreas Bartschat, Ralf Mikut, and Markus Reischl. Influence of synthetic label image object properties on gan supported segmentation pipelines. In *Proceedings 29th Workshop Computational Intelligence*, pages 289–305, 2019.
132. Kenneth W Dunn, Chichen Fu, David Joon Ho, Soonam Lee, Shuo Han, Paul Salama, and Edward J Delp. Deepsynth: Three-dimensional nuclear segmentation of biological images using neural networks trained with synthetic data. *Scientific reports*, 9(1):1–15, 2019.
133. Casey Chu, Andrey Zhmoginov, and Mark Sandler. Cyclegan, a master of steganography. *arXiv preprint* arXiv:1712.02950, 2017.
134. Kai Yao, Kaizhu Huang, Jie Sun, and Curran Jude. Ad-gan: End-to-end unsupervised nuclei segmentation with aligned disentangling training. *arXiv preprint* arXiv:2107.11022, 2021.
135. David Svoboda, Michal Kozubek, and Stanislav Stejskal. Generation of digital phantoms of cell nuclei and simulation of image formation in 3d image cytometry. *Cytometry Part A: The Journal of the International Society for Advancement of Cytometry*, 75(6):494–509, 2009.
136. Leander Lauenburg, Zudi Lin, Ruihan Zhang, Márcia dos Santos, Siyu Huang, Ignacio Arganda-Carreras, Edward S Boyden, Hanspeter Pfister, and Donglai Wei. Instance segmentation of unlabeled modalities via cyclic segmentation gan. *arXiv preprint* arXiv:2204.03082, 2022.
137. Carsen Stringer, Tim Wang, Michalis Michaelos, and Marius Pachitariu. Cellpose: a generalist algorithm for cellular segmentation. *Nature methods*, 18(1):100–106, 2021.
138. Martin Weigert, Uwe Schmidt, Robert Haase, Ko Sugawara, and Gene Myers. Star-convex polyhedra for 3d object detection and segmentation in microscopy. In *Proceedings of the IEEE/CVF Winter Conference on Applications of Computer Vision*, pages 3666–3673, 2020.
139. Fei Chen, Paul W Tillberg, and Edward S Boyden. Expansion microscopy. *Science*, 347(6221):543–548, 2015.
140. Yaroslav Ganin and Victor Lempitsky. Unsupervised domain adaptation by backpropagation. In *International conference on machine learning*, pages 1180–1189. PMLR, 2015.
141. Eric Tzeng, Judy Hoffman, Kate Saenko, and Trevor Darrell. Adversarial discriminative domain adaptation. In *Proceedings of the IEEE conference on computer vision and pattern recognition*, pages 7167–7176, 2017.
142. Dongnan Liu, Donghao Zhang, Yang Song, Fan Zhang, Lauren O'Donnell, Heng Huang, Mei Chen, and Weidong Cai. Pdam: A panoptic-level feature alignment framework for unsupervised domain adaptive instance segmentation in microscopy images. *IEEE Transactions on Medical Imaging*, 40(1):154–165, 2020.
143. Holger R Roth, Le Lu, Ari Seff, Kevin M Cherry, Joanne Hoffman, Shijun Wang, Jiamin Liu, Evrim Turkbey, and Ronald M Summers. A new 2.5 d representation for lymph node detection using random sets of deep convolutional neural network observations. In *International*

conference on medical image computing and computer-assisted intervention, pages 520–527. Springer, 2014.

144. Rushil Anirudh, Jayaraman J Thiagarajan, Timo Bremer, and Hyojin Kim. Lung nodule detection using 3d convolutional neural networks trained on weakly labeled data. In *Medical Imaging 2016: Computer-Aided Diagnosis*, volume 9785, pages 791–796. SPIE, 2016.
145. Gregor Urban, M Bendszus, F Hamprecht, and J Kleesiek. Multi-modal brain tumor segmentation using deep convolutional neural networks. *MICCAI BraTS (brain tumor segmentation) challenge. Proceedings, winning contribution*, pages 31–35, 2014.
146. Qi Dou, Lequan Yu, Hao Chen, Yueming Jin, Xin Yang, Jing Qin, and Pheng-Ann Heng. 3d deeply supervised network for automated segmentation of volumetric medical images. *Medical image analysis*, 41:40–54, 2017.
147. Christian F Baumgartner, Lisa M Koch, Marc Pollefeys, and Ender Konukoglu. An exploration of 2d and 3d deep learning techniques for cardiac mr image segmentation. In *International Workshop on Statistical Atlases and Computational Models of the Heart*, pages 111–119. Springer, 2017.

Analysis of GAN-Based Data Augmentation for GI-Tract Disease Classification

Muhammad Nouman Noor, Imran Ashraf, and Muhammad Nazir

Abstract Gastro-Intestinal (GI) disorders are a significant problem for the humans' digestive system. GI disorders are on the rise worldwide. The United States has the highest rates of GI cancer. Before the onset of symptoms, routine screening for patients at average risk can help with early identification and treatment. The use of automated technologies by doctors is one technique to enhance diagnosis. Convolutional Neural Network (CNN) models have been used by automated systems based on Deep Learning (DL) to produce noteworthy breakthroughs in the field of image classification. A hurdle in the field of medical imaging is the requirement for a sizeable amount of annotated data to increase the results' quality. Furthermore, the class imbalance exacerbates the problem and adds bias towards classes with more images. Data augmentation is typically used to address this problem. Generative Adversarial Networks (GANs) have recently demonstrated significant outcomes in data augmentation. In this chapter, we analyze the use of GAN-based data augmentation and geometric transformation-based data augmentation for the classification of GI tract illnesses. According to our findings, GAN-based data augmentation keeps the model from being overly tailored to the dominant class. Additionally, training with this enriched data improves performance across classes by regularising training.

1 Introduction

GI diseases, including colorectal cancer, are a significant global health issue and a leading cause of cancer-related deaths [1]. Despite progresses in treatment, the five years' survival rate for colorectal cancer is relatively high at 68% [2] but that for stomach cancer is much lower at 44%. Early detection and removal of lesions

M. N. Noor · I. Ashraf (✉) · M. Nazir
HITEC University Cantt Taxila, Rawalpindi, Punjab 47080, Pakistan
e-mail: imran.ashraf@hitecuni.edu.pk

M. N. Noor
e-mail: nouman.noor@hitecuni.edu.pk

M. Nazir
e-mail: muhammad.nazir@hitecuni.edu.pk

H. Ali et al. (eds.), *Advances in Deep Generative Models for Medical Artificial Intelligence*, Studies in Computational Intelligence 1124,
https://doi.org/10.1007/978-3-031-46341-9_2

can prevent cancer from developing and improve survival rates to nearly 100% [3]. Regular inspection for patients at average risk before symptoms appear can facilitate early diagnosis and treatment. Endoscopic processes are considered the high-quality processes for the diagnosis of GI abnormalities and cancers [4]. In light of this, there is a need to develop an automated Computer Aided system that can be incorporated into medical procedures [5]. However, this involves attentive assessment of the methods on a benchmark dataset, as well as assessing their clinical applicability in terms of patient variability and instantaneous processing capability.

The integration of AI-based systems in medical imaging has led to a surge of research in the field of GI endoscopy. One of the key challenges in this area is to accurately identify and classify diseases in order to improve the chances of early detection. This entails the incorporation of expert gastroentologists' awareness and the development of efficient automated systems that can aid in instantaneous decision making during the endoscopic procedure. This can help to reduce the workload of expert endoscopists, and aid less experienced endoscopists in identifying clinically relevant markers and regions. Additionally, automated reporting spawned by automated methods can help to improve productivity and focus on critical cases [6].

The utilization of computer vision and AI in the field of gastrointestinal endoscopy has seen significant progress in recent years. However, a major limitation of these methods and datasets is that they tend to focus on a narrow range of lesions and are typically restricted to a single organ. In reality, routine monitoring of the gastrointestinal tract often involves multiple organs such as the esophagus, stomach, duodenum, small intestine, and large intestine, each with their own unique set of diseases. This complexity makes it challenging to detect all types of lesions across multiple locations within the gastrointestinal tract, highlighting the need for a more comprehensive approach to GI surveillance [6].

Automated systems based on Deep Learning (DL) have achieved notable breakthroughs and successes in image classification tasks by utilizing Convolutional Neural Network (CNN) models. However, improved quality of the results demands significant amount of annotated data, which is a challenge in the field of medical imaging. Another challenge is that the available datasets are quite unbalanced, making it hard to train a CNN model to accurately classify diseases across classes. To solve this issue, data augmentation is generally performed. Recently, Generative Adversarial Networks (GANs) have shown impressive results in performing data-augmentation. In this chapter, we present an analysis of geometric transformations-based as well as GAN-based data augmentation and studied its impact for the classification of GI-Tract disease which is the main contribution. Our analysis shows that GAN-based data augmentation prevents the model from over-fitting to the dominant class. Moreover, training on this augmented data helps to regularize the training and improve performance across classes.

2 Related Work

We discussed here various techniques for data augmentation in the area of computer-vision, particularly in the context of image classification. Data augmentation techniques aim to increase the size of the dataset and reduce over-fitting when training a CNN or deep networks. One of the initial applications of data augmentation was the use of data warping in LeNet-5 [9], a CNN model for handwritten digit classification.

Oversampling is one method for addressing the issue of class-imbalance in a dataset. To balance the distribution of classes, this method increases the number of samples in the smaller class. A straightforward technique called random oversampling (ROS) involves randomly reproducing photos from the minority class. Another technique is called Synthetic-Minority-Oversampling-Technique, which creates new samples by interpolating between minority class samples already present. This method attempts to address the issue of class imbalance and is often applied to datasets in the form of tables or vectors.

Using convolutional-networks on the ImageNet dataset, the CNN architecture of AlexNet has a tremendous impact on the field of image categorization. They used Data Augmentation techniques to increase the dataset size by randomly cropping the original photos to 224×224 pixels, flipping them horizontally, and altering the R, G, and B channel intensities through colour augmentation. According to the authors [10], these augmentations were able to enhance the model's performance by lowering the error rate by more than 1%.

Over time, numerous data augmentation techniques have been developed to enhance the performance of medical image analysis tasks. These techniques include GANs [11], Neural Style Transfer, and Neural Architecture Search (NAS). In particular, GAN-based image synthesis data augmentation was utilized in 2018 for liver lesion classification. This approach led to a significant improvement in classification performance compared to traditional augmentation methods. In the study by Ianjamasimanana et al. [12], GAN-based data augmentation was employed for liver lesion classification. The results showed that the use of GAN-based data augmentation improved the sensitivity from 78.6% to 85.7% and the specificity from 88.4% to 92.4% when compared to classic augmentation techniques. This indicates a substantial enhancement in the accuracy and reliability of the classification task.

By using relationships between segmentation labels to direct the shape generation process, the authors of [37] developed a unique method for producing convincing retinal OCT pictures. Through uncertainty sampling, diversity is incorporated into the image production process. Comparative results demonstrate that when used to segment problematic regions (fluid filled areas) in retinal OCT images, the enhanced dataset using GAN outperforms standard data augmentation and other competing approaches. Another study [38] looked into the viability of using generative adversarial networks to produce realistic-looking dermoscopic images (GANs). Then, in an effort to improve the performance of a deep convolutional neural network on the skin lesion classification task, these images are used to supplement our current training set. Results show that GAN-based augmentation yields sizable performance increases when compared to traditional data augmentation techniques. The authors' in the study [56] presented the GAN-based data augmentation for brain images in contrast with the classical augmentation and enhanced their work towards 3-D imaging. Conditional Generative Adversarial Networks (cGAN) are used in this study [57] to generate signals artificially. For identifying the respiratory signals, publicly accessible repositories like the ICBHI 2017 challenge, RALE, and Think Labs Lung Sounds Library are taken into account. Similarity measurements between the original and augmented signals are computed in order to evaluate the effectiveness of the artificially generated signals produced by the DA technique. Following that, scalogram representations of generated signals are provided as input to various pre-trained deep learning architectures, including Alexnet, GoogLeNet, and ResNet-50, in order to quantify the performance of augmentation in classification. The experimental findings are calculated, and performance outcomes are contrasted with currently used conventional augmentation methods. According to the research's findings, the proposed cGAN technique offers superior accuracy for the two data sets utilising the ResNet-50 model, with scores of 92.50% and 92.68%, respectively.

Data augmentation techniques have come a long way since the introduction of AlexNet CNN architecture in 2012, which used convolutional networks on the ImageNet dataset. Innovations include the use of GAN [11], Transfer learning, and neural-architecture-search to enhance the performance of image classification. One such technique, data augmentation on the basis of GAN, was applied for the classification of liver-lesion was proposed in 2018 and resulted in improved classification performance, with sensitivity and specificity increasing from 78.6% and 88.4% respectively using traditional techniques to 85.7 and 92.4% [12].

Data augmentation techniques have been traditionally used to improve image recognition models, such as those that predict labels for input images. However, these techniques have also been applied to other computer-vision tasks, like object-detection and semantic-segmentation, to enhance their performance [13–15].

2.1 Data Augmentation Approaches for Medical Imaging

Various techniques have been employed in numerous studies to augment brain MR images, including rotation, noise addition, shearing, and translation. These methods have proven to be effective in increasing the number of images and enhancing the performance of various tasks. For example, Khan et al. [39] utilized noise addition and sharpening techniques for image augmentation, leading to improved accuracy in tumor segmentation and classification. Similarly, Dufumier et al. [40] employed translation, random rotation, cropping, multiple blurring, as well noise-addition to augment images, achieving high performance in tasks such as age-prediction, and gender-classification. Furthermore, Isensee et al. [41] utilized random-rotation, multiple-scaling, as well elastic-deformation to augment images, resulting in improved accuracy for tumor segmentation. In addition to these techniques, researchers have explored advanced approaches to further enhance image augmentation. Wang et al. [42] introduced a modified version of Mixup called TensorMixup, which combines two image patches using a tensor in a voxel-based approach. This method significantly improved tumor segmentation accuracy. Moreover, a recent study by Kossen et al. [43] and Li et al. [44] employed a GAN-based augmentation technique for cerebrovascular segmentation.

The utilization of computerized methods for medical tasks, such as nodule or lung-parenchyma-segmentation as well classification, and disease-diagnosis (e.g., COVID-19), often involves the application of CT lung image augmentation. Traditional techniques like random-rotation, flipping, and random-scaling are commonly employed in this augmentation process. For instance, Hu et al. [45] enhanced the automated diagnosis of COVID-19 by employing flipping, translation, rotation, and brightness adjustments as part of their image augmentation strategy. Similarly, Alshazly et al. [46] applied various augmentations, including Gaussian noise addition, cropping, flipping, blurring, brightness changes, shearing, and rotation, to improve the performance of COVID-19 diagnosis. In addition to traditional techniques, GAN models have also been utilized to generate synthetic images for augmenting lung CT images. When applying GAN-based augmentation to lung CT scans, generating the specific area that displays lung nodules within the entire image is often preferred due to its cost-effectiveness compared to generating a larger background area. Wan et al. [47] employed guided GAN structures to produce synthetic images highlighting the region containing lung nodules. On the other hand, Nishimura et al. [48] used information about the size of nodules and guided GANs to generate images with diverse sizes of lung nodules.

In the domain of mammography images, augmentation methods are commonly employed to enhance the automated-recognition, localization, and detection of breast-lesions. Typically, positive patches containing marked lesions by radiologists and random regions from the same image representing negative patches are extracted as training samples. To improve performance, it is preferable to refine and segment the lesion regions before applying augmentation methods. Various techniques such as random-scaling, noise-addition, mirroring, random-rotation, and shearing, either individually or in combinations, are commonly used for augmentation in this context [49, 50]. In addition to traditional augmentation techniques, GAN models have also been utilized to generate synthetic images for augmentation purposes. For instance, Alyafi et al. [51] combined flipping and deep-convolutional-GAN to perform binary classification of mammography images as normal or with a mass. Similarly, contextual-GAN has been employed to improve binary classification (normal vs. malignant) by generating new images that synthesize lesions based on the context of the surrounding tissue. This approach aims to capture the characteristics of lesions in their natural context. Furthermore, in another study, both contextual-GAN and deep-convolutional-GAN were used to generate synthetic images of lesions, incorporating margin and texture information. This approach resulted in improved performance in lesion detection and segmentation tasks [52].

In [53], authors applied geometric transformations for data augmentation in gastrointestinal disease classification and achieved 96.43% accuracy. Similarly, another [54] researcher applied geometric transformation on gastro diseases and achieved

Table 1 Summary of augmentation techniques on medical imaging

Reference	Augmentation technique	Implementation area	Results
[39]	Geometric transformation and noise addition	Brain Tumor recognition	94.06 % Accuracy
[40]	Geometric transformation and noise addition	Schizophrenia recognition and sex classification	83.01% Accuracy for schizophrenia recognition and 83.01% Accuracy for sex classification
[41]	Geometric transformation and elastic deformation	Brain Tumor segmentation	88.95% Dice score
[42]	TensorMixup	Brain tumor segmentation	91.32% Dice score
[43]	Wasserstein GAN	Vessel segmentation	91.00% Dice score
[44]	Image to image translation based on GAN	Tumor segmentation	76.00% dice score
[45]	Geometric transformation	COVID-19 diagnosis	91.21% accuracy
[46]	Geometric transformation ,noise addition, blurring and brightness changing	COVID-19 detection	92.90% accuracy
[47]	Co-guided GAN	Prediction of malignancy level	84.03% F1 score
[48]	GAN	Nodule classification	87.50% accuracy
[49]	Geometric transformation	Breast lesion classification	96.53% accuracy
[50]	Shifting	Breast lesion detection and segmentation	0.897 Auc
[51]	Deep GAN	Breast classification	0.09 F1 score
[52]	Deep convolutional and contextual GAN	Breast lesion detection	0.172 Auc
[53]	Geometric transformations	Gastrointestinal disease classification	96.43% accuracy
[54]	Geometric transformations	GI-tract disease classification	96.40% accuracy
[55]	Deep convolutional GAN	Gastro disease classification	97.25% accuracy

96.40% accuracy. In [55], deep-convolutional-GAN are applied for gastrointestinal disease classification and achieved 97.25% accuracy. The summary of the augmentation techniques for medical imaging discussed in literature is shown in Table 1.

3 Data Augmentation

The advancements in deep learning, specifically the development of CNNs, have greatly improved the ability to tackle discriminatory tasks in computer vision. The use of parameterized, sparsely connected kernels in CNNs allows for the preservation of spatial characteristics in images, and the convolutional layers in these networks effectively reduce the spatial clarity while increasing the deepness of feature-maps, resulting in more informative representations of the images. This has led to increased interest and optimism in using deep learning for various computer-vision tasks such as image-classification, object-detection, and image-segmentation [7].

Large datasets, the creation of potent architectures, accessibility to potent computing resources, and the growth of deep learning have all contributed to substantial breakthroughs in computer vision. CNNs have demonstrated their superior performance in a variety of tasks, including image segmentation, object detection, and classification. The 3-D characteristics of images are preserved by these networks' parameterized kernels. These networks' convolutional layers gradually decrease the 3-D resolution of the images while enhancing the deepness of the feature-maps. Compared to hand-crafted representations of the same photos, the ones produced this way are less three-dimensional and more informational. Despite these advances, the generalizability of these models-the difference in performance when a model is assessed on data it has previously seen (training data) against data it has never seen before—is still being worked on (testing data). Models that are difficult to generalize over—fit the training set of data.

Convolutional Neural Networks (CNNs) and the accessibility of big datasets have both contributed to the advancement of deep learning models in applications involving image identification. The capacity of these models to perform well on untested data, or generalise, is a significant hurdle in these activities. Data augmentation is a technique that solves this problem by generating synthetic data instances using methods like mixing-images, feature-space-augmentations, and GAN [7] or by artificially growing the training dataset using techniques like adversarial training, neural style transfer, geometric and colour changes, random erasing, and random erasing.

As it must deal with challenges like viewpoint, illumination, occlusion, scale, and more, picture recognition is a difficult process. By incorporating translational invariances into the dataset, data augmentation seeks to overcome these difficulties and produce models that are effective in spite of them.

In the field of medical image analysis, limited datasets are a common challenge [8]. The manual effort and expense required for collecting and labeling data, as well as patient privacy and rarity of diseases, make it difficult to build large datasets. This has led to a focus on data augmentation techniques, particularly GAN-based oversampling, to improve the performance of medical-image classification models.

Popular images datasets including CIFAR-10, CIFAR-100, and ImageNet have been utilised in prior research on the effectiveness of data-augmentation to compare results. However, several of these experiments used a portion of the dataset to simulate issues with insufficient data. Additionally, data augmentation techniques have been used to address the issue of class imbalance, which arises when a dataset has an unbalanced ratio of majority to minority samples. Since data augmentation enables the model to "imagine" changes to images and obtain a deeper knowledge of them, it might be compared to human imagination or dreaming.

4 Types of Image Data Augmentation Techniques

Simple manipulations like flipping, changing the colour space, and randomly cropping images have been used in early research to show how data augmentation techniques might be used to enhance the performance of image recognition models. These methods work well for tackling the invariances that often complicate picture recognition jobs. Various data augmentation techniques are utilized in literature as depicted nicely in Fig. 1. Geometric transformations and GAN-based augmentations are only a couple of the strategies for data augmentation that have been researched. This section will describe these two augmentation algorithms. We provide experimental findings and highlight the limitations of these approaches.

4.1 Geometric Transformations Based Augmentation

In this section, various techniques for augmenting data through geometric transformations and image processing functions will be examined. These methods are simple to implement and can serve as a starting point for further exploration into data augmentation techniques.

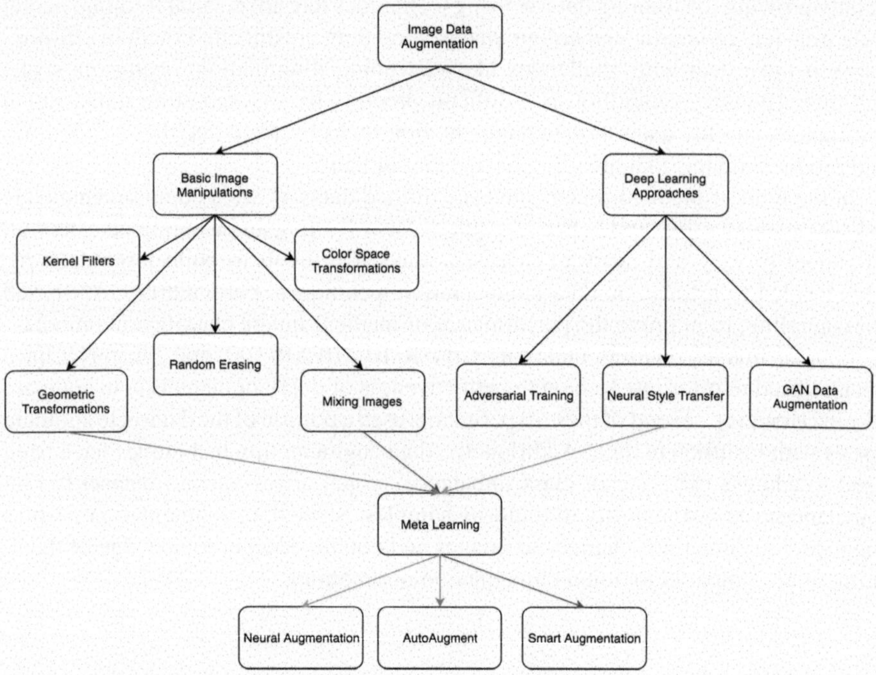

Fig. 1 Augmentation techniques [58]

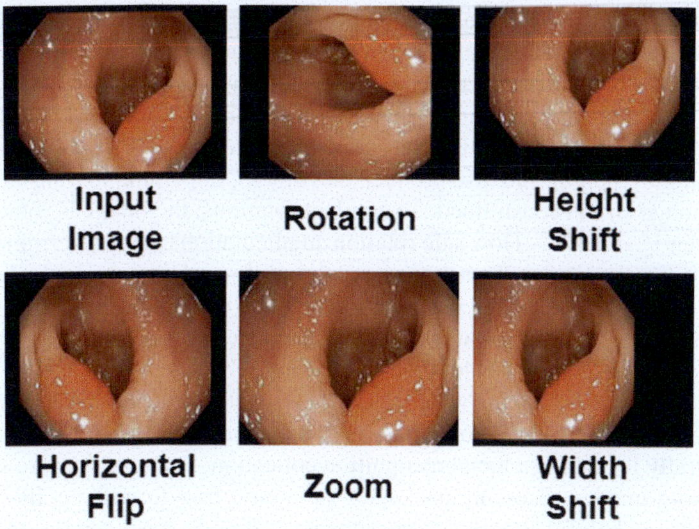

Fig. 2 Data augmentation using geometric transformation on gastrointestinal disease image

This section looks at several data augmentation approaches that use geometric transformations and other image processing techniques. These augmentations can be used as a jumping off point for additional research on data augmentation because they are easy to apply. We will also assess the safety of these augmentations, which refers to their capacity to preserve the correctness of the original label following the transformation. For example, rotations and flips may be useful for picture classification tasks like detecting cats and dogs but not for tasks requiring the recognition of digits like 6 and 9. It is important to keep in mind that employing non-label preserving transformations may enhance a model's capacity to output a response indicating that it is unsure about its prediction, but this would necessitate more computation to refine labels after the augmentation [16].

Several different types of geometric augmentations, including flipping, color space, cropping, rotation, translations, and scaling are discussed here. Each of these augmentations has its own strengths and weaknesses, and the choice of which augmentation to use will depend on the specific dataset and task at hand. The augmentation of such images on gastrointestinal disease dataset is shown in Fig. 2. It's also important to keep in mind that the choice of augmentation is somewhat domain-dependent and therefore developing generalizable augmentation policies is a challenging task. However, some recent works such as AutoAugment, try to solve this problem by finding generalizable augmentations [17].

Flipping is a straightforward augmentation technique that includes horizontally flipping an image. This is a simple method that has been shown effective on datasets like CIFAR-10 and ImageNet. In text recognition datasets like "MNIST" or "SVHN", it is not a label-preserving transformation, though. Enhancements in colour space require changing an image's colour channels. The brightness of the image can be changed by focusing on a specific colour channel, such as red, green, or blue, and adjusting the RGB values. Deriving a colour histogram and altering the intensity values are two more sophisticated colour augmentation techniques. Cropping is a helpful step in the processing of images with mismatched width and height dimensions. Random cropping can also produce outcomes comparable to translations, but the input image size is constrained. To conduct rotations, the image is rotated on an axis between 1° and 359° . How safe rotation augmentations are is determined by the variation degree constraint. Translations involve shifting the image to the left, right, up, or down in order to prevent positional bias in the data. Noise injection involves injecting a matrix of random values, often derived from a Gaussian distribution, to help CNNs acquire more durable features [18–20].

Geometric modifications are widely used to eliminate positional biases in the training data [21–23]. One of the numerous probable sources of these biases is images being centrally located in a facial recognition collection. Because they are simple to execute using image processing packages, geometric transformations like flipping and rotation are helpful in these circumstances. They do have certain drawbacks, though, such higher memory utilization, higher processing costs, and lengthier training times. It's also crucial to manually verify that the label of the image hasn't changed as a result of these adjustments. The range of where and when geometric alterations can be used is constrained in many application domains, including medical image analysis, by the biases between the training and testing data, which are more complex than positional and translational variances.

4.2 Data Augmentation with GANs

A technique for data augmentation known as generative modelling produces fake instances from a dataset that share properties with the original set. Generative Adversarial Networks (GANs), a framework for generative modelling through adversarial training, are one well-known generative modelling method. Due to their quick calculation times and excellent output quality, GANs have grown in prominence. They function by teaching a generator network to generate fictitious data that a discriminator network cannot distinguish from genuine data [24]. This generates fresh training data that can help categorization models perform better. The GAN architecture is depicted in Fig. 3.

Generative techniques like Variational Autoencoder (VAE) [25] can also be used to augment data sets [26]. VAE works by learning a low-dimensional representation of data points, which can be used to generate new instances of data by performing vector operations. For example, a 3D rotation of an image [27] can be simulated by adding and subtracting vectors in the low-dimensional representation. These generated images can be further improved by inputting them into GANs. Additionally, bidirectional GANs can be used to perform vector manipulation on the noise inputs to GANs [28].

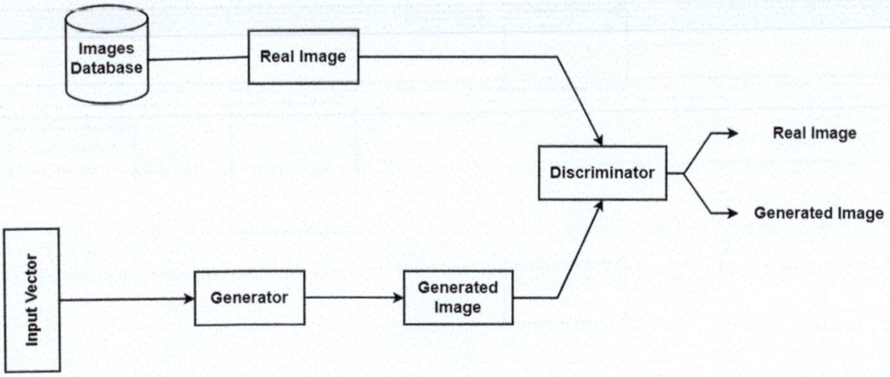

Fig. 3 Generative adversarial network architecture

It's important to keep in mind that while GANs are a well-liked and effective method, they are not the sole choice for generative modelling. Additionally, GANs can be made even better by including VAEs or other techniques to produce images that are more realistic and varied [29]. The generator and discriminator neural networks that make up GANs are trained concurrently in a two-player minimax game. The discriminator learns to discriminate between the created samples and the actual samples while the generator learns to generate new data samples that are comparable to the training data. The discriminator's goal is to accurately identify the generated samples, whereas the generator's goal is to "trick" the discriminator [30].

GANs is a potent method for generative modelling that is distinguished by its capacity to generate excellent, realistic images. The method is based on a strategy influenced by game theory, in which a generator network creates images and a discriminator network determines the veracity of those images. As a result, a *minimax* game is created, in which the generator seeks to make deceptive images while the discriminator strives to properly detect deceptive images. The discriminator's objective is for the generator to finally produce images that are identical to genuine photographs. The generator and discriminator networks of the original GAN design, also referred to as *vanilla GAN*, are built using straightforward architectures such multilayer perceptron networks. While this architecture can produce good results on simpler datasets such as MNIST, it struggles to produce high-quality results on more complex and high-resolution datasets like ImageNet or CIFAR-10.

Numerous research articles have been published that suggest alterations to the GAN architecture, including adjustments to the network topology, loss functions, and evolutionary techniques, to get around this constraint. The quality of the samples produced by GANs has greatly improved as a result of these adjustments. The designs *Deep-Convolutional-GANs*, *Progressively-Growing-GANs*, *CycleGANs*, and *Conditional-GANs* have all demonstrated potential for generating output images with better resolution.

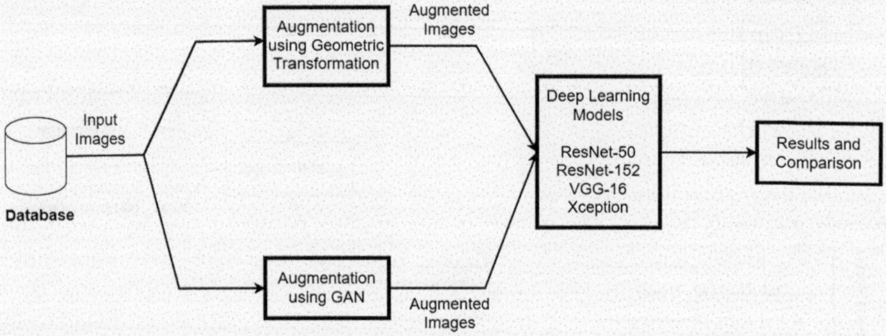

Fig. 4 Methodology step

The ability of GANs to produce fresh, never-before-seen data is one of their primary advantages. These networks are made up of the discriminator and generator neural networks, which compete with one another to provide data of higher quality. GANs' design has changed over time to accommodate larger, higher-resolution datasets. The *Deep-Convolutional-GANs* is one such architecture that makes use of CNNs in both the generator and discriminator networks. This architecture has been demonstrated to produce $64 \times 64 \times 3$ pixel high-resolution photos using the LSUN dataset (interior bedroom image dataset). DCGANs are designed to make the generator network more complicated so that it can project the input into a high-dimensional tensor. The spatial dimensions of the image are then expanded using deconvolutional layers, producing output images with a higher resolution.

5 Methodology

In this section we have explained the methodology steps we have followed. Overall, we have augmented the data using multiple geometric transformations as well as Deep-Convolutional-GAN-based data augmentation separately and then analyzed the produced results on classification accuracy separately. Initially, we have taken the input dataset known as Kvasir-V1 which has 8 different classes like *ulcerative-colitis*, *esophagitis*, *polyp*, *dyed-lifted-polyps*, *dyed-resection-margins*, *normal-cecum*, *normal-pylorus* and *normal-z-line*. Each class has 500 images in the dataset with total of 4000 images. For a better generalization, we increase the size of dataset by applying different augmentation techniques. Then we have applied geometric transformations on the dataset by applying multiple different transformations. In a parallel step, GAN-based data augmentation is performed and separately placed. Subsequently, the deep learning models named as ResNet-50, ResNet-152, VGG-16 as well as Xception model is applied for the training and checking the classification accuracy separately on both augmented datasets. The steps followed for our methodology are shown in Fig. 4.

The process of training a model using data augmentation begins by loading the dataset and dividing the images into two sets: training examples and testing examples. The ratio of images allocated to each set is typically 70% for training and 30% for testing. Once the dataset has been divided, data augmentation is applied to the training images by randomly applying various transformations to them. The purpose of this step is to prevent the model from seeing similar images multiple times during training, which can lead to overfitting. One of the major transformations applied to the training images is rotation, which is done by rotating the images by a randomly chosen angle between 10, 20 and 30 °C. This helps the model to learn to recognize objects in different orientations. Additionally, we applied random shifting of width and height of the images by 0.1, 0.2 and 0.3 values. This is done to simulate the object being in different positions within the image. Zoom-in and out, Shear transformation, Rescaling and horizontal and vertical flip also been applied to the images, which helps the model to learn to recognize objects in different scales, sizes and perspectives. All these augmentation techniques help to generalize the model, by training it to recognize objects in different variations, which in turn improves its ability to generalize to new unseen images. With the help of these augmentation techniques, the model is able to learn more robust features that can generalize well to new images. Total images after performing augmentation are 40,000.

In parallel, Deep-Convolutional-GAN-based data augmentation is applied to the input images and generated images are placed in separate place then geometric transformed images. For augmenting the images, only generator module of GAN is utilized. The Deep-Convolutional-GAN is a type of adversarial network that employs convolutional networks. It operates on the same principle as GAN but uses CNN techniques in GAN mode. The generator utilizes deconvolution to reconstruct the original image when generating data, and the discriminator uses convolutional techniques to identify image features and distinguish between real and fake images. To improve the quality of generated images and network convergence speed, some modifications were made to the CNN structure. These include using sigmoid as the activation function in the last layer and tanh in other layers. Also, batch normalization is applied. The architecture of applied GAN is shown in Fig. 5. Initially, each input image to GAN is added with a noise like gaussian-noise, salt&pepper-noise as well as z-noise.

The total number of images after augmentation are 40,000. The results showed that Deep-Convolutional-GAN may be used to effectively augment the endoscopic data. The augmented dataset also resulted in varying degrees of performance improvement for numerous detection networks. Samples Images obtained from proposed architecture of GAN are shown in Fig. 6.

After performing the data augmentation, four deep learning models i.e. ResNet-50, ResNet-152, VGG-16 and Xception are applied to the augmented dataset separately for training as well as testing the model. In the end, the softmax classifier is applied to all models for classification.

The ResNet-50 model is a deep neural network architecture that is composed of more than 50 layers. The number 50 in the name of the model refers to the total number of layers in the network. This deep layered architecture allows the model to have a

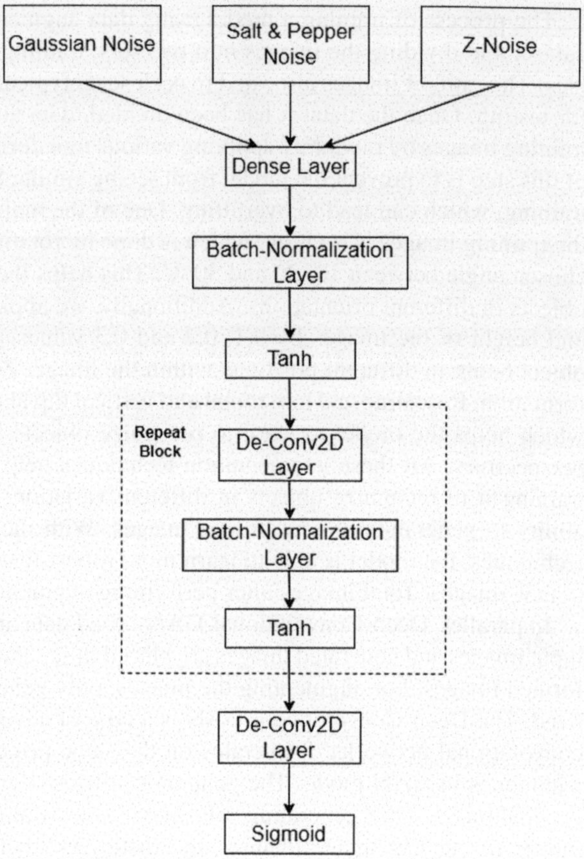

Fig. 5 Deep convolutional GAN architectures

large capacity to learn and represent complex data patterns. The ResNet-50 model is also equipped with a large number of trainable parameters, which are the values that are adjusted during the training process to optimize the model's performance. Specifically, this model has more than 23 million trainable parameters, which means that there are over 23 million values that can be adjusted during training to fine-tune the model's ability to classify or predict based on the given data. This large number of trainable parameters allows the model to learn a wide variety of features and representations from the input data, which in turn enables the model to perform well on complex and diverse datasets [31, 32].

ResNet-152 is a deep neural network model with 152 layers [33], each of which serves a particular purpose in the processing and analysis of the input data. By changing the values of its trainable parameters, this model can be trained to carry out a specific task, such as object detection or image categorization. More than 60 million trainable parameters-values that can be changed during the training process to enhance the performance of the model-are available in ResNet-152. The model can learn from the input data and produce predictions thanks to these trainable parameters.

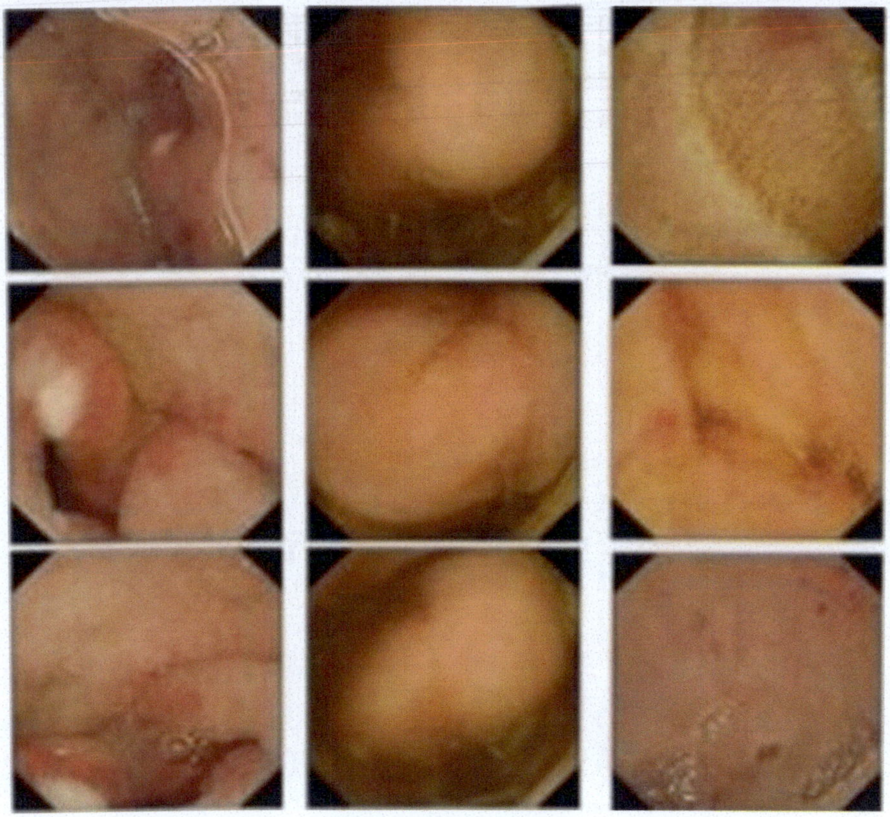

Fig. 6 GAN generated images

The model is more expressive and able to extract more intricate characteristics from the data thanks to the large number of trainable parameters, which can enhance performance. However, if insufficient data is provided or the model is not regularized correctly, it also increases the danger of over-fitting, which is when a model performs well on the training data but badly on the unseen data.

The VGG-16 model is a neural network architecture that consists of 16 layers [34]. These layers are made up of a combination of convolutional layers, pooling layers, and fully connected layers. The architecture is designed in such a way that it extracts features at different scales and resolutions, allowing the model to learn increasingly complex representations of the input data. One of the key characteristics of this model is its large number of trainable parameters, which is greater than 138 million. These parameters are the values that are learned during the training process and are used to make predictions on new input data. The large number of parameters in the VGG-16 model allows it to learn highly complex representations of the input data, but also makes the model more computationally expensive to train and requires larger amount of data to generalize well.

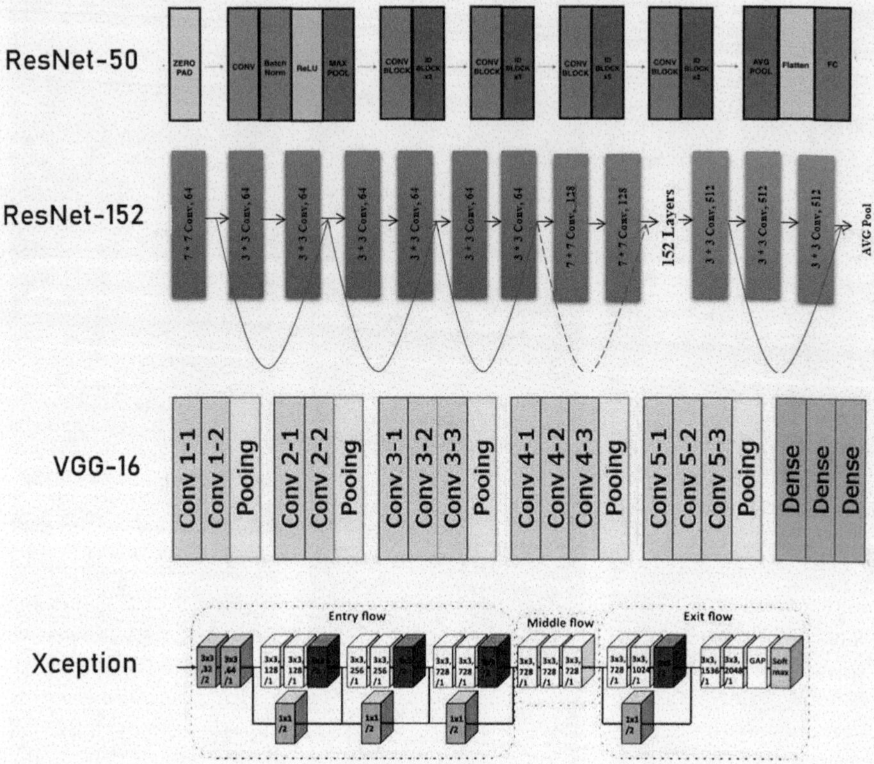

Fig. 7 Deep learning model architectures

An image categorization task-specific convolutional neural network architecture is called Xception. The model has 71 layers [35], with convolutional layers making up the majority of them. The goal of these convolutional layers is to learn hierarchical representations of the input image, starting with basic features like edges and progressing to more intricate features like textures and object pieces. The inclusion of depthwise separable convolutional layers, which are intended to lessen the computational complexity of the model while keeping its capacity to learn useful representations of the input, is one of the distinguishing characteristics of the Xception model. As a result, the model can have a lot of layers-71-while still being computationally effective. The fact that the Xception model has a lot of trainable parameters-that is, parameters whose values the model may learn during training-is another crucial feature of the model. The model includes more than 22.8 million trainable parameters specifically. Due to the huge number of parameters, the model may learn a complex mapping from the input image to the desired output, enabling it to perform image classification tasks with high accuracy. To create predictions, it also needs a lot of data to train on and powerful computing power.

The architectures of these four deep learning models are shown in Fig. 7.

6 Results and Discussion

This section elaborates the experimental setup, evaluation criteria, actual results as well as the discussion of results in the end. The primary tools and libraries used in this study for conducting experiments are Python, Keras, PyTorch, Tensorflow, and Matplotlib. The experiments were run on a computer system with a 4 GB AMD Radeon graphics card and 16 GB of RAM. Stochastic gradient descent with a learning rate of 0.0001 is the optimization approach used to train the model. A loss function is a key component of deep learning and it helps in measuring the difference between the predicted label and the target label. The loss function used in this study is Categorical Cross Entropy (CCE). CCE is a commonly used loss function in deep learning that compares two discrete probability distributions, and it helps the model to adjust its weights to better fit the data [36]. The model was trained for a total of 600 epochs with a batch size of 30. An epoch is a complete pass of the entire dataset through the model, and a batch size is the number of samples used in one forward/backward pass. By using a batch size of 30, the model is updated after every 30 samples, and by using 600 epochs, the model is trained on all the samples in the dataset multiple times. The model's performance is evaluated using the metric of accuracy, which is a commonly used and reliable measure for assessing the performance of a classification model. This is particularly useful in situations where the data is balanced across classes, meaning that the number of examples in each class is roughly equal, and where there is no significant class imbalance present. The accuracy metric calculates the proportion of correctly classified examples out of the total number of examples, providing a value between 0 and 1, with a higher value indicating better performance. It is a simple and straightforward metric that gives a clear idea of how well the model is performing in classifying the examples in the dataset.

Initially, classification results are collected on the original input dataset without any augmentation, and the results of the models are shown in Table 2. Afterward classification results are collected on the geometric augmented dataset which are also shown in Table 2. By looking at the results it can be seen that on this augmented Kvasir dataset, ResNet-50 performed better with 88.67% accuracy with an increase of 7.01% from the original dataset. On the second best, Xception performance remained better. Testing accuracy graph can on the stated models are shown in Fig. 8.

Classification results on the GAN-based augmented dataset are shown in Table 2. By looking at the result it can be seen that on this augmented Kvasir dataset, ResNet-50 performed better with 92.21% accuracy. On the second best, ResNet-152 performance remained better. Testing accuracy graph can on the stated models are shown in Fig. 9.

It is clear from an analysis of the findings shown in Table 2 that the ResNet-50 model had the highest accuracy of all the models tried. This model is a deep learning architecture that has been specifically adjusted for the Kvasir dataset after being pre-trained on a sizable dataset. However, all models performed more accurately when applied to a GAN-based enhanced dataset. A GAN, or generative adversarial network, is a machine learning system that creates new data that is comparable to the

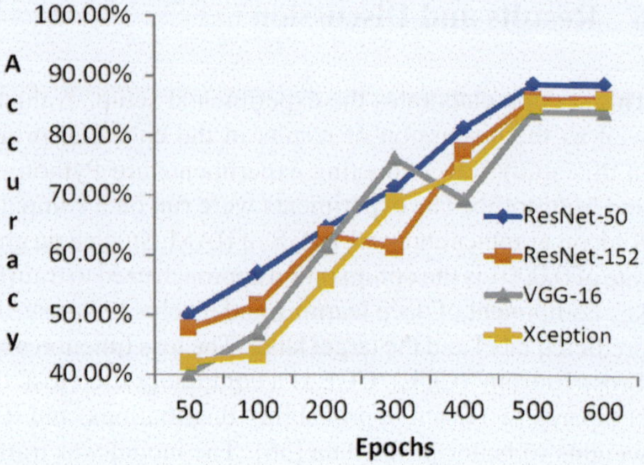

Fig. 8 Testing accuracy graph on geometric augmented dataset

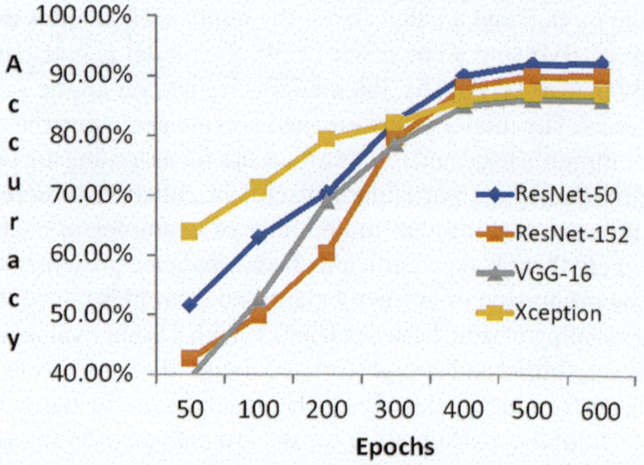

Fig. 9 Testing accuracy graph on GAN-based augmented dataset

original dataset using two neural networks: a generator and a discriminator. In this instance, the original Kvasir dataset was supplemented with additional images created using the GAN. It is evident from comparing the ResNet-50 model's performance on the geometric augmented dataset and the GAN-augmented dataset that employing the GAN-augmented dataset resulted in a notable accuracy gain of 3.54%. Upon comparison with original input dataset, it can be seen that the overall accuracy is increased by 10.55%. This implies that a GAN-based augmentation technique can enhance the model's performance on the Kvasir dataset. Overall, it can be concluded that utilizing a GAN-based augmentation strategy can increase the model's accuracy and that the ResNet-50 model performed well on the Kvasir dataset.

By obliging the arrangement of expansions and mutilations accessible to a GAN, it can figure out how to create increases that outcome in misclassifications, in this way shaping a successful pursuit calculation. These expansions are significant for reinforcing points of concern in the grouping model. In this manner, GAN can be a compelling quest procedure for Information Expansion. This is in weighty difference

Table 2 Classification results

Performance measure	Sr.	Model	Without augmentation (%)	Geometric transformation-based augmentation (%)	GAN-based augmentation (%)
Accuracy	1.	ResNet-50	**81.66**	**88.67**	**92.21**
	2.	ResNet-152	79.36	86.31	90.41
	3.	VGG-16	76.04	84.12	86.13
	4.	Xception	78.66	85.96	87.22
Precision	1.	ResNet-50	**85.24**	**91.45**	**94.36**
	2.	ResNet-152	82.44	89.08	93.42
	3.	VGG-16	80.13	87.49	87.61
	4.	Xception	81.01	89.02	89.96
Recall	1.	ResNet-50	**83.03**	**90.14**	**92.99**
	2.	ResNet-152	81.31	88.07	91.82
	3.	VGG-16	78.32	86.61	86.98
	4.	Xception	79.11	87.63	88.84

Bold mean the best-achieved performance values

to the conventional expansion methods portrayed beforehand. GAN expansions may not address models prone to happen in the test set, however they can work on points of weakness in the learned choice limit. Also, DCGAN works on the nature of result images and creates higher-quality yield images. These contentions legitimize the better outcomes of GANs.

7 Conclusion

In this chapter, we assessed how data augmentation methods affected the classification accuracy of deep learning models. On the Kvasir dataset, we specifically looked at the effects of applying geometric modifications like translation, rotation, and cropping as well as employing Generative Adversarial Networks (GANs). The dataset was initially enhanced using geometric transformations and independently with GANs in order to conduct the analysis. Deep learning models were then trained and tested on the supplemented datasets before being placed in their relevant directories. Comparison of the classification results showed that the GAN-based augmentation strategy produced superior performance as compared to the traditional geometric transformations. In the future, we intend to look at the effects of feature selection and contrast enhancement on the performance of deep learning models on the Kvasir dataset.

Acknowledgements The authors have no conflict of interest and all have contributed equally to the preparation of this book chapter. Furthermore, no funding is received for this study.

References

1. F. Bray, J. Ferlay, I. Soerjomataram, R.L. Siegel, L.A. Torre, A. Jemal "Global cancer statistics 2018: GLOBOCAN estimates of incidence and mortality worldwide for 36 cancers in 185 countries" CA Cancer J. Clin., 68 (6) (2018), pp. 394–424.
2. J. Asplund, J.H. Kauppila, F. Mattsson, J. Lagergren "Survival trends in gastric adenocarcinoma: a population-based study in Sweden" Ann. Surgi. Oncol., 25 (9) (2018), pp. 2693–2702.
3. B. Levin, et al. "Screening and surveillance for the early detection of colorectal cancer and adenomatous polyps, 2008: a joint guideline from the american cancer society, the us multi-society task force on colorectal cancer, and the american college of radiology" CA Cancer J. Clin., 58 (3) (2008), pp. 130–160.
4. K. Pogorelov, et al. "Medico multimedia task at mediaeval 2018" Proc. CEUR Worksh. Multim. Bench. Worksh. (MediaEval) (2018).
5. K. Suzuki "A review of computer-aided diagnosis in thoracic and colonic imaging" Quant. Imaging Med. Surg., 2 (3) (2012), pp. 163–176.
6. K. Suzuki "A review of computer-aided diagnosis in thoracic and colonic imaging" Quant. Imaging Med. Surg., 2 (3) (2012), pp. 163–176.
7. Debesh Jha, Sharib Ali, Steven Hicks, Vajira Thambawita, et al. "A comprehensive analysis of classification methods in gastrointestinal endoscopy imaging" Medical Image Analysis, Volume 70, 2021, 102007.
8. Shorten, C., Khoshgoftaar, T.M. A survey on Image Data Augmentation for Deep Learning. J Big Data 6, 60 (2019). https://doi.org/10.1186/s40537-019-0197-0
9. Halevy A, Norvig P, Pereira F. The unreasonable effectiveness of data. IEEE Intell Syst. 2009;24:8–12.
10. LeCun Y, Bottou L, Bengio Y, Haffner P. Gradient-based learning applied to document recognition. Proc IEEE. 1998;86(11):2278–324.
11. Krizhevsky A, Sutskever I, Hinton GE. ImageNet classification with deep convolutional neural networks. Adv Neural Inf Process Syst. 2012;25:1106–14.
12. Ian JG, Jean PA, Mehdi M, Bing X, David WF, Sherjil O, Aaron C, Yoshua B. Generative adversarial nets. NIPS. 2014.
13. Maayan F-A, Eyal K, Jacob G, Hayit G. GAN-based data augmentation for improved liver lesion classification. arXiv preprint. 2018.
14. Joseph R, Santosh D, Ross G, Ali F. You only look once: unified, real-time object detection. In: CVPR'16. 2016.
15. Ross G, Jeff D, Trevor D, Jitendra M. Rich feature hierarchies for accurate object detection and semantic segmentation. In: CVPR '14. 2014.
16. Olaf R, Philipp F, Thomas B. U-Net: convolutional networks for biomedical image segmentation. In: MICCAI. Springer; 2015, p. 234–41.
17. Hessam B, Maxwell H, Mohammad R, Ali F. Label refinery: improving imagenet classification through label progression. arXiv preprint. 2018.
18. Quanzeng Y, Jiebo L, Hailin J, Jianchao Y. Robust image sentiment analysis using progressively trained and domain transferred deep networks. In: AAAI. 2015, pp. 381–8.
19. Pereira S, Pinto A, Alves V, Silva CA. Brain tumor segmentation using convolutional neural networks in MRI images. IEEE Trans Med Imaging 2016; 35: 1240–51.
20. Zhang L, Wang X, Yang D et al. Generalizing deep learning for medical image segmentation to unseen domains via deep stacked transformation. IEEE Trans Med Imaging 2020; 39: 2531–40.
21. Huang X, Shan J, Vaidya V. Lung nodule detection in CT using 3D convolutional neural networks. In: 2017 IEEE 14th International Symposium on Biomedical Imaging (ISBI 2017), 2017; 379–83.
22. Herzog L, Murina E, Durr O, Wegener S, Sick B. Integrating uncertainty in deep neural networks for MRI based stroke analysis. Med Image Anal 2020; 65: 101790.
23. Hua W, Xiao T, Jiang X et al. Lymph-vascular space invasion prediction in cervical cancer: exploring radiomics and deep learning multilevel features of tumor and peritumor tissue on multiparametric MRI. Biomed Signal Process Control 2020; 58: 101869.

24. Kumar R, Wang WenYong, Kumar J et al. An Integration of blockchain and AI for secure data sharing and detection of CT images for the hospitals. Comput Med Imaging Graph 2020; 87: 101812.
25. Christopher B, Liang C, Ricardo GPB, Roger G, Alexander H, David AD, Maria VH, Joanna W, Daniel R. GAN augmentation: augmenting training data using generative adversarial networks. arXiv preprint. 2018.
26. Doersch C. Tutorial on Variational Autoencoders. ArXiv e-prints. 2016.
27. Ian JG, Jean PA, Mehdi M, Bing X, David WF, Sherjil O, Aaron C, Yoshua B. Generative adversarial nets. NIPS. 2014.
28. Jeff D, Philipp K, Trevor D. Adversarial feature learning. In: CVPR'16. 2016.
29. Lin Z, Shi Y, Xue Z. IDSGAN: Generative Adversarial Networks for Attack Generation against Intrusion Detection. arXiv preprint; 2018.
30. William F, Mihaela R, Balaji L, Andrew MD, Shakir M, Ian G. Many paths to equilibrium: GANs do not need to decrease a divergence at every step. In: International conference on learning representations (ICLR); 2017.
31. H. Jung, B. Lodhi and J. Kang, "An automatic nuclei segmentation method based on deep convolutional neural networks for histopathology images," BMC Biomedical Engineering, vol. 1, pp. 1–12, 2019.
32. Noor M, Nazir M, Rehman S, Tariq J. Sketch-Recognition using Pre-Trained Model. InProc. of National Conf. on Engineering and Computing Technology 2021.
33. Nguyen, Long & Lin, Dongyun & Lin, Zhiping & Cao, Jiuwen. (2018). Deep CNNs for microscopic image classification by exploiting transfer learning and feature concatenation. 1-5. https://doi.org/10.1109/ISCAS.2018.8351550.
34. J. Tao, Y. Gu, J. Sun, Y. Bie and H. Wang, "Research on vgg16 convolutional neural network feature classification algorithm based on Transfer Learning," 2021 2nd China International SAR Symposium (CISS), Shanghai, China, 2021, pp. 1-3, https://doi.org/10.23919/CISS51089.2021.9652277.
35. Rahimzadeh M, Attar A. A modified deep convolutional neural network for detecting COVID-19 and pneumonia from chest X-ray images based on the concatenation of Xception and ResNet50V2. Informatics in medicine unlocked. 2020 1;19:100360.
36. Y. Ho and S. Wookey, "The real-world-weight cross-entropy loss function: modeling the costs of mislabeling," IEEE Access, vol. 8, pp. 4806–4813, 2019.
37. Mahapatra, D., Bozorgtabar, B., & Shao, L. (2020). Pathological retinal region segmentation from oct images using geometric relation based augmentation. In Proceedings of the IEEE/CVF Conference on Computer Vision and Pattern Recognition (pp. 9611–9620).
38. H. Rashid, M. A. Tanveer and H. Aqeel Khan, "Skin Lesion Classification Using GAN based Data Augmentation," 2019 41st Annual International Conference of the IEEE Engineering in Medicine and Biology Society (EMBC), Berlin, Germany, 2019, pp. 916–919, https://doi.org/10.1109/EMBC.2019.8857905.
39. Khan AR, Khan S, Harouni M, Abbasi R, Iqbal S, Mehmood Z (2021) Brain tumor segmentation using K-means clustering and deep learning with synthetic data augmentation for classification. Microsc Res Tech 84:1389–1399.
40. Dufumier B, Gori P, Battaglia I, Victor J, Grigis A, Duchesnay E (2021) Benchmarking cnn on 3d anatomical brain mri: architectures, data augmentation and deep ensemble learning. arXiv preprint, pp 1–25. arXiv:2106.01132
41. Isensee F, Jäger PF, Full PM et al (2020) nnu-Net for brain tumor segmentation. In: International MICCAI brainlesion workshop. Springer, Cham, pp 118-132.
42. Wang Y, Ji Y, Xiao H (2022) A Data Augmentation Method for Fully Automatic Brain Tumor Segmentation. arXiv preprint, pp 1-15. arXiv:2202.06344
43. Kossen T, Subramaniam P, Madai VI, Hennemuth A, Hildebrand K, Hilbert A, Sobesky J, Livne M, Galinovic I, Khalil AA, Fiebach JB (2021) Synthesizing anonymized and labeled TOF-MRA patches for brain vessel segmentation using generative adversarial networks. Comput Biol Med 131:1-9

44. Li Q, Yu Z, Wang Y et al (2020) Tumorgan: a multi-modal data augmentation framework for brain tumor segmentation. Sensors 20:1–16
45. Hu R, Ruan G, Xiang S, Huang M, Liang Q, Li J (2020) Automated diagnosis of covid-19 using deep learning and data augmentation on chest CT. medRxiv, pp 1–11.
46. Alshazly H, Linse C, Barth E et al (2021) Explainable covid-19 detection using chest ct scans and deep learning. Sensors 21:1–22.
47. Wang Q, Zhang X, Zhang W, Gao M, Huang S, Wang J, Zhang J, Yang D, Liu C (2021) Realistic lung nodule synthesis with multi-target co-guided adversarial mechanism. IEEE Trans Med Imaging 40:2343–2353
48. Nishio M, Muramatsu C, Noguchi S, Nakai H, Fujimoto K, Sakamoto R, Fujita H (2020) Attribute-guided image generation of three-dimensional computed tomography images of lung nodules using a generative adversarial network. Comput Biol Med. https://doi.org/10.1016/j.compbiomed.2020.104032
49. Karthiga R, Narasimhan K, Amirtharajan R (2022) Diagnosis of breast cancer for modern mammography using artificial intelligence. Math Comput Simul 202:316–330.
50. Kim YJ, Kim KG (2022) Detection and weak segmentation of masses in gray-scale breast mammogram images using deep learning. Yonsei Med J 63:S63.
51. Alyafi B, Diaz O, Marti R (2020) DCGANs for realistic breast mass augmentation in X-ray mammography. IN: Medical imaging 2020: computer-aided diagnosis, International Society for Optics and Photonics, pp 1–4. https://doi.org/10.1117/12.2543506
52. Shen T, Hao K, Gou C, Wang FY (2021) Mass image synthesis in mammogram with contextual information based on GANS. Comput Methods Programs Biomed. https://doi.org/10.1016/j.cmpb.2021.106019
53. M. Alhajlah, M. N. Noor, M. Nazir, A. Mahmood, I. Ashraf et al., Gastrointestinal diseases classification using deep transfer learning and features optimization, Computers, Materials & Continua, vol. 75, no.1, pp. 2227–2245, 2023.
54. Nouman Noor, M.; Nazir, M.; Khan, S.A.; Song, O.-Y.; Ashraf, I. Efficient Gastrointestinal Disease Classification Using Pretrained Deep Convolutional Neural Network. Electronics 2023, 12, 1557. https://doi.org/10.3390/electronics12071557
55. Xiao, Z., Lu, J., Wang, X., Li, N., Wang, Y., Zhao, N.: WCE-DCGAN: A data augmentation method based on wireless capsule endoscopy images for gastrointestinal disease detection. IET Image Process. 17, 1170–1180 (2023). https://doi.org/10.1049/ipr2.12704
56. Minne, P., Fernandez-Quilez, A., Aarsland, D., Ferreira, D., Westman, E., Lemstra, A. W. & Oppedal, K. (2022, April). A study on 3D classical versus GAN-based augmentation for MRI brain image to predict the diagnosis of dementia with Lewy bodies and Alzheimer's disease in a European multi-center study. In Medical Imaging 2022: Computer-Aided Diagnosis (Vol. 12033, pp. 624–632).
57. Jayalakshmy S, Sudha GF. Conditional GAN based augmentation for predictive modeling of respiratory signals. Comput Biol Med. 2021 Nov;138:104930. https://doi.org/10.1016/j.compbiomed.2021.104930.Epub 2021 Oct 8. PMID: 34638019; PMCID: PMC8501269.
58. Luis P, Jason W. The effectiveness of data augmentation in image classification using deep learning. In: Stanford University research report, 2017.

Deep Generative Adversarial Network-Based MRI Slices Reconstruction and Enhancement for Alzheimer's Stages Classification

Venkatesh Gauri Shankar and Dilip Singh Sisodia

Abstract Alzheimer's disease (AD) is a neurodegenerative brain disorder that leads to a steady decline in brain function and the death of brain cells. AD condition causes dementia, which cannot be treated. Deep learning techniques have quickly become one of the most essential ways to analyse MRI images in recent times. However, they often require a significant amount of data, and medical data is frequently unavailable. The latest discovery in machine learning, known as the "generative adversarial network" or GAN, has the potential to solve the issue of limited data availability by creating realistic images. In this paper, we implement a Vanilla-GAN initiated model for enhancing and reconstructing brain magnetic resonance imaging (MRI). Vanilla-GAN uses the power of CNN, also known as Deep Convolutional GAN (DCGAN), which is also used in classification. After generating the enhanced images, we performed a classification task to identify the stages of Alzheimer's. To conduct our experiment, we used the dataset collected by the Alzheimer's Disease Neuroimaging Initiative. We evaluated and validated the proposed model's performance using assessment and evaluation metrics. Our study shows that GAN frameworks can enhance both the performance of AD classification and the quality of images.

1 Introduction

Alzheimer's disease (AD) is a brain disorder that results in the death of nerve cells, worsens over time, and is incurable [1]. AD is a widespread type of dementia that typically suffers patients in their late 60s or early 80s [1, 2]. AD kills nerve cells, which makes it difficult to remember things and think clearly. By 2050, it is expected

V. G. Shankar (✉)
Department of Information Technology, Manipal University Jaipur, Jaipur, Rajasthan, India
e-mail: venkateshgaurishankar@gmail.com

V. G. Shankar · D. S. Sisodia
Department of Computer Science and Engineering, National Institute of Technology Raipur, Raipur, Chhattisgarh, India
e-mail: dssisodia.cs@nitrr.ac.in

H. Ali et al. (eds.), *Advances in Deep Generative Models for Medical Artificial Intelligence*, Studies in Computational Intelligence 1124,
https://doi.org/10.1007/978-3-031-46341-9_3

that the number of people with AD will increase to the point where it affects one person in every 85 in the general population [3, 4]. The clinical diagnosis of AD is based on the structural changes that occur in nerve cells over time. Patients with AD have TAU protein that undergoes a chemical shift and manages to clump together, leading to the structure of neurofibrillary tangles [4, 5]. TAU protein is normally treated to maintain the internal arrangement of cells. It initially causes cells to malfunction and ultimately leads to their death. On an MRI, the areas of the brain known as the medial temporal and hippocampal lobes are the first to show signs of damage when AD is present. The hippocampus is a brain region that is connected to another region responsible for cognition and decision-making. The hippocampus is also responsible for our ability to recall information [1, 2, 5].

In most cases, the stages of AD are classified based on the degree of cognitive decline experienced by patients. People in the early stages of AD disease have difficulty remembering things, may feel uneasy around others, and may lose interest in activities they previously enjoyed. In the middle stages, they may begin to show renewed interest in things, but they may also experience increasing forgetfulness and confusion [4, 6]. As the disease progresses, patients may become incontinent and lose the ability to care for themselves. Complications almost always result in the patient's death. While it is easy to identify someone with AD in the late stages of the disease, it can be more challenging to do so in the mild to moderate stages [7, 8].

Approximately 60–70% of AD cases are caused by brain cell dead condition, which leads to severe problems with thinking, memory, and behaviour [4, 5, 9]. The progression and severity of the disease are influenced by a wide scale of reasons, including environmental and hereditary factors. The diagnosis of AD can be made using the patient's medical history, clinical observations, and information from people who are familiar with the patient. AD consists of six stages that range from very debilitating to somewhat manageable. However, clinical, or survey-based assessments of AD stages may be unreliable or unhelpful, as some individuals may be reluctant to discuss their illness due to fear or social stigma [1, 3–5]. The following are the six stages of AD progression [1, 2, 5, 10]:

- Cognitive normal (CN) is the first stage where individuals have no significant cognitive decline, and their cognitive functions are within normal limits for their age and education level.
- Significant memory concern (SMC) is a second stage of subjective cognitive decline, in which individuals experience noticeable memory loss or cognitive decline but have no objective evidence of MCI.
- Early mild cognitive impairment (EMCI) is the diagnosis given to individuals who are in the early stages of MCI and have only minor cognitive impairment, which is not severe enough to affect their daily activities.
- Mild cognitive impairment (MCI) is the fourth stage of AD, which is a transitional stage between normal age-related memory decline and Alzheimer's dementia. In this stage, individuals may experience mild memory loss and difficulty in decision-making, but they can still perform their daily activities independently.

- Late mild cognitive impairment (LMCI) is a diagnosis given to individuals who are in the later stages of MCI and have more noticeable cognitive impairment than early MCI. They may experience more memory loss, language problems, and difficulty in performing complex tasks.
- The last stage of AD is Alzheimer's dementia, which is the most severe stage of the disease. It is characterized by significant memory loss, difficulty communicating, confusion, and mood changes. This stage is often diagnosed when a person's symptoms interfere with daily life activities.

When attempting to diagnose Alzheimer's, imaging is the most common way to detect signs of the disease [11, 12]. These techniques make it easier to look inside the body without any intervention or surgery, and as a result, they have changed how diseases are diagnosed [6, 13, 14]. Earlier in history treating Alzheimer's disease was difficult when the disease could only be identified after death. However, nowadays, medical imaging plays a significant role in determining if someone has AD and how to treat it [6, 14]. Alzheimer's disease can be detected with imaging tests such as computed tomography (CT), magnetic resonance imaging (MRI), diffusion tensor imaging (DTI), and positron emission tomography (PET). MRI and PET scans are usually the most used methods for viewing the inside of the body [13, 15].

Imaging studies can rule out cerebrovascular disease, syphilis, and many other potential causes of dementia [13]. In addition to blood tests, electroencephalograms (EEG), and genotyping, there are other available tests. In most cases, the brain's CT scan shows that the brain is shrinking, and the third ventricle is expanding. These symptoms indicate AD, but it does not provide a definitive diagnosis [13, 16]. An MRI shows a decrease in the size of the middle temporal lobe. Operational brain imaging methods, such as PET, fMRI, and SPECT, are used to represent dysfunctional relationships in the medial temporal and parietal lobes, which are shorter [13, 16, 17]. Researchers have found that clinical trials need to focus on patients at an earlier stage before the brain begins to shrink significantly. However, it can be difficult to clinically diagnose the disease in the early stage [13, 17].

PET scans and cerebral spinal fluid (CSF) tests are more expensive than MRI data, which is why most studies concentrate on MRI data. In current days, machine learning and deep learning models have been employed with CT and MRI scans [8, 18–20]. Deep neural networks can automatically extract features from MRI images, analyse the MRI of the brain, and determine the stages of AD. Rapid advancements in neuroimaging methods, such as magnetic resonance imaging (MRI), have made it easier to detect Alzheimer's disease-related neurodegeneration (AD). Examining the pathophysiological changes in an MRI can help physicians, patients, and their families discover novel therapies. The signal-to-noise (SN) ratio of the input data, which is entirely dependent on instrument features such as magnetic field intensity, is crucial for accurately detecting Alzheimer's disorder using MR images [16, 21, 22].

The latest advancements in deep neural networks have made it possible to effectively handle the inverse problem of MR image reconstruction. Deep learning-based methodologies have been used in computer vision applications, such as image super resolution, noise reduction, and inpainting, for quite some time, but they are still in their infancy in medical imaging. To reconstruct an MR image, these methods find the right transformation between the source (a zero-filled, under-sampled k-space) and the destination (a fully sampled k-space) by training to minimize a particular loss function. In recent years, several network types have been used to autonomously assemble medical images [8, 20, 21]. In the past, meaningful tasks were taught to machine learning models by hand-designing features derived from raw data or by allowing other rudimentary machine learning models to teach them features. In deep learning, computers automatically discover meaningful representations and characteristics from raw data, eliminating this laborious phase. There are various types of artificial neural networks, but deep learning approaches emphasize feature learning, which is the process of learning how to represent data automatically. This is the key difference between deep learning and conventional machine learning.

The integration of finding features and accomplishing a task into a single challenge is a key aspect of deep learning. During training, both skills increase concurrently [18, 23–25]. However, training deep neural networks requires hundreds of examples, which may not always be possible. To overcome the issue of insufficient data, one-shot learning algorithms have been developed to train models with just a handful of instances. With these strategies, each class requires only a few training examples, and the model can be applied to other classes with little further instruction. Therefore, the primary objectives of few-shot learning are to become adept at generalizing to new scenarios and to achieve correct results with a small amount of data [20, 24, 26].

In modern days, there has been substantial importance in the use of deep learning to automatically detect and diagnose the early stages of AD [19, 27]. This is due to the rapid improvement of neuroimaging methods, which has resulted in a wealth of multimodal neuroimaging data. A thorough review of articles that used deep learning algorithms and neuroimaging data was conducted to determine how to identify Alzheimer's disease. Deep learning techniques appear to be improving in their ability to identify AD by grouping different types of neuroimaging data. Deep learning research in AD continues to evolve and improve as more hybrid data sources are added. However, finding early signs of Alzheimer's can be challenging due to a lack of training, resources, or datasets, or insufficient high-quality data. Researchers have shown that using MRI data and deep learning could be a way to automatically detect early signs of Alzheimer's disease [20, 24–26, 28].

There are several ways to increase the amount of data in the training set. One of these is called "data augmentation," which contains scaling of image, cropping of image, zooming image, flipping image, and rotating the original image. This technique works well for nature photos but not for medical photos [29, 30]. Translating and inverting the original image can remove the helpful patterns that doctors use to diagnose medical conditions, which can result in lower accuracy of machine learning algorithms. Creating synthetic (programmable) images is another way to generate new information, making it easier to analyze medical images. Since the dataset includes both positive and negative examples of each class, this strategy can help create a more general model [29, 31]. Using a neural network to generate training data for fake images is an active area of research. Image-to-image translation and other methods have produced amazing results in creating fake images by changing the way the image is shown, such as turning a black-and-white image into an RGB image or vice versa. There are supervised and unsupervised ways to translate images. Generative adversarial networks (GANs) are a way to generate new data samples from the existing ones by using random noise from a latent space to create new images that resemble the features of the original dataset.

Generative adversarial learning is a novel machine learning method in which two neural networks compete against each other in a "zero-sum" game. This approach is one way to address insufficient or imbalanced problems. Ever since its inception, there has been great interest in how GAN frameworks can be used to study the brain. Some of the ways in which they can be utilized include improving image resolution or quality, adding data, segmenting, recreating images, changing one image into another, and fixing motion. While these important studies have demonstrated how fascinating it can be to use GAN architectures, not much research has been conducted on how to use the generated images for other purposes, such as classifying diseases.

Here, we investigated whether a generative adversarial network (GAN) could enhance the performance of a classifier trained on images created by the GAN [29, 30]. GANs are a vital component of generating synthetic images, and they have been found to reduce the time required for training to identify issues [9, 22, 29]. GANs compete with discriminative and generative classifiers to improve detection performance. Typically, a GAN consists of two components: the generator generates an image and tests to convince the discriminator that it is real, while the discriminator evaluates both the synthetic and genuine images and learns to distinguish between them. The size of the training sets and the GAN network architectures were compared using a baseline discriminative network and Bayes' classifiers. The findings indicate that neither the network configuration nor the size of the training sets had a significant impact on the algorithm's effectiveness. Discriminator classifiers were trained using more network nodes and iterations than GANs [30–32].

DCGAN [33, 34] is a common GAN network architecture that works well. It is mostly made up of convolution layers and doesn't have any fully linked or maximum pooling layers. For down sampling and up sampling, convolutional stride and transposed convolution are used. The generator's network setup is shown in Fig. 1 below. DCGAN is a deep convolutional generative adversarial network that utilizes deep convolutional networks to enhance its stability and performance. DCGAN uses a transposed convolutional network to increase the size of images, while GAN uses a fully connected network for the generator [33–36].

In the Vanilla GAN configuration [37], there are two types of models: those that generate new ideas and those that select the best ideas. Discriminative models are commonly employed to address classification problems, where a decision boundary is learned to predict which class a data point belongs to. Vanilla GAN is the simplest type of GAN, with both the generator and discriminator being multilayer perceptrons. The method employed in vanilla GAN is stochastic gradient descent to discover the optimal solution to the mathematical problem [37, 38].

In this proposed work, we talk about a supervised generative modeling technique that uses Deep Convolutional Generative Adversarial Networks (DCGANs) to make

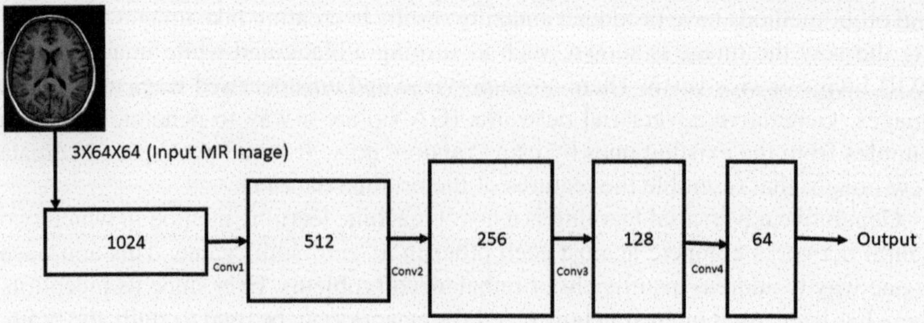

Fig. 1 DCGAN layered architecture on MRI dataset

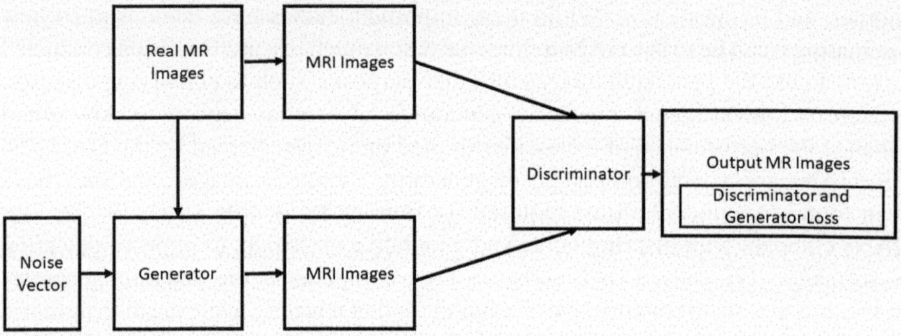

Fig. 2 Vanilla GAN process flowchart on MRI dataset

synthetic images that don't exist in the real world. A way to use labeled Magnetic Resonance Imaging (MRI) dataset and then apply DCGAN to the small amount of data to augment and reconstruct them. This makes the dataset bigger, enhanced, and more varied. Vanilla-GAN uses the power of CNN, also known as Deep Convolutional GAN (DCGAN), which is also used in classification. Finally, the synthetic images and training dataset are put together to the same DCGAN extended as Vanilla GAN to classification of the four stages of AD.

2 Related Work

Using GANs to translate from one image to another has worked well in several computer vision research initiatives [7, 9, 14, 39]. It can be used to make images with higher resolution or better quality, as well as for data augmentation, segmentation, image reconstruction, image-to-image translation, and classification [6, 8, 40, 41]. Shin et al. [17] used a GAN model and integrated tumor MRI images to address the issue of imbalance in brain MRI datasets. This resulted in improved segmentation of tumors. Goodfellow et al. [21] initially suggested the generative adversarial network (GAN) a short time ago. GAN has shown effective in recent years for identifying

Alzheimer's disease (AD) by assisting with image processing and enhancing the quality of low-quality MRI images with insufficient or imbalanced data [16, 23, 32]. GANs have been put to good use in medical imaging, namely for the reconstruction of MRI and CT scans as well as unconditional synthesis [19, 31]. Lin et al. [27] published a study in which they used GAN to analyze genomic data from a mouse model of Alzheimer's disease. Both investigations were limited in scope and did not contain any kind of data evaluation about the identification of AD. Hosseini et al. [42] used 3D CNN to detect morphological alterations associated with Alzheimer's disease (AD), such as differences in hippocampal volume and brain volume. The complete PET volume was used by Liu et al. [22] to encode spatial volume information using 3D CNN. The paper [28] describes inceptionV3, a system built for the initial finding of Alzheimer's disease with a ROC of 95% and a sensitivity of 100%. Alzheimer's illness was classified using ResNet-50 and the GD boost algorithm, both with and without images [28]. As a way of transfer learning, the authors of the study [26] used a smart choice of data from MRI scans for VGG16. In the end, they had an overall multi-classification accuracy of 99.20%. Researchers rebuilt a single medical image using GANs [20, 24], Autoencoder (AEs), or both, given that GANs can generate realistic images and AEs, particularly Variational AEs, may directly map data onto its latent representation [25, 43]. They are unable to distinguish between diseases like Alzheimer's that are made up of many small anatomical problems right away because they don't look at the continuity between many images next to each other (AD) [44, 45]. A good method for filling in missing data that uses the generative adversarial network to rebuild the PET images [46].

3 Dataset

The proposed model was applied to ADNI (Alzheimer's Disease Neuroimaging Initiative) data [1, 2]. ADNI brings together experts and studies data to evaluate the development of Alzheimer's disorder (AD). ADNI scholars gather, evaluate, and utilize data like MRI and PET scans, CSF, and blood biomarkers to predict the disorder. This offers study materials and information from the North American project, which featured comparison groups comprised of persons with AD, MCI, and CN [1, 2, 5]. The dataset with individual subjects is given in Table 1.

Table 1 Data collection and information

Alzheimer's stages	Male	Female	Total
AD	255	245	500
MCI	280	220	500
SMC	270	230	500
CN	290	210	500

(*Source* ADNI [2])

4 Methodology

In this work, we first collected the MRI dataset from the ADNI and augment, reconstruct, and enhance them using DCGAN and then processed images to Vanilla GAN. Vanilla-GAN uses the power of CNN, also known as Deep Convolutional GAN (DCGAN), which is also used in classification. Finally, the synthetic images and training dataset are put together to the same DCGAN extended as Vanilla GAN to classify the four stages of Alzheimer's disorder. Figure 5 depicts the whole methodology of the proposed model. Algorithm 1 shows the pseudo-code of the proposed model. The whole methodology is explained below covering each subsection wise.

4.1 Deep Convolutional GAN (DCGAN)

Utilizing generative adversarial learning is one of the potential solutions that solve the problem of image augmentation, reconstruction, and enhancement of MR images. In this work, we investigated the possibility of using a GAN to improve the implementation of a classifier, which is trained using an image that was made. To reach this objective, we looked at MR images from the ADNI dataset that were taken at different magnetic field strengths, such as 1.5T and 3T. The framework for deep learning needs to be able to make more accurate predictions about the class label than the original scans could. To do this, we used 1.5T and 3T scans of the same group of people taken around the same time to train a GAN model. We have used DCGAN for the same proposed model. DCGAN is one of the most well-known and widely used network designs for GAN. It doesn't use max pooling or fully linked layers and is mostly made up of convolution layers. The downsampling and the upsampling are both done with the help of a convolutional stride and a transposed convolution. Figure 1 shows the DCGAN architecture used for the augmentation, reconstruction, and enhancement of MR images. It follows a few rules, the most essential of which are: Pooling layers are replaced with stride convolutions (discriminator) and fractional-stride convolutions (generator). The batch norm is used by both the generator and the discriminator. Getting rid of hidden layers that are connected so that deeper structures can be made. The generator applies the ReLU function with each layer except the output, which utilizes the Tanh. Using a LeakyReLU activation in each of the discriminator's layers.

4.2 Vanilla GAN (VGAN)

Vanilla-GAN uses the power of CNN, also known as Deep Convolutional GAN (DCGAN), which is also used in classification. Finally, the synthetic images and training dataset are put together to the same DCGAN extended as Vanilla GAN to

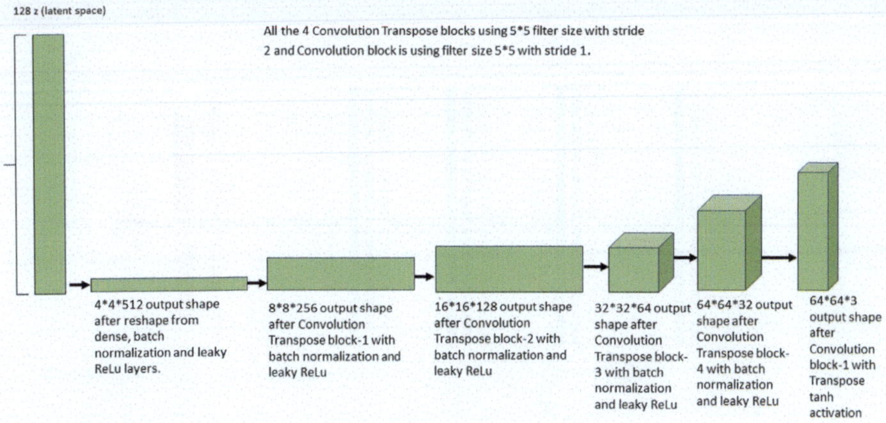

Fig. 3 Generator model for Alzheimer's stages classification

classify the four stages of Alzheimer's disease. Vanilla GAN is the simplest type of GAN. The Generator and the Discriminator are both multilayer simple perceptron's in this case. The method is simple in vanilla GAN. It uses a method called stochastic gradient descent to find the best answer to the math problem. Since a generator is just a neural network, we must tell it what to do and then choose what the network will do. The input is a sample of random noise from a distribution with values in a narrow range. This is the simplest way to show what the input is. This is what we call latent space, which is also sometimes called continuous space. When we say "random," it means that the vector sample I get from a random distribution will be different every time I take a sample from that distribution. This is the most important thing to know about chance. When we use this kind of input, we get something that is not set in stochastic. Both the discriminator and the classifier are the same. On the other hand, we won't be focusing on putting images in the right category. Instead, we'll be looking at how the class is split up (for example, creating photographs of buildings). Since this is the case, and since the target class is already known, we want the classifier to be able to tell us how close the class is to the real class distribution. Because of this, discriminators only give one probability, where 0 means that fake images have been made and 1 means that real samples from our distribution have been taken. As for Alzheimer's stages, classification VanillaGAN is categorized as 0 as CN, 1 as AD, 2 as SMC, and 3 as MCI. Figure 2 shows the VanillaGAN architecture used for Alzheimer's stages classification. The proposed generator and discriminator model are presented in Figs. 3 and 4. The generated, reconstructed, and enhanced sample is shown in Fig. 6.

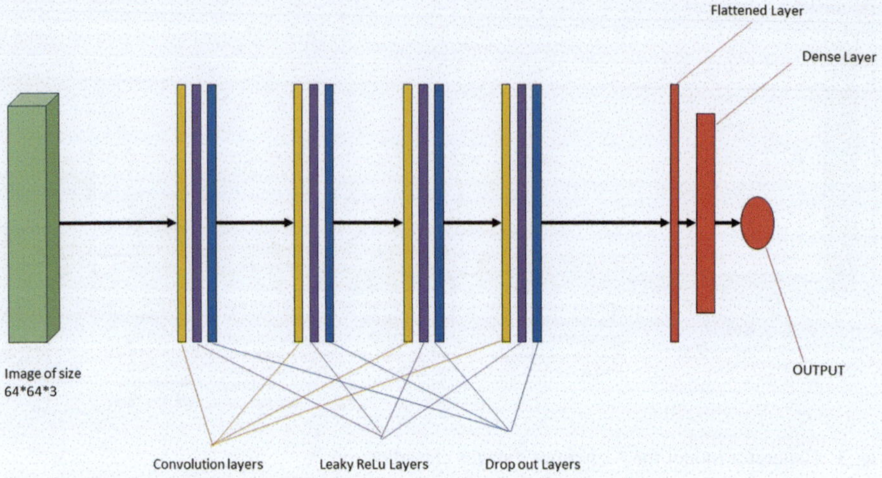

Fig. 4 Discriminator model for Alzheimer's stages classification

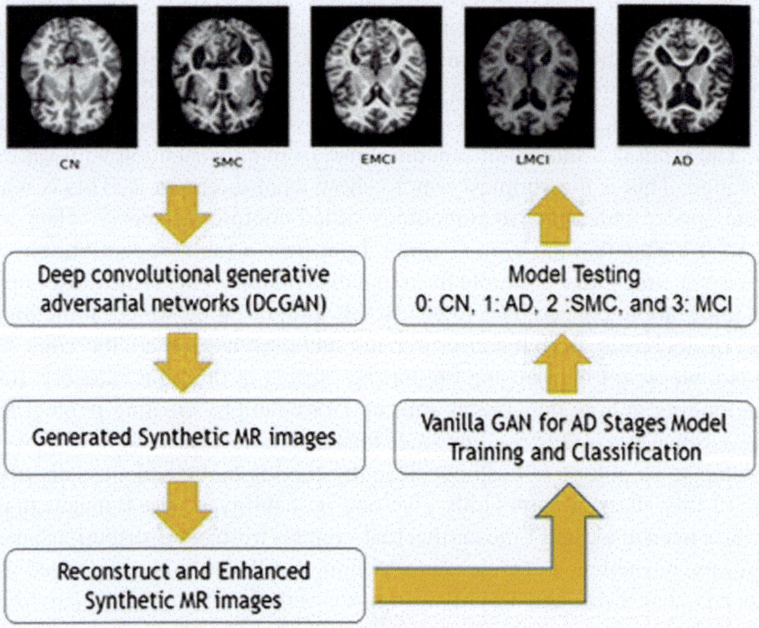

Fig. 5 Whole methodology of the proposed model

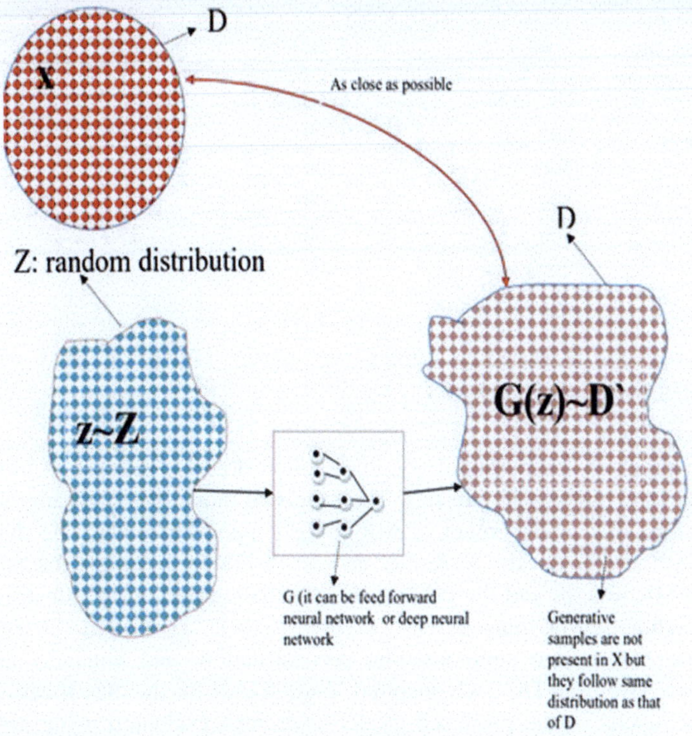

Fig. 6 Proposed model for reconstructed, and enhanced sample generation

---

Algorithm 1 Pseudo code of the proposed model

INPUT I_M: MR images (AD, CN, MCI, SMC)
INTERMEDIATE OUTPUT: Augmented, Reconstructed, and Enhanced MR Images
OUTPUT: AD stages classification (AD, CN, MCI, SMC)
while $I_M \neq \emptyset$ **do**
  for ($I_M \rightarrow 1$ to A) **do**
    if $I_A \neq$ (Augmented, Reconstructed, and Enhanced (I_M)) **then**
      Perform DCGAN as generator
      Perform DCGAN as discriminator
    else
      $I_A \leftarrow$ (Augmented, Reconstructed, and Enhanced (I_M))
      Perform Vanilla GAN for classification
      Classification $\leftarrow (I_M, I_A)$
    end if
  end for
end while
return (Output: AD stages classification (AD, CN, MCI, SMC))

Table 2 Data augmentation results after DCGAN

Alzheimer's stages	Total before augmentation using DCGAN	Total after augmentation using DCGAN	Reconstruction and enhancement (%)
AD	500	1700	69
MCI	500	1700	61
SMC	500	1700	55
CN	500	1700	43
Total	2000	6800	

5 Results and Discussion

After description of the methodology, this section presents the results in the form of evaluation and assessment metrics. The proposed model has used augmentation, reconstruction, and enhancement of MR images using DCGAN. The description and process of DCGAN are presented in Sect. 4. Table 2 depicts the number of augmented MR images and the percentage of enhancement and reconstruction for producing synthetic MR images.

After the MR image augmentation, reconstruction, and enhancement using DCGAN, we have used DCGAN-inspired VanillaGAN for the classification of AD stages. The results of the proposed model have been evaluated using assessment metrics such as precision, recall, and F1-score. The proposed model has been evaluated before cross-validation and after cross-validation. The valuable assessment in Fig. 7 presents the comparative assessment metrics before cross-validation, whereas Fig. 8 shows the comparative assessment metrics after cross-validation. The proposed model has used 10-fold cross-validation.

We have evaluated the accuracy of the model in terms of training and validation. Other than assessment metrics training and validation accuracy for model performance and testing score. In our proposed model, validation accuracies are slightly greater than the training accuracy. It shows that the model performs well in the given dataset. Table 3 presents validation, training, and test accuracy for the classification of Alzheimer's stages before data augmentation, whereas Table 4 shows validation and training, and test accuracy for the classification of Alzheimer's stages after data augmentation.

Finally, the proposed study attained a training, validation, and testing accuracy of 94.87%, 95.32%, and 95.55% respectively. As for assessment metrics before cross-validation achieved precision of 95.61%, recall of 92.45%, and F1 score of 94.03%. The train, test, and validation accuracy are shown in Fig. 9 and loss is also visualized in Fig. 10.

In our proposed work test accuracy is higher than training and validation accuracy because the model is underfitting during training, and the test set helps the model generalize better and reduces the underfitting. The test loss is less than training and

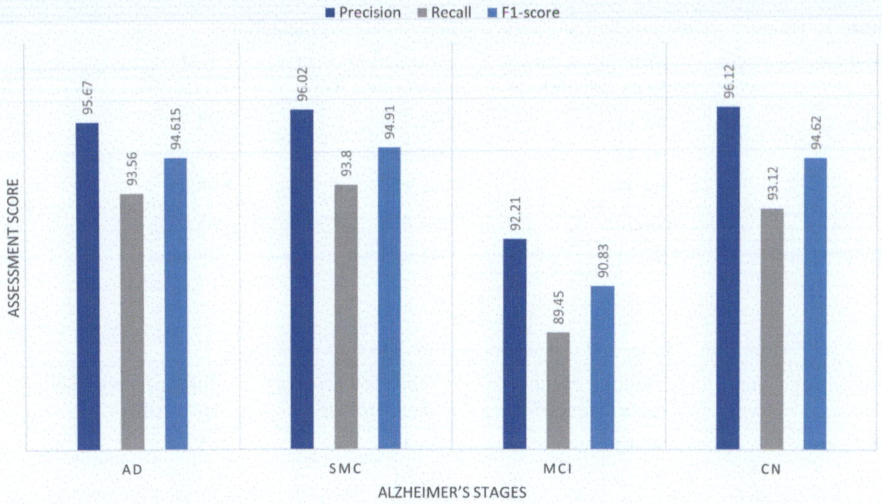

Fig. 7 Assessment metrics before cross-validation

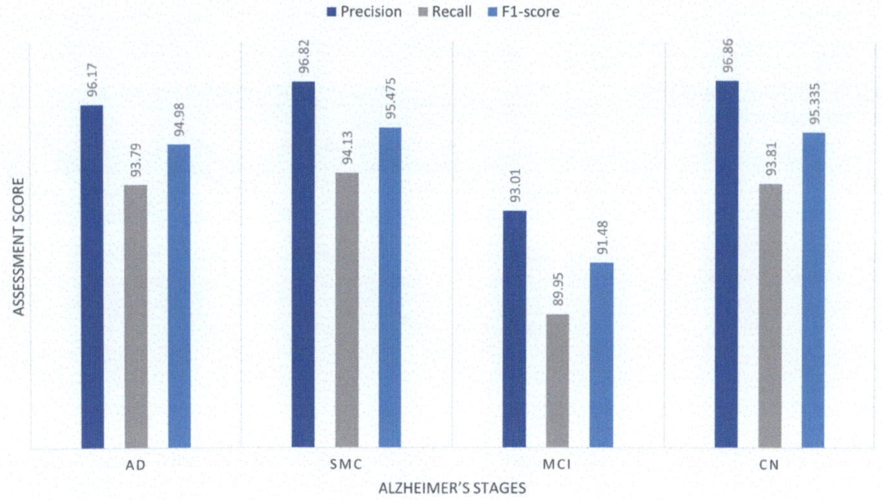

Fig. 8 Assessment metrics after cross-validation

validation loss. The test loss is less due to the data in the test set could be more like the data the model has already seen during training. As a comparison from Tables 3 and 4, the proposed model after augmented MR images performs better than before augmentation. We have also reported the computational cost of model by selecting the number of FLOPs per epoch and elapsed time, and the same computed cost is shown in Table 5. The computational cost of model during training can be measured in terms of the number of floating-point operations (FLOPs) required to perform forward and

Table 3 Training, validation, and test accuracy before data augmentation

Alzheimer's stages	Training accuracy (data size: 60%)	Validation accuracy (data size: 20%)	Test accuracy (data size: 20%)
AD	94.11	94.22	94.71
MCI	91.12	92.01	92.24
SMC	94.37	94.81	95.41
CN	94.52	94.81	95.07
Total	94.31	94.81	95.89

Table 4 Training, validation, and test accuracy after data augmentation

Alzheimer's stages	Training accuracy (data size: 60%)	Validation accuracy (data size: 20%)	Test accuracy (data size: 20%)
AD	95.15	95.38	95.79
MCI	93.14	94.01	94.27
SMC	95.56	95.91	96.01
CN	95.61	95.97	96.11
Total	94.87	95.32	95.55

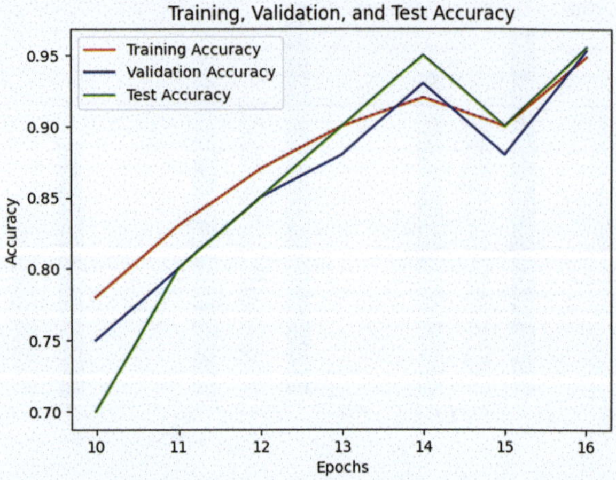

Fig. 9 Training, validation, and test accuracy

backward passes through the model. FLOPs provide a measure of the number of arithmetic operations (such as additions and multiplications) required to perform a given computation. The proposed model shows the augmented, reconstructed, and enhanced images as a part of the extended dataset and scored higher accuracy and low loss in the same cohorts of work.

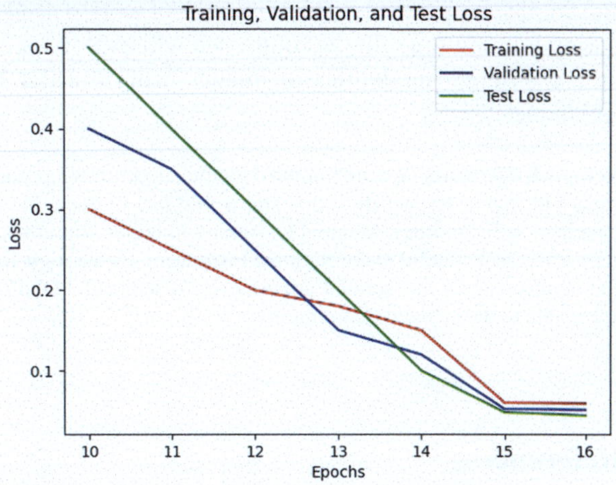

Fig. 10 Training, validation, and test loss

Table 5 Computational cost of the model

Architecture/model	Number of FLOPs per epoch	Time elapsed (HH:MM:SS)
Vanilla GAN	$O(W \times n)$, where W is the number of weights and n is the number of training samples	00:45:34
Deep convolutional GAN (DCGAN)	$O(W \times k^2 \times d \times h \times n)$, where W is the number of weights, k is the kernel size, d is the number of input channels, h is the number of output channels, and n is the number of training samples	00:57:12
Vanilla GAN + DCGAN	-	01:47:00
DCGAN + pre-processing + vanilla GAN	-	01:25:10

6 Conclusion

In the domain of disease classification, Alzheimer's disease classification is prominent in the current era. We have used DCGAN as a part of image augmentation, reconstruction, and image enhancement. Later, the proposed model used the flavor of DCGA as Vanilla GAN used for the classification of stages of Alzheimer's. Vanilla-GAN uses the power of CNN, also known as Deep Convolutional GAN (DCGAN), which is also used in classification. After generating the enhanced images, we performed a classification task to classify the stages of Alzheimer's. To experiment, this study makes use of the dataset that was collected by the ADNI. The proposed model's performance has been evaluated and validated using assessment and evaluation metrics. We have reported training, validation, and testing accuracy of 94.87%, 95.32%, and 95.55% respectively. The limitation of work it needed a high computing machine during training time. In the future, we will explore or extend more datasets to work on the different modalities of images using transfer learning and soft computing techniques.

Acknowledgements We are humbled by the opportunity to conduct this research at Manipal University in Jaipur, Rajasthan, India, and would like to thank the CIDCR Lab-103-2AB, School of Information Technology, Manipal University in Jaipur, Rajasthan, India, for making it possible. We are particularly grateful to the National Institute of Technology, Raipur, India, for the assistance and encouragement for this study. Furthermore, we applaud ADNI's generosity in making the dataset accessible to the scholarly community.

References

1. Petersen RC, Aisen PS, Beckett LA, et al. Alzheimer's Disease Neuroimaging Initiative (ADNI): Clinical characterization. Neurology 2010; 74(3): 201–9. http://dx.doi.org/10.1212/WNL.0b013e3181cb3e25
2. LONI-ADNI. Alzheimer's Disease Neuroimaging Initiative (ADNI) Available from: http://adni.loni.usc.edu/data-samples/access-data/ (Accessed on: January 20, 2022).
3. Clinically relevant changes for cognitive outcomes in preclinical and prodromal cognitive stages: Implications for clinical alzheimer trials. (2023). Neurology. https://doi.org/10.1212/wnl.0000000000206876
4. Bondi MW, Edmonds EC, Salmon DP. Alzheimer's disease: Past, present, and future. J Int Neuropsychol Soc 2017; 23(9-10): 818–31. http://dx.doi.org/10.1017/S135561771700100X
5. Ulrich, J. (1985). Alzheimer changes in nondemented patients younger than sixty-five: Possible early stages of alzheimer's disease and senile dementia of alzheimer type. Annals of Neurology, 17(3), 273–277. https://doi.org/10.1002/ana.410170309
6. Wang J, Chen Y, Wu Y, Shi J, Gee J. Enhanced generative adversarial network for 3D brain MRI super-resolution. In: 2020 IEEE Winter Conference on Applications of Computer Vision (WACV); 2020. p. 3616–25.
7. Porkodi, S. P., Sarada, V., Maik, V., I& Gurushankar, K. (2022). Generic image application using Gans (generative adversarial networks): A Review. Evolving Systems. https://doi.org/10.1007/s12530-022-09464-y
8. Shaul, R., David, I., Shitrit, O., I& Riklin Raviv, T. (2020). Subsampled Brain MRI reconstruction by Generative Adversarial Neural Networks. Medical Image Analysis, 65, 101747. https://doi.org/10.1016/j.media.2020.101747
9. Gareev, D., Glassl, O., I& Nouzri, S. (2022). Using Gans to generate lyric videos. IFAC-PapersOnLine, 55(10), 3292–3297. https://doi.org/10.1016/j.ifacol.2022.10.126
10. Shankar, V.G., Sisodia, D.S., Chandrakar, P. (2023). An intelligent hierarchical residual attention learning-based conjoined twin neural network for Alzheimer's stage detection and prediction. Computational Intelligence, 39(5), 783–805. https://doi.org/10.1111/coin.12594
11. Shankar, VG, Sisodia, DS, Chandrakar, P. A novel discriminant feature selection-based mutual information extraction from MR brain images for Alzheimer's stages detection and prediction. International Journal of Imaging Systems and Technology. 2022; 32(4): 1172–1191. https://doi.org/10.1002/ima.22685
12. Shankar Venkatesh Gauri*, Sisodia Dilip Singh and Chandrakar Preeti, A Novel Continuous-time Hidden Markov Model Based on a Bag of Features Extracted from MR Brain Images for Alzheimer's Stage Progression and Detection, Current Medical Imaging 2023. https://dx.doi.org/10.2174/1573405619666230213111047

13. Wada, N., I& Kobayashi, M. (2022). Unsupervised image-to-image translation from MRI-based simulated images to realistic images reflecting specific color characteristics. Proceedings of the 15th International Joint Conference on Biomedical Engineering Systems and Technologies. https://doi.org/10.5220/0010916300003123
14. Rizvi, S. K., Azad, M. A., I& Fraz, M. M. (2021). Spectrum of advancements and developments in multidisciplinary domains for generative adversarial networks (Gans). Archives of Computational Methods in Engineering, 28(7), 4503–4521. https://doi.org/10.1007/s11831-021-09543-4
15. Shankar, V.G., Sisodia, D.S., Chandrakar, P. (2023). An Efficient MR Images Based Analysis to Predict Alzheimer's Dementia Stage Using Random Forest Classifier. Lecture Notes in Networks and Systems, vol 521. Springer, Cham. https://doi.org/10.1007/978-3-031-13150-9_9
16. Kim, H. W., Lee, H. E., Lee, S., Oh, K. T., Yun, M., I& Yoo, S. K. (2020). Slice-selective learning for alzheimer's disease classification using a generative adversarial network: A feasibility study of external validation. European Journal of Nuclear Medicine and Molecular Imaging, 47(9), 2197–2206. https://doi.org/10.1007/s00259-019-04676-y
17. Shin, H.-C., Tenenholtz, N. A., Rogers, J. K., Schwarz, C. G., Senjem, M. L., Gunter, J. L., Andriole, K. P., I& Michalski, M. (2018). Medical image synthesis for data augmentation and anonymization using generative adversarial networks. Simulation and Synthesis in Medical Imaging, 1–11. https://doi.org/10.1007/978-3-030-00536-81
18. Helaly, H. A., Badawy, M., I& Haikal, A. Y. (2021). Deep Learning Approach for early detection of alzheimer's disease. Cognitive Computation, 14(5), 1711–1727. https://doi.org/10.1007/s12559-021-09946-2
19. Wolterink, J. M., Dinkla, A. M., Savenije, M. H., Seevinck, P. R., van den Berg, C. A., I& Išgum, I. (2017). Deep MR to CT synthesis using unpaired data. Simulation and Synthesis in Medical Imaging, 14–23. https://doi.org/10.1007/978-3-319-68127-62
20. Schlegl, T., Seeböck, P., Waldstein, S. M., Langs, G., I& Schmidt-Erfurth, U. (2019). F-anogan: Fast unsupervised anomaly detection with generative adversarial networks. Medical Image Analysis, 54, 30–44. https://doi.org/10.1016/j.media.2019.01.010
21. Goodfellow, I. J., Pouget-Abadie, J., Mirza, M., Xu, B., Warde-Farley, D., Ozair, S., et al. (2014). Generative adversarial networks. Adv. Neural Inform. Process. Syst. 3, 2672–2680.
22. Liu M, Cheng D, Wang K, Wang Y. Multi-modality cascaded convolutional neural networks for Alzheimer's disease diagnosis. Neuroinformatics. 2018;16:295–308.
23. Logan, R., Williams, B. G., Ferreira da Silva, M., Indani, A., Schcolnicov, N., Ganguly, A., I& Miller, S. J. (2021). Deep Convolutional Neural Networks with ensemble learning and generative adversarial networks for alzheimer's Disease Image Data Classification. Frontiers in Aging Neuroscience, 13. https://doi.org/10.3389/fnagi.2021.720226
24. Uzunova, H., Schultz, S., Handels, H., I& Ehrhardt, J. (2018). Unsupervised pathology detection in medical images using conditional variational autoencoders. International Journal of Computer Assisted Radiology and Surgery, 14(3), 451–461. https://doi.org/10.1007/s11548-018-1898-0
25. Sahu, S., Gupta, R., Sivaraman, G., AbdAlmageed, W., I& Espy-Wilson, C. (2017). Adversarial auto-encoders for speech based emotion recognition. Interspeech 2017. https://doi.org/10.21437/interspeech.2017-1421
26. Khan, N. M., Abraham, N., I& Hon, M. (2019). Transfer learning with intelligent training data selection for prediction of alzheimer's disease. IEEE Access, 7, 72726–72735. https://doi.org/10.1109/access.2019.2920448
27. Lin E., Lin C. H., Lane H. Y. (2021). Deep learning with neuroimaging and genomics in Alzheimer's disease. Int. J. Mol. Sci. 22:7911. 10.3390/ijms22157911
28. Fulton, L., Dolezel, D., Harrop, J., Yan, Y., I& Fulton, C. (2019). Classification of alzheimer's disease with and without imagery using gradient boosted machines and resnet-50. Brain Sciences, 9(9), 212. https://doi.org/10.3390/brainsci9090212
29. Data augmentation for intelligent contingency management using generative Adversarial Networks. (2022). https://doi.org/10.2514/6.2022-0622.vid

30. Aggarwal, A., Mittal, M., I& Battineni, G. (2021). Generative Adversarial Network: An overview of theory and applications. International Journal of Information Management Data Insights, 1(1), 100004. https://doi.org/10.1016/j.jjimei.2020.100004
31. Yi, X., Walia, E., I& Babyn, P. (2019). Generative Adversarial Network in medical imaging: A Review. Medical Image Analysis, 58, 101552. https://doi.org/10.1016/j.media.2019.101552
32. Zhou, X., Qiu, S., Joshi, P. S., Xue, C., Killiany, R. J., Mian, A. Z., et al. (2021). Enhancing magnetic resonance imaging−driven Alzheimer's disease classification performance using generative adversarial learning. Alzheimers Res. Ther. 13:60. https://doi.org/10.1186/s13195-021-00797-5
33. Bathla, A., I& Gupta, A. (2021). Image formation using deep convolutional generative Adversarial Networks. Predictive Analytics, 81–88. https://doi.org/10.1201/9781003083177-5
34. Alec Radford, Luke Metz, Soumith Chintala. (2016), Unsupervised Representation Learning with Deep Convolutional Generative Adversarial Networks, arXiv. https://doi.org/10.48550/arXiv.1511.06434
35. Liu, B., Lv, J., Fan, X., Luo, J., I& Zou, T. (2021). Application of an improved DCGAN for image generationapplication of an improved DCGAN for image generation. https://doi.org/10.21203/rs.3.rs-266104/v1
36. Kim, J. S. (2021). Validation model of land price adequacy by applying DCGAN. APPRAISAL STUDIES, 20(2), 67-98. https://doi.org/10.23843/as.20.2.3
37. Cai, Likun, Yanjie Chen, Ning Cai, Wei Cheng, and Hao Wang. 2020. "Utilizing Amari-Alpha Divergence to Stabilize the Training of Generative Adversarial Networks" Entropy 22, no. 4: 410. https://doi.org/10.3390/e22040410
38. van Rhijn, J., Oosterlee, C. W., Grzelak, L. A., I& Liu, S. (2022). Monte Carlo simulation of sdes using Gans. Japan Journal of Industrial and Applied Mathematics. https://doi.org/10.1007/s13160-022-00534-x
39. Pavan Kumar, M. R., I& Jayagopal, P. (2020). Generative Adversarial Networks: A survey on applications and challenges. International Journal of Multimedia Information Retrieval, 10(1), 1–24. https://doi.org/10.1007/s13735-020-00196-w
40. Delannoy, Q., Pham, C.-H., Cazorla, C., Tor-Díez, C., Dollé, G., Meunier, H., Bednarek, N., Fablet, R., Passat, N., I& Rousseau, F. (2020). Segsrgan: Super-resolution and segmentation using generative adversarial networks - application to neonatal brain MRI. Computers in Biology and Medicine, 120, 103755. https://doi.org/10.1016/j.compbiomed.2020.103755
41. Fahimi, F., Dosen, S., Ang, K. K., Mrachacz-Kersting, N., I& Guan, C. (2021). Generative adversarial networks-based data augmentation for Brain-computer interface. IEEE Transactions on Neural Networks and Learning Systems, 32(9), 4039–4051. https://doi.org/10.1109/tnnls.2020.3016666
42. Hosseini-asl E, Keynton R, El-baz A, Drzezga A, Lautenschlager N, Siebner H, et al. Alzheimer's disease diagnostics by adaptation of 3D convolutional network electrical and computer engineering department , University of Louisville , Louisville , KY, USA. Eur J Nucl Med Mol Imaging. 2016;30:1104–13.
43. Liang, J., Chen, S., I& Jin, Q. (2019). Semi-supervised Multimodal Emotion Recognition with improved Wasserstein Gans. 2019 Asia-Pacific Signal and Information Processing Association Annual Summit and Conference (APSIPA ASC). https://doi.org/10.1109/apsipaasc47483.2019.9023144
44. Mukherjee, T., Sharma, S., I& Suganthi, K. (2021). Alzheimer detection using deep convolutional gan. 2021 IEEE Madras Section Conference (MASCON). https://doi.org/10.1109/mascon51689.2021.9563368
45. Khaled, A., I& Han, J.-J. (2021). Multi-model medical image segmentation using multi-stage generative Adversarial Network. https://doi.org/10.20944/preprints202112.0025.v1
46. Hu, S., Yu, W., Chen, Z., I& Wang, S. (2020). Medical image reconstruction using generative adversarial network for alzheimer disease assessment with class-imbalance problem. 2020 IEEE 6th International Conference on Computer and Communications (ICCC). https://doi.org/10.1109/iccc51575.2020.9344912

Evaluating the Quality and Diversity of DCGAN-Based Generatively Synthesized Diabetic Retinopathy Imagery

Cristina-Madalina Dragan, Muhammad Muneeb Saad, Mubashir Husain Rehmani, and Ruairi O'Reilly

Abstract Publicly available diabetic retinopathy (DR) datasets are imbalanced, containing limited numbers of images with DR. This imbalance contributes to overfitting when training machine learning classifiers. The impact of this imbalance is exacerbated as the severity of the DR stage increases, affecting the classifiers' diagnostic capacity. The imbalance can be addressed using Generative Adversarial Networks (GANs) to augment the datasets with synthetic images. Generating synthetic images is advantageous if high-quality and diverse images are produced. To evaluate the quality and diversity of synthetic images, several evaluation metrics, such as Multi-Scale Structural Similarity Index (MS-SSIM), Cosine Distance (CD), and Fréchet Inception Distance (FID), are used. Understanding the effectiveness of each metric in evaluating the quality and diversity of synthetic images is critical to select images for augmentation. To date, there has been limited analysis of the appropriateness of these metrics in the context of biomedical imagery. This work contributes an empirical assessment of these evaluation metrics as applied to synthetic Proliferative DR imagery generated by a Deep Convolutional GAN (DCGAN). Furthermore, the metrics' capacity to indicate the quality and diversity of synthetic images and their correlation with classifier performance are examined. This enables a quantitative selection of synthetic imagery and an informed augmentation strategy, which are often lacking in the literature. Results indicate that FID is suitable for evaluating the quality, while MS-SSIM and CD are suitable for evaluating the diversity of synthetic imagery. Furthermore, the superior performance of Convolutional Neural Network (CNN) and EfficientNet classifiers, as indicated by the F_1 and AUC scores, for the

---

C.-M. Dragan (✉) · M. M. Saad · M. H. Rehmani · R. O'Reilly
Munster Technological University, Cork, Ireland
e-mail: cristina.madalina.dragan@gmail.com

M. M. Saad
e-mail: muhammad.saad@mycit.ie

M. H. Rehmani
e-mail: mubashir.rehmani@mtu.ie

R. O'Reilly
e-mail: ruairi.oreilly@mtu.ie

H. Ali et al. (eds.), *Advances in Deep Generative Models for Medical Artificial Intelligence*, Studies in Computational Intelligence 1124,
https://doi.org/10.1007/978-3-031-46341-9_4

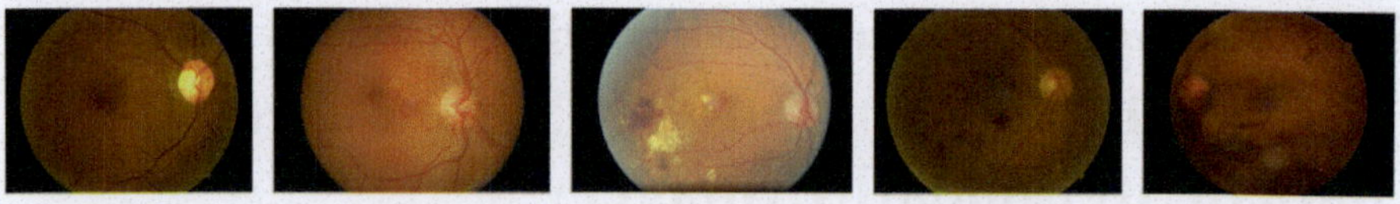

(a) (b) (c) (d) (e)

Fig. 1 Retinal fundus images with different stages of DR: **a** no DR, **b** mild NPDR, **c** moderate NPDR, **d** severe NPDR, **e** PDR

augmented datasets compared to the original dataset demonstrate the efficacy of synthetic imagery to augment the imbalanced dataset while improving the classification scores

Keywords Diabetic retinopathy · Retinal fundus imagery · Generative adversarial networks · Convolutional neural networks · Multi-scale structural similarity index · Cosine distance · Fréchet inception distance

1 Introduction

Diabetic retinopathy (DR) is a complication caused by high blood sugar levels over a prolonged period that is estimated to affect 415 million people globally [1] and can lead to blindness if it is not treated timely. The diagnosis of DR is made based on the analysis of retinal fundus imagery, where lesions specific to DR are identified. The severity of DR is evaluated using the international severity grading scale (ISGR) [2], which has four stages: Mild Non-Proliferative DR (Mild NPDR), Moderate NPDR, Severe NPDR, and Proliferative DR (PDR) (see Fig. 1). The increasing prevalence of the disease and the lack of medical personnel capable of diagnosing it highlight the need for computer-aided diagnostics to assist healthcare professionals [3–5].

Artificial intelligence (AI) techniques have become important in finding solutions to modern engineering problems. AI has been utilized in the domain of biomedical imagery for disease analysis and the interpretation of clinical data [6]. Healthcare has become increasingly dependent on computer-aided diagnosis (CAD), a computer-based application that assists clinicians [7]. There is a vast contribution made by AI-based classifiers, including Support Vector Machine (SVM), Logistic Regression (LR), Artificial Neural Networks (ANNs), and deep learning models such as Convolutional Neural Networks (CNNs), to assist clinicians through automated analysis of numerous diseases such as diabetes, cancer, and COVID-19 using biomedical imagery [3–5, 8]. Deep learning models can provide more effective disease analysis than alternate techniques. However, these models require large quantities of training data to enable effective classification, which is a challenging problem in the domain of biomedical imagery [9, 10].

Table 1 Publicly available datasets containing retinal fundus images at different stages of DR

Dataset	No. image	No DR	Mild NPDR	Moderate NPDR	Severe NPDR	PDR
Kaggle [12]	88,702	65,343	6205	13,153	2087	1914
APTOS [13]	3662	1805	370	999	193	295
FGADR [14]	2842	244	337	1161	752	348
Messidor-2 [15, 16]	1744	1017	270	347	75	35
Messidor[a] [15]	1200	546	153	247	254	–
IDRID [17]	516	168	25	168	93	62
DR2 [18]	435	98	337	–	–	–
1000 fundus [19]	144	38	18	49	39	–
STARE [20]	113	41	51	21	–	–
HRFID [21]	30	15	15	–	–	–
Total[a]	98,188	68,769	7628	15,898	3239	2654
As %		70	7.8	16.2	3.3	2.7

DR: Diabetic Retinopathy; NPDR: Non-Proliferative DR; PDR: Proliferative DR
[a] Messidor excluded from total as 1058 images overlap with the Messidor-2 dataset

Publicly available retinal fundus image datasets are imbalanced, containing significantly more images without DR than images with DR, as indicated in Table 1. The availability of images decreases as the severity of DR increases, with severe NDPR and PDR accounting for a total of 6% of the available images. Imbalanced datasets contain images with skewed classes. The skewness in imbalanced datasets refers to the asymmetry distribution of images across different classes [10]. Therefore, when the severity of DR disease increases then this imbalance causes overfitting of the classifiers to the class representing the most severe stage of the disease [11]. The Kaggle [12] dataset (see Table 1) is highly imbalanced and has the largest number of images as compared to the other datasets. This dataset is important as it contains images from patients of different ethnicities.

In the domain of biomedical imagery, data imbalance is a challenging problem as it deals with imagery that contains salient features indicative of diseases that directly impact human lives [7]. As such, addressing the issue of data imbalance is considered a worthwhile endeavor. One potential solution is to augment training data with synthetic imagery belonging to the underrepresented classes [22].

Synthetic biomedical imagery can be derived from generative models. Several generative models such as variational autoencoders [23], diffusion models [24], and Generative Adversarial Networks (GANs) [25] have been utilized to generate retinal fundus synthetic images. For generating synthetic images, autoencoders produce blurry images while diffusion models are trained slowly with high-computational cost as compared to GANs [26]. GANs are generative models consisting of two neural networks, a generator, and a discriminator. The generator aims to produce realistic synthetic images, and the discriminator's aim is to distinguish between real and synthetic images.

The GAN-based generated synthetic images are evaluated using two critical criteria, the quality of the images, indicating how representative they are of real images of that class, and the diversity of the images, indicating how broad and uniform the coverage of their feature distribution is compared to the real images. The quality of synthetic imagery is characterized by an alignment of its feature distribution with the class label [25, 27, 28] and a low level of noise, blurriness, and distortions [29]. The diversity of synthetic images is characterized by the level of similarity to each other [30].

The quality and diversity of synthetic images have a significant impact on the performance of classifiers when these images are used for augmenting limited and imbalanced datasets. A classifier will not learn the features representative of different classes if the training dataset is augmented with low-quality synthetic images. Similarly, the classifier will incorrectly classify images containing feature distributions that belong to the less represented areas if the training dataset is augmented with less diversified synthetic images. When synthetic images are used in training a classifier, it is essential that they are of high quality and that the features representative of a class are sufficiently diverse.

The quality of synthetic imagery represents the level of similarity to the real imagery and the diversity represents the level of dissimilarity between the synthetic imagery. There are several metrics used for evaluating the similarity between images such as peak signal-to-noise ratio (PSNR) [31], structural similarity index (SSIM) [31, 32], multi-scale structural similarity index (MS-SSIM) [32, 33], cosine distance (CD) [34], and Fréchet inception distance (FID) [35].

In the literature, these metrics are categorized based on qualitative and quantitative measures [31]. Qualitative measures require subjective information such as visual examination of synthetic images by humans which is time-consuming and cumbersome [31]. It includes evaluation metrics such as nearest neighbors [36], rapid scene categorization [37], and preference judgment [38]. On the other hand, quantitative measures do not require subjective information and only rely on objective information such as the diversity and quality of images, when evaluating synthetic images using quantitative evaluation metrics [31].

In this work, quantitative metrics such as MS-SSIM, CD, and FID are used. A combination of these metrics provides quantitative measures using perceptual features (MS-SSIM) and the distance between image pixels (CD and FID) to evaluate the quality and diversity of synthetic images.

PDR is the most severe stage of DR with the lowest quantity of publicly available imagery, as such this work narrows its focus to the generation of synthetic PDR imagery. PDR is a serious eye complication of diabetes that can lead to severe vision loss or even blindness. It occurs when abnormal blood vessels grow in the retina, the light-sensitive tissue at the back of the eye, in response to high blood sugar levels. It is important for people with diabetes to have regular eye exams to detect PDR

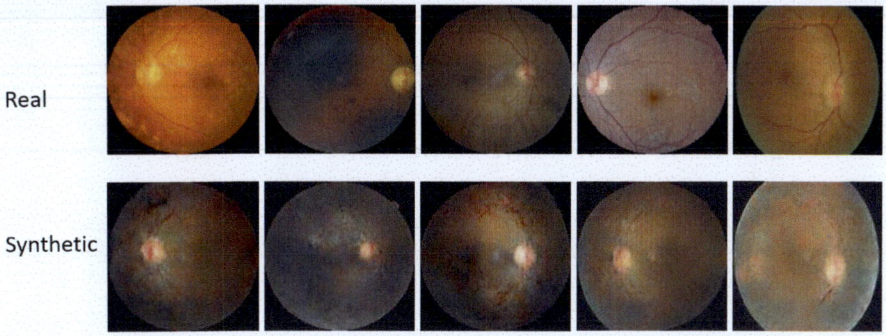

Fig. 2 Real and synthetically generated PDR image samples of deep convolutional GAN depicting lesions of different size, shape, and location

at early stages and prevent vision loss [1]. In the context of PDR, a high-quality synthetic image depicts the presence of valid lesions specific to PDR, and a high level of diversity is indicated by the presence of lesions of different sizes, shapes, and locations, as shown in Fig. 2.

There are a few evaluation metrics, such as SSIM and PSNR, that evaluate the quality of generated images by comparing them to ground truth images using image pixel values. Other evaluation metrics, such as SWD and FID, quantify the distance between images to evaluate the quality of images. However, it is important to evaluate the diversity of images because GANs should generate synthetic images that are as diverse as real images. Therefore, evaluation metrics that can quantify the quality and diversity of synthetic images should be used. Several methods, such as classification scores achieved through neural networks and the analysis of radiologists, for evaluating synthetic images have been adopted, as indicated in Table 2. It is challenging to find evaluation metrics that explicitly evaluate the quality and diversity of synthetic images using significant image features by comparing synthetic images to real images.

Technical discussions on the selection and suitability of metrics for evaluating the quality and diversity of GAN-based synthetic retinal fundus images are lacking in the literature. A limiting factor in existing works is that the method of selecting the synthetic images used for data augmentation is not specified. In the works indicated in Table 2, it is not assessed whether the metrics used are suitable to evaluate the quality and diversity of the synthetic imagery.

In this work, an empirical assessment of MS-SSIM, CD, and FID metrics is conducted to assess the suitability of these metrics in evaluating the quality and diversity of synthetic DR images generated by the DCGAN. Moreover, this work contributes to: (i) a critical analysis of quantitative evaluation metrics' capacity to identify if imagery contains features corresponding to its class label; (ii) an investigation of DCGAN's capacity to generate diversified and high-quality synthetic PDR images; (iii) an assessment of DCGAN's synthetic images to improve the classification performance of classifiers such as CNN and EfficientNet; and (iv) an evaluation of the

Table 2 Generation of biomedical imagery utilizing GANs

Medical img.	Ref. year	GANs	Dataset	Img. res.	Clf.	Clf. (gain)	Quality	Div.
DR retinal fundus	[25] 2020	CGAN	Kaggle	1280 × 1280	VGG-16, ResNet-50, I-v3	Acc: (0.01) Kappa: (0.01–0.02)	FID, SWD, visualized by ophthalmologists	N/A
	[39] 2020	DCGAN	Kaggle	128 × 128	CNN	Mac-aver Prec: (– 0.01 to 0) Mac-aver Rec: (0.01) Mac-aver F1: (0–0.01)	CD	CD
Retinal fundus	[40] 2020	StyleGAN	Kaggle	512 × 512	ResNet-50	N/A	N/A	N/A
	[41] 2019	ProGAN	AREDS	512 × 512	ResNet-50	N/A	Visualized by eye specialists	N/A
	[42] 2020	CGAN	DRIVE [43]	512 × 512	N/A	N/A	N/A	N/A
	[27] 2018	CGAN	Messidor	256 × 256	N/A	N/A	ISC score	N/A
	[28] 2019	Pix2pix, Cycle-GAN	DRISHTI-GS [44], DRIVE	512× 512, 256× 256	N/A	N/A	SSIM, PSNR	N/A
	[45] 2019	SS-DCGAN	Irrelevant	128 × 128	SS-DCGAN	N/A	LSE, T-SNE	AVP, MSE
DR lesions	[46] 2019	DCGAN	Irrelevant	32 × 32	CNN	Sens: (0.05–0.2) Spec: (0.07–0.23)	N/A	N/A
Brain PET	[47] 2020	DCGAN	Irrelevant	128 × 128	CNN	Acc: (0.1)	PSNR, SSIM	N/A
Liver CT	[48] 2018	DCGAN, AC-GAN	Irrelevant	64 × 64	CNN	Sens: (0.02–0.13) Spec: (– 0.01 to 0.07)	Visualized by radio	N/A
Brain MR	[49] 2019	Cond. PGGAN	Irrelevant	256 × 256	YOLOv3 CNN [50]	Sens: (0.01–0.1)	VTT	T-SNE
	[51] 2019	PGGAN, SimGAN	Irrelevant	224 × 224	ResNet-50	Acc: (– 0.08 to 0.1) Sens: (– 0.08 to 0.08) Spec: (– 0.11 to 0.14)	VTT, T-SNE	T-SNE

The classification performance gain is noted where generated images were used in training a classifier
Acc: Accuracy; Clf: Classifier; Cond: Conditional; Div: Diversity; DR: Diabetic Retinopathy; Img: Image; Mac-aver: Macro-averaged; Prec: Precision; Ref: Reference; Res: Resolution; Rec: Recall; Radio: Radiologists; Sens: Sensitivity; Spec: Specificity; VTT: Visual Turing Test

Table 3 CNN-based classification of DR stages based on the ISGR

Ref. year	Model	Dataset	Acc.	Mac. F1	Data augment.	Image res.
[54] 2020	CNN and DT	Kaggle	99.99	0.999[a]	–	227 × 227
[55] 2019	Inception V4	Private	88.4	0.678[a]	–	779 × 779
[56] 2019	Siamese CNN	Kaggle	84.25[a]	0.603[a]	Trad.	299 × 299
[4] 2017	CNN/denoising	Kaggle	85	0.566[a]	Trad.	512 × 512
[57] 2019	Ensemble/TL	Kaggle	80.8	0.532	Trad.	512 × 512
[58] 2018	Deep CNN	Kaggle	50.8	0.482[a]	Trad.	224 × 224
[59] 2016	Deep CNN	Kaggle	73.76[a]	0.335[a]	Trad. (+ CW)	512 × 512
[39] 2020	Deep CNN	Kaggle	0.693[a]	0.268[a]	GANs	128 × 128
[3] 2019	CNN	Kaggle	74	–	Trad.	128 × 128
[5] 2019	Deep CNN	Kaggle	87.2	–	Sampling and IW	600 × 600
[25] 2020	VGG-16, ResNet-50, I-v3, AFN, Zoom-in	Kaggle, FGARD	82.45–89.16	–	GANs	1280 × 1280

Augment: Augmentation; Acc: Accuracy; CW: Class Weights; DT: Decision Trees; IW: Instance Weights; Mac. F1: Macro F1; Ref: Reference; Res: Resolution; Trad: Traditional; TL: Transfer Learning

[a] Denotes the derived performance from confusion matrix

relationship between diversity and quality of the synthetic imagery as indicated by MS-SSIM, CD, FID, and classification performance.

It is envisaged that understanding which evaluation metrics are suitable for evaluating the quality and diversity of synthetic retinal fundus imagery will enable an improved selection of synthetic imagery to augment the training dataset of a classifier.

2 Related Work

Several state-of-the-art works that use CNNs for automatically classifying DR via retinal fundus imagery are denoted in Table 3. In order for CNNs to generalize across DR stages whilst achieving a performant classification accuracy, these classifiers need to be trained on a large and balanced dataset [52, 53].

In detailing the CNNs in Table 3 macro-averaged F1 score (mac. F1) was used to compare their performance, as all classes are treated equally [60]. This is particularly important due to the data imbalance and the minority class (PDR) being the most severe stage of DR. The macro-averaged F1 score was calculated based on the mean of the F1 scores for every class [61].

Data augmentation is one approach to address data imbalance when training a CNN. It consists of adding synthetic or modified versions of the original images from the underrepresented classes to the dataset [3, 54, 62, 63]. Modified versions of the original images can be obtained with rotation, flipping, or random cropping techniques [10]. The limitation of these techniques is that the diversity of the resulting dataset is limited [25, 40]. An alternate technique is the generation of synthetic imagery using GANs to augment the training data.

2.1 GAN-Based Approaches to Addressing Data Imbalance for DR

Medical datasets are often imbalanced [9, 64], as such, there has been extensive work carried out on the generation of synthetic medical imagery (see Table 2). The quality and diversity of synthetic medical imagery are evaluated manually by physicians and quantitatively with evaluation metrics such as SSIM, FID, etc. It can be seen in Table 2 that there is no consensus for evaluating the quality and diversity of generated imagery.

However, the quality of synthetic images is evaluated more significantly than diversity measures. The diversity evaluation is important as it indicates the degree of mode collapse, a potential problem of training GANs consisting in generating similar synthetic images for diverse input images.

In this work, these perspectives have acted as motivating factors, for enabling a more transparent assessment of a GAN's capacity to generate suitably diversified retinal fundus images with PDR.

To demonstrate the benefits of generating synthetic imagery, in several works the training dataset is augmented with the synthetic images, and classification performance is calculated with evaluation metrics like accuracy, sensitivity, precision, kappa, and specificity.

In [25] a conditional GAN (CGAN) is used to generate retinal fundus images for each DR stage. Quality is evaluated using three methods: manual evaluation, FID, and Sliced Wasserstein distance (SWD). Five hundred real and five hundred synthetic images are mixed, and two experiments are undertaken. Three ophthalmologists labeled each image as real or synthetic and assigned a severity level of DR. FID and SWD were calculated between the real and synthetic images.

In [39] a DCGAN is used to generate retinal fundus images of PDR. Quality and diversity are evaluated using an average CD. The synthetic images are added to the training dataset. The InceptionV3 model [65] pre-trained on the ImageNet database [66] extracts features from the images with PDR from the augmented dataset. The CDs between the extracted features are calculated and their average is compared to the average of the CDs between the features extracted only from the real images with PDR.

In [40] a MixGAN is proposed based on progressive layers and Style transfer to generate retinal fundus images of different DR stages such as moderate NPDR, severe NPDR, and PDR. It is not specified how synthetically generated images were evaluated.

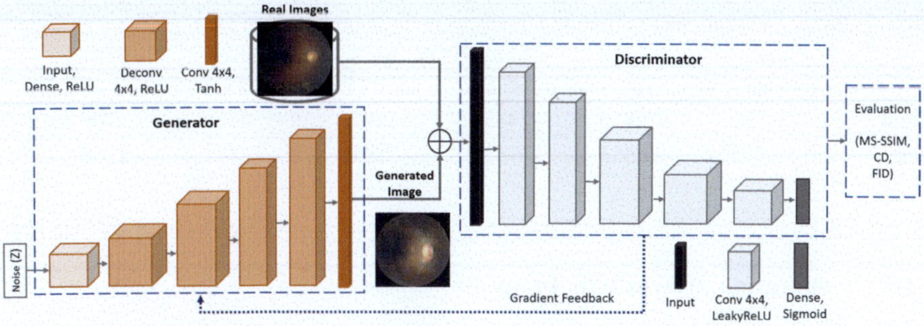

Fig. 3 Architecture of DCGAN for PDR image synthesis. DCGAN generates synthetic PDR images using five convolutional layers in the discriminator and four deconvolutional layers in the generator

3 Methodology

In this work, the suitability of evaluation metrics for assessing the quality and diversity of GAN-based retinal fundus synthetic images is analyzed. For this purpose, the methodology of GANs architectures, dataset, evaluation metrics, and the proposed idea of identifying suitable evaluation metrics is discussed as follows.

3.1 DCGAN Architecture

It is important to understand the characteristics of GANs so that these models can easily be reimplemented and fine-tuned for generating high-quality synthetic images [67]. For generating synthetic images, DCGAN [68] is considered a baseline model due to its simple architecture. DCGAN architecture can easily be adopted and reimplemented for any type of imagery to address the data imbalance problem [69]. Therefore, this work adopted DCGAN for synthesizing PDR fundus images.

The architecture of DCGAN is depicted in Fig. 3. Initially, the DCGAN from [39] was adopted and reimplemented using the same parameter settings for generating PDR images. The DCGAN produced noisy images and was unable to generate realistic synthetic images. This could be due to batch normalization layers with upsampling and convolution layers in the generator and discriminator models of the DCGAN. Sometimes, batch normalization layers cannot reduce overfitting but explode gradients due to the usage of rescaling layers repeatedly [70]. So, the layers of the generator and discriminator models were redesigned with deconvolution and convolution layers only as reported in [8].

The DCGAN is fine-tuned with a learning rate of 0.0001 for the Adam optimizer. A Gaussian latent random value of 100 is used for input z to the generator as adopted in [39, 46, 47]. The DCGAN is trained with a batch size of 16 for 500 epochs because both generator and discriminator models converge to a balanced state at this stage.

Table 4 Image distributions of different DR stages in the Kaggle dataset [12]

	Total no. images	No DR	Mild NPDR	Moderate NPDR	Severe NPDR	PDR
Train	35,126	25,810	2443	5292	873	708
Test	53,576	39,533	3762	7861	1214	1206

3.1.1 Generation of Synthetic Images

In GANs, synthetic images are generated without directly observing real data [34]. Real images are used for training the discriminator, while the generator generates the synthetic images. During the training of GANs [67], the generator model takes input from random values and generates noisy synthetic images. These images are passed to the discriminator. The discriminator also takes real images as input and distinguishes them from synthetic images. The discriminator backpropagates its feedback as gradients to the generator model. The generator model learns from that feedback and ideally enhances its capacity to generate realistically looking synthetic images. Once the generator is well-trained, it can generate several synthetic images by taking random input values. This is a baseline methodology used in GAN architectures to generate synthetic images.

3.2 *Retinal Fundus Imagery*

Publicly available retinal fundus imagery is imbalanced and increasingly limited as the severity of DR increases. As denoted in Table 1, PDR is the minority class associated with DR. This work focuses on generating imagery of a minority class representative of the PDR.

In this work, the Kaggle dataset [12] is used, which is the largest publicly available dataset containing retinal fundus images from patients with different DR stages. Table 4 denotes the number of images per stage of DR available in the training and test datasets. The distribution of retinal fundus images within the classes varies significantly across training and test datasets.

PDR images were rescaled to a resolution of 128×128 for training the DCGAN. Generally, the DCGAN model works with a resolution of 128×128 as it is considered an intermediate size which is not too low to degrade the pixel information and not too high such that it is difficult to handle the training of the DCGAN [45]. In the domain of biomedical imagery, this resolution is commonly adopted to train GANs for generating synthetic images [8, 25, 39, 45, 47].

For the classification of PDR images, the size of the images depends upon the type of classifier. A complex classifier, such as variants of CNNs, requires high-resolution images for learning salient image features. In contrast, a traditional classifier, such as a support vector machine (SVM) [71], can efficiently work with lower image resolutions. In this work, images were rescaled to a resolution of 227 $\times$ 227 for the CNN model [54] and 224 $\times$ 224 for the EfficientNet model [72].

3.2.1 Selection of Images for the Classifiers and GANs

When training a multi-class classifier, images from each class are required to be diversified significantly as compared to the images of alternate classes. Therefore, it is essential to analyze the distribution of all images to decide the selection of diversified images for the classifier. To that end, MS-SSIM, CD, and FID are used to evaluate the similarity of images of each class to alternate classes for the training and test datasets as indicated in Table 5.

To find the correlation among images of different classes from the training dataset and test dataset, 708 image samples from the training dataset and 1206 image samples from the test dataset were randomly selected for each class to measure the similarity scores. The 708 and 1206 samples were selected because these are the upper bounds that can be used for all classes. Table 5 indicates that the distribution of images of all classes follows a relatively similar pattern in the training as compared to the test sets. It shows that the existing distribution of images is significant and should be used.

This work focuses on augmenting the PDR class using GAN-based synthetic images. Therefore, 708 images of PDR are used for training the DCGAN.

3.3 Evaluation of GAN-Based Synthetic Imagery

3.3.1 MS-SSIM

The MS-SSIM metric evaluates the quality and diversity of synthetic images using perceptual similarities between images. It computes the similarity between images based on pixels and structural information of images. A higher value of MS-SSIM indicates higher similarity while a lower value of MS-SSIM indicates higher diversity between images of a single class [33]. MS-SSIM is measured between two images a and b using Eq. 1.

$$MS{-}SSIM(a,b) = I_M(a,b)^{\alpha_M} \prod_{j=1}^{M} C_j(a,b)^{\beta_j} S_j(a,b)^{\gamma_j} \quad (1)$$

In Eq. 1 [31], structure (S) and contrast (C) image features are computed using the j scale. M indicates the coarsest scale for measuring luminance (I). Weight parameters such as α β, and γ are used for measuring S, C, and I values.

In this work, 708 image pairs (real-synthetic) are selected randomly from real and synthetic datasets to measure the MS-SSIM score for the quality of synthetically generated images. However, 354 image pairs (real-real) from the real dataset and 354

Table 5 Similarity between sampled retinal fundus images with different stages of DR measured via MS-SSIM, CD, and FID with 95% confidence interval

EM, dataset	Class	No DR	Mild NPDR	Mod. NPDR	Sev. NPDR	PDR
FID, training data	No DR	**1**	0.389 ± 0.019	0.196 ± 0.009	0	0.054 ± 0.002
	Mild NPDR	0.389 ± 0.019	> **0.999**	0.359 ± 0.017	0.261 ± 0.013	0.110 ± 0.005
	Mod. NPDR	0.196 ± 0.09	0.359 ± 0.017	> **0.999**	0.391 ± 0.019	0.226 ± 0.011
	Sev. NPDR	0	0.261 ± 0.013	0.391 ± 0.019	> **0.999**	0.096 ± 0.004
	PDR	0.054 ± 0.002	0.110 ± 0.005	0.226 ± 0.011	0.096 ± 0.004	> **0.999**
FID, test data	No DR	**1**	0.409 ± 0.020	0.253 ± 0.012	0.140 ± 0.007	0
	Mild NPDR	0.409 ± 0.020	> **0.999**	0.390 ± 0.019	0.290 ± 0.014	0.023 ± 0.001
	Mod. NPDR	0.253 ± 0.012	0.390 ± 0.019	> **0.999**	0.453 ± 0.022	0.142 ± 0.007
	Sev. NPDR	0.140 ± 0.007	0.290 ± 0.014	0.453 ± 0.022	> **0.999**	0.102 ± 0.005
	PDR	0	0.023 ± 0.001	0.142 ± 0.007	0.102 ± 0.005	> **0.999**
CD, training data	No DR	0.543 ± 0.027	0.634 ± 0.032	0.341 ± 0.017	**1**	0.426 ± 0.021
	Mild NPDR	0.634 ± 0.032	0.364 ± 0.018	0.118 ± 0.006	**0.659 ± 0.033**	0
	Mod. NPDR	0.341 ± 0.017	0.118 ± 0.006	0.18 ± 0.009	**0.714 ± 0.036**	0.088 ± 0.004
	Sev. NPDR	**1**	0.659 ± 0.033	0.714 ± 0.036	0.818 ± 0.041	0.462 ± 0.023
	PDR	0.426 ± 0.021	0	0.088 ± 0.004	**0.462 ± 0.023**	0.318 ± 0.016
CD, test data	No DR	**0.772 ± 0.039**	0.714 ± 0.036	0.685 ± 0.034	0.654 ± 0.033	0.58 ± 0.029
	Mild NPDR	**0.714 ± 0.036**	0.258 ± 0.013	0.387 ± 0.019	0.62 ± 0.031	0.013 ± 0.001
	Mod. NPDR	**0.685 ± 0.034**	0.387 ± 0.019	0.193 ± 0.01	0.624 ± 0.031	0
	Sev. NPDR	0.654 ± 0.033	0.62 ± 0.031	0.624 ± 0.031	**1**	0.474 ± 0.024
	PDR	**0.58 ± 0.029**	0.013 ± 0.001	0	0.474 ± 0.024	0.45 ± 0.023
MS-SSIM, training data	No DR	**1**	0.02 ± 0.001	0.04 ± 0.002	0.039 ± 0.002	0.018 ± 0.001
	Mild NPDR	0.02 ± 0.001	**1**	0.036 ± 0.002	0.053 ± 0.003	0
	Mod. NPDR	0.04 ± 0.002	0.036 ± 0.002	**1**	0.029 ± 0.001	0.009
	Sev. NPDR	0.039 ± 0.002	0.053 ± 0.003	0.029 ± 0.001	**1**	0.003
	PDR	0.018 ± 0.001	0	0.009	0.003	**1**
MS-SSIM, test data	No DR	**1**	0.009	0.01 ± 0.001	0.021 ± 0.001	0.002
	Mild NPDR	0.009	**1**	0	0.007	0.003
	Mod. NPDR	0.01 ± 0.001	0	**1**	0.015 ± 0.001	0.014 ± 0.001
	Sev. NPDR	0.021 ± 0.001	0.007	0.015 ± 0.001	**1**	0.009
	PDR	0.002	0.003	0.014 ± 0.001	0.009	1

EM: Evaluation Metric; Mod: Moderate; Sev: Severe Note: The numbers in bold indicate the highest similarity scores for images of each class

image pairs (synthetic-synthetic) from the synthetic dataset are selected randomly to measure the MS-SSIM scores for the diversity of synthetically generated images.

3.3.2 CD

CD is used to assess the quality and diversity of images. The cosine distance is computed by extracting the feature vectors of images using deep neural networks [34]. CD for two images is computed using the feature vectors *f1* and *f2* as defined in Eq. 2.

$$CD(f1, f2) = 1 - \frac{f1 \cdot f2}{||f1|| \times ||f2||} \tag{2}$$

In Eq. 2 [34], *f1* and *f2* refer to the feature vectors extracted from 2 images. A higher value of CD indicates higher diversity between images of a single class. In this work, feature vectors are extracted from an InceptionV3 model pre-trained on the ImageNet dataset. The CD is computed using 708 real and 708 synthetic images.

3.3.3 FID

FID is an evaluation metric used for assessing the quality and diversity of synthetic images. It computes the quality of images using the Wasserstein-2 distance between real and synthetic images. FID uses an Inception-V3 model pre-trained on the ImageNet dataset to measure the distance [31]. FID is computed between two sets of images x and y as defined in Eq. 3.

$$FID(x, y) = ||m_1 - m_2||^2 + Tr\left(C_1 + C_2 - 2 \cdot \sqrt{C_1 \times C_2}\right) \tag{3}$$

In Eq. 3 [31], m_1 and m_2 denote the vectors containing the mean of every feature from sets of images x and y, respectively. However, *Tr* indicates a trace representing the sum of the elements from the main diagonal of a matrix. C_1 and C_2 represent covariance matrices for the feature vectors from the sets of images x and y, respectively.

In this work, 708 real and 708 synthetic images are selected to measure the FID score. A lower value of FID indicates a higher quality of synthetic images as compared to real images.

3.4 Normalization of Evaluation Metrics

The evaluation metrics MS-SSIM, CD, and FID are computed differently using perceptual features and distance-based measures. These evaluation metrics have different scales for similarity measures. The resultant values are presented in a non-uniform manner such that higher MS-SSIM scores indicate higher similarity while higher CD and FID distance scores indicate lower similarity.

Therefore, it is significant to normalize these metrics so that all these metrics evaluate the quality and diversity of synthetic images using similarity measures with a uniform scale. For this purpose, Eqs. 4, 5, and 6 are proposed.

$$Normalized\ MS{-}SSIM = \frac{(MS{-}SSIM) - min\ (MS{-}SSIM)}{max\ (MS{-}SSIM) - min\ (MS{-}SSIM)} \tag{4}$$

$$Normalized\ CD = 1\ -\ \frac{CD\ -\ min\ CD}{max\ CD - min\ CD} \tag{5}$$

$$Normalized\ FID = 1\ -\ \frac{FID\ -\ min\ FID}{max\ FID - min\ FID} \tag{6}$$

The returned values are normalized to a 0–1 range. A high similarity between two sets of images is indicated by high values of the normalized evaluation metrics.

In Eqs. 4, 5, and 6, *max* MS-SSIM, *max* CD and *max* FID indicate the highest MS-SSIM, CD, and FID values respectively between two sets of images from the dataset. Similarly, *min* MS-SSIM, *min* CD, and *min* FID indicate the lowest MS-SSIM, CD, and FID values respectively between two sets of images from the dataset.

Normalization is performed individually for each metric, each dataset (training and test), and each experiment. The normalized results obtained in different experiments or for different evaluation metrics are therefore not comparable.

3.5 Classification of PDR Images

To assess the capacity of synthetically generated PDR images by DCGAN, these images are used to augment the minority class of PDR in the imbalanced dataset of [12]. Augmentation is undertaken in order to improve the classification performance of PDR disease. To this end, a state-of-the-art multi-class classifier from [54] is reimplemented for comparing the PDR classification results. The architecture of the classifier is designed with a CNN for feature extraction and a Random Forest model for classification as depicted in Fig. 4. In [54], a single training dataset [12] is used. The CNN classifier is trained with 10-fold cross-validation using a batch size of 64 and stochastic gradient descent (SGD) optimizer with a learning rate of 0.003 as reported in [54]. In this work, a CNN is trained with 10-fold cross-validation using the same approach as in [54] for all the training dataset classes except PDR. For the PDR class, PDR images from the test dataset [12] are used for 10-fold cross-validation. This approach is used to avoid any biasing as the PDR images from the training dataset were used for training the DCGAN for generating synthetic images.

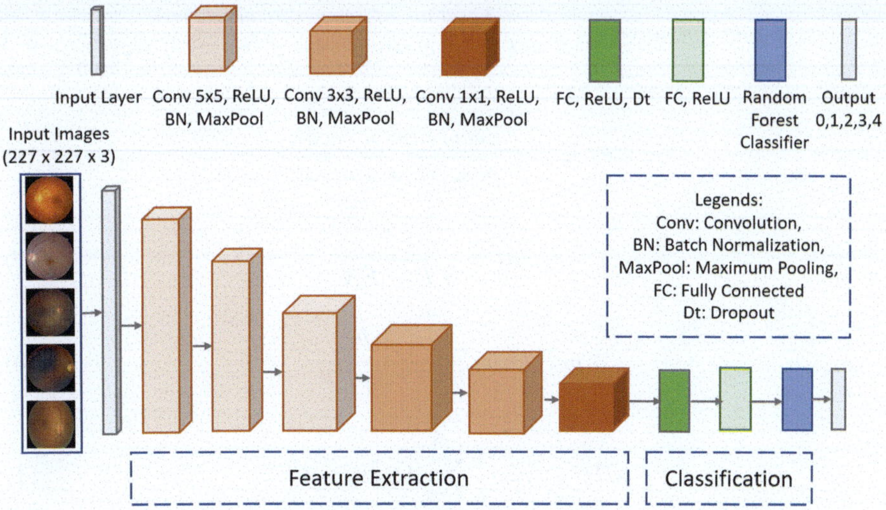

Fig. 4 Classification of PDR images using CNN model

The CNN classifier required a high computational time of approximately hundreds of hours for training the whole dataset. Therefore, CNN is trained on one batch of images from each fold only. However, an additional classifier such as EfficientNet [72] is also trained for 20 epochs using pretrained weights of the ImageNet dataset [66] on the whole dataset including all batches of images. The EfficientNet classifier required a low computational cost of 9 minutes to train all batches of images in the dataset.

In [54], the training dataset is highly imbalanced and there is no discussion of alleviating bias in the trained model. Consequently, this work uses class weights in the loss computation to address potential bias in the model. Class weights penalize the classifier for the instances that are misclassified. Class weight values are selected using a formula defined in Eq. 7 [73], corresponding to the "balanced" value of the *class_weight* parameter from the scikit-learn library [74].

Classification performance is evaluated with the F_1 score and Area Under the Curve (AUC), using the formulas denoted in Eqs. 8 and 11. F_1 score is calculated based on recall and precision. The recall of class PDR indicates the proportion of patients with PDR that were diagnosed as having PDR. The precision of class PDR indicates the proportion of patients diagnosed with PDR that have PDR. It is important that patients with PDR are diagnosed correctly, in order to get the treatment required. It is also important that patients are only diagnosed with PDR if they have the disease, in order to prevent unnecessary/incorrect treatments. AUC measures how accurately the border between the classes is identified by the classifier. The one-versus-rest (OVR) approach [75] is used for calculating AUC.

$$Class\ weight\ for\ class\ x = \frac{Total\ no.\ of\ images\ of\ all\ classes}{Total\ no.\ of\ classes \times No.\ of\ images\ of\ class\ x} \tag{7}$$

$$F_1 = 2 \times \frac{precision \times recall}{precision + recall} \tag{8}$$

$$recall = \frac{TP}{TP + FN} \tag{9}$$

$$precision = \frac{TP}{TP + FP} \tag{10}$$

$$AUC_{OVR} = \frac{1}{c}\sum_{i=0}^{c-1} AUC(C_i, C_i^C) \tag{11}$$

The F_1 score, recall and precision are calculated separately for each class. In Eqs. 9 and 10, *TP* denotes the true positives. *TP* of class x represents the number of images belonging to class x that are classified correctly. *FN* denotes the false negatives. *FN* of class x represents the number of images belonging to class x that are classified as belonging to other classes. *FP* denotes the false positives. *FP* of class x represents the number of images classified as class x, that belong to other classes.

3.6 Correlation of Quality, Diversity, and Classification Performances

The synthetically generated PDR images are used to augment the dataset for improving the classification performance of the classifier. The classification performance is higher when the training images are of high quality. Therefore, a metric is considered suitable for evaluating the quality of synthetic imagery if a high-quality score indicated by that metric correlates with a high classification performance. If the classification performance is lower with high-quality scores, then it shows that either the quality evaluation metric does not correctly assess the quality of images or the images still lack the level of quality to improve the classifier's score. Similarly, classification performance is higher when the training images are diverse. Therefore, a metric is considered suitable for evaluating the diversity of synthetic imagery if a high diversity score indicated by that metric aligns with a high classification performance. A lower classification score with highly diversified images indicates that either the evaluation metric does not correctly assess the diversity of images or the desired level of diversity is not achieved. Therefore, the quality and diversity scores are analyzed using each evaluation metric and correlated against the classification performance. The intent is to assess the metrics' suitability for evaluating the quality and diversity of synthetic imagery.

4 Results and Discussion

4.1 Critical Analysis of Quantitative Evaluation Metrics

The similarity scores between retinal fundus images with different stages of DR are derived using MS-SSIM, CD, and FID, as denoted in Table 5. FID and MS-SSIM produce the most performant similarity scores, as values between images of the same class are greater than values between images of alternate classes. However, CD does not provide a utilizable similarity score as values derived for the images of one class are more similar to the images of alternate classes.

Consequently, FID and MS-SSIM are considered suitable metrics for evaluating synthetic images, if these images are representative of the real images of the targeted class. The quantitative measures of FID and MS-SSIM enable the selection of suitable synthetic imagery for data augmentation when training a classifier.

CD is unsuitable for evaluating synthetic imagery representative of its class because it is calculated based on the angle between the extracted features. If the angle between two feature vectors is zero, they are not necessarily identical.

4.2 Evaluation of Synthetic PDR Imagery

4.2.1 Quality of Synthetic PDR Imagery

The quality of synthetic images generated is calculated via the evaluation metrics MS-SSIM, CD, and FID (see Sect. 3.3). The quality of synthetic images is evaluated using the unnormalized and normalized values of MS-SSIM, CD, and FID as depicted in Figs. 5 and 6. An improvement in quality with unnormalized metrics values is denoted as follows: higher MS-SSIM, lower CD, and lower FID when compared synthetic to real images as depicted in Fig. 5. In Fig. 5, the decrease in FID indicates that the imagery generated in the last epochs of training is of higher quality than that generated in the early epochs. MS-SSIM indicates an improvement in quality up to epoch 200 and then oscillates with inconsistent behavior. CD indicates consistent behavior in the quality of images generated throughout training.

An improvement in quality with normalized metrics values is denoted as follows: higher MS-SSIM, higher CD, and higher FID when comparing synthetic to real images as depicted in Fig. 6. In Fig. 6, normalized FID indicates an increase in the quality indicating that the last epochs of training have higher-quality images. The normalized MS-SSIM and normalized CD indicate a significant improvement in quality for the first few epochs and then oscillate inconsistently.

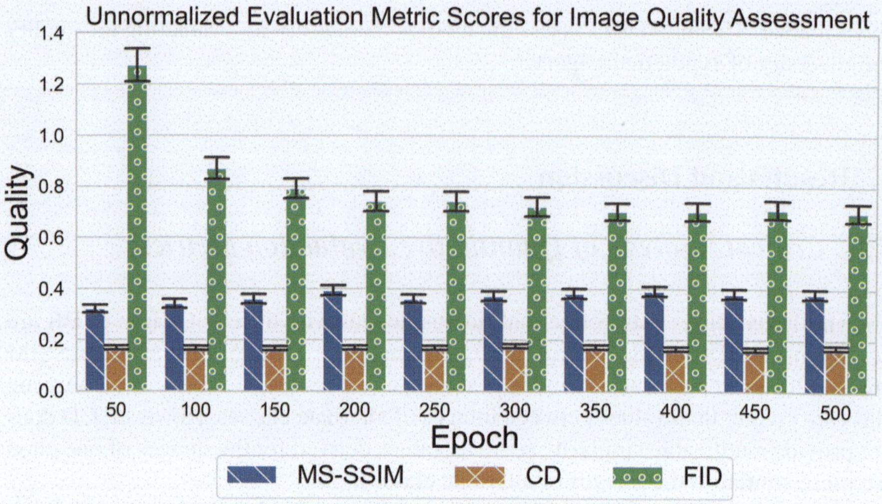

Fig. 5 Quality scores for each evaluation metric indicate the comparison of quality between synthetic and real imagery. Quality is evaluated using unnormalized scores of MS-SSIM, CD, and FID metrics

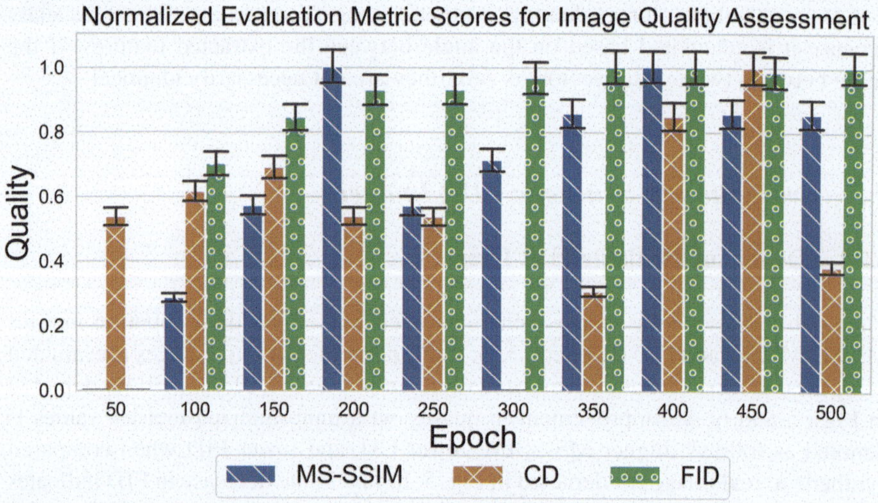

Fig. 6 Quality scores for each evaluation metric indicate the comparison of quality between synthetic and real imagery. Quality is evaluated using normalized scores of MS-SSIM, CD, and FID metrics

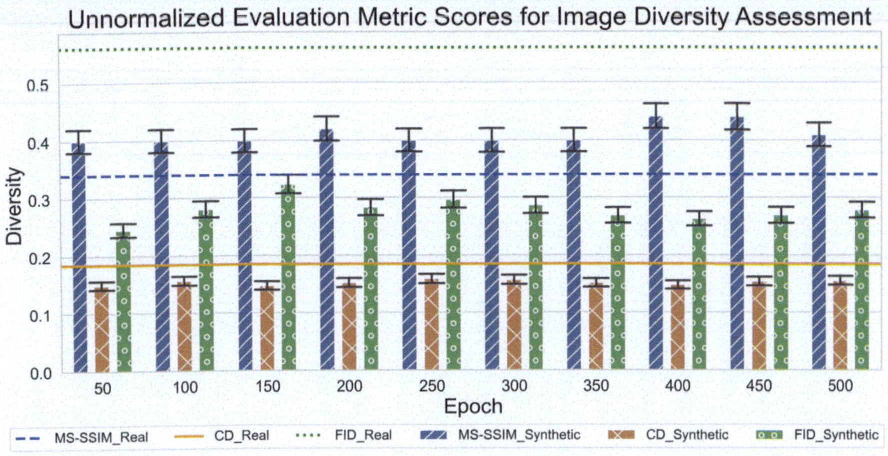

Fig. 7 Diversity scores for each evaluation metric indicate the comparison of diversity between (synthetic: synthetic) and (real: real). Diversity is evaluated using unnormalized scores of MS-SSIM, CD, and FID metrics

FID is used to evaluate the quality of synthetic images as compared to real images significantly as evidenced by FID analysis in Figs. 5 and 6. MS-SSIM and CD do not enable meaningful analysis of the quality of images as they measure the similarity and distance between image pairs respectively. Synthetic images may have different statistical properties than real images, such as different color distributions or noise characteristics, which can lead to a lower MS-SSIM score even if the synthetic images are of high quality. Similarly, CD does not consider the spatial relationships between the pixels in the image, which can be important for the overall visual quality between real and synthetic images. Therefore, MS-SSIM and CD are not suitable metrics for evaluating the quality of synthetic images.

4.2.2 Diversity of Synthetic PDR Imagery

The diversity of synthetic images generated is calculated via the evaluation metrics MS-SSIM, CD, and FID (see Sect. 3.3). The diversity of synthetic images is evaluated using the unnormalized and normalized values of MS-SSIM, CD, and FID as depicted in Figs. 7 and 8. An improvement in diversity unnormalized metrics values is denoted as follows: lower MS-SSIM, higher CD, and higher FID when comparing synthetic to real images as depicted in Fig. 7.

In Fig. 7, FID indicates a significant drop in diversity throughout the training of the DCGAN. MS-SSIM indicates relatively consistent diversity for synthetic images until epoch 350. The diversity of synthetic images starts decreasing from epoch 350 to 400 and then improving from epochs 400 and onwards. The CD indicates consistent

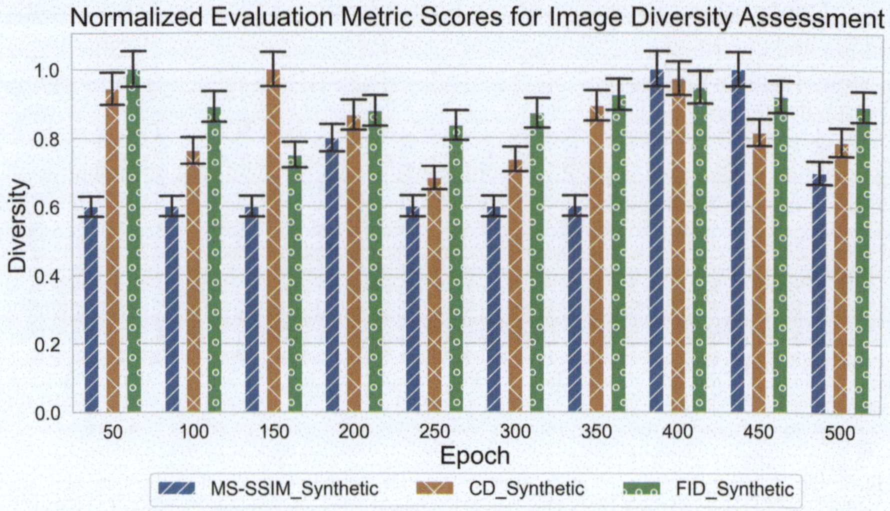

Fig. 8 Diversity scores for each evaluation metric indicate the comparison of diversity between (synthetic: synthetic) and (real: real). Real images have higher diversity (metric scores = 0). Diversity is evaluated using normalized scores of MS-SSIM, CD, and FID metrics

behavior of diversity of synthetic images compared to real images throughout the training of the DCGAN.

An improvement in diversity with normalized metric values is denoted as follows: lower MS-SSIM, lower CD, and lower FID when comparing synthetic to real images as depicted in Fig. 8. In Fig. 8, all three metrics indicate inconsistent behavior for the diversity of synthetic images as compared to real images. MS-SSIM indicates that real images are more diverse than synthetic images at various epochs because synthetic images lack the distribution of structure features as compared to real images. The CD indicates that real imagery is more diverse than most sets of synthetic imagery because the features extracted from real imagery are less dependent on each other. FID indicates that the features from the real imagery are spread over a larger area as it uses embedding layers of a pre-trained model.

MS-SSIM and CD metrics are used to evaluate the diversity of synthetic images as compared to real images. This work also depicts the significance of using these metrics to evaluate diversity, as depicted in Figs. 7 and 8. FID is unsuitable for diversity evaluation as it provides inconsistent analysis for the diversity of synthetic images that is significantly away from the MS-SSIM and CD analysis.

4.2.3 Selection of Synthetic Imagery for Augmenting Imbalanced Datasets

The DCGAN-based synthetic images are ranked based on the quality and diversity scores measured by the MS-SSIM, CD, and FID evaluation metrics as indicated in

Table 6 Selection of DCGAN-based synthetic images based on quality and diversity ranking using MS-SSIM, CD, and FID metric scores to augment the original dataset

Characteristic	Ranking metric	Epoch									
		50	100	150	200	250	300	350	400	450	500
Diversity	MS-SSIM	1	1	1	**3**	**1**	1	1	4	4	**2**
	CD	8	3	10	**6**	**1**	2	7	9	5	**4**
Quality	FID	7	6	5	**4**	**4**	3	1	1	2	**1**

Bold values indicate the top-ranked and moderate-ranked scores

Table 6. A significant variance is observed in the metric values for evaluating the quality and diversity of synthetic images. Therefore, it is important to find a suitable set of synthetic images that can be used for augmenting datasets. The ranking of synthetic images generated from each epoch enables the selection of synthetic images significantly, which helps in improving the performance of classifiers for augmented datasets. A rank of 1 indicates the most promising high-quality images while a rank of 7 indicates the lower-quality images. Similarly, a rank of 1 indicates higher diversity, while rank 10 indicates a lower diversity of synthetic images.

The synthetic images with top-ranked and moderate-ranked scores are selected to assess the quality and diversity measures. FID scores at epochs 350, 400, and 500 achieved rank 1. However, synthetic images with epoch 500 are selected because this rank is also consistent with the best ranks of MS-SSIM and CD. Similarly, MS-SSIM and CD with epoch 250 achieved rank 1 scores. Therefore, synthetic images of epoch 250 are selected. The moderate-ranked quality and diversity scores of each epoch are also analyzed to select the synthetic images. The images of epoch 200 are selected as indicated by moderate-ranked scores in Table 6.

The detailed analysis of the synthetic images' best-ranked quality and diversity scores is compared using unnormalized and normalized metric scores as indicated in Table 7. In Table 7, a higher normalized FID score of 1 for epoch 500 indicates that the synthetic images preserve the best quality compared to the real images. In contrast, the moderate scores of MS-SSIM and CD for epoch 500 do not reflect the best diversity of synthetic images as compared to real images. Similarly, higher normalized values of MS-SSIM and CD for epoch 250 indicate that the synthetic images have the best diversity while the moderate score of FID at epoch 250 indicates the poor quality of synthetic images as compared to real images.

PDR images contain several salient features such as the structure, shape, color, and size of blood vessels and lesions as depicted in Fig. 2. It is important to learn and generate these features when synthesizing PDR images using GANs. In this work, DCGAN has generated synthetic PDR images that are representative of real images. FID has evaluated the quality of synthetic images compared to real images. In Table 7, the best quality of synthetic images is achieved at epoch 500 with an unnormalized value of 0.70 and the normalized value of 1. However, the suppressed structural features of vessels in synthetic PDR images are indicative of the DCGAN's limitation to generate high-quality synthetic images as depicted in Fig. 2.

Table 7 Comparing best-ranked DCGAN-based synthetic image datasets using unnormalized and normalized metric scores for quality and diversity measures

Epoch	MS-SSIM			CD			FID			Comment
	Rank	Unnorm	Norm	Rank	Unnorm	Norm	Rank	Unnorm	Norm	
200	3	0.42	0.8	6	0.152	0.868	4	0.74	0.93	Moderate diversity, moderate quality
250	1	0.4	0.6	1	0.159	0.684	4	0.74	0.93	Higher diversity, moderate quality
500	2	0.41	0.7	4	0.155	0.789	1	0.70	1	Moderate diversity, higher quality

MS-SSIM and CD values refer to the synthetic datasets

Table 8 Assessment of synthetically generated PDR images using the classifiers' F_1 scores and AUC scores in augmenting the original imbalanced dataset

Classifier	k-fold	CW	No DR	Mild NPDR	Mod. NPDR	Severe NPDR	PDR	AUC	Tr. Tm. (Min)	No. image batches
$CNN_{Ref.}$ [54]	10-fold	N/A	0.999	0.999	1	0.974	0.981	N/A	N/A	548
$CNN_{Reimp.}$	10 fold	Yes	0.744	0.001	0.0003	0	0	0.542	60	1
$CNN_{Ep.500}$	10 fold	Yes	0.744	0	0	0	0	0.549	61	1
Effi. Net	N/A	Yes	0.690	0.156	0.338	0.290	0.395	0.760	9	1097
Effi. $Net_{Ep.200}$	N/A	Yes	0.598	0.158	0.336	0.302	0.408	0.764	9	1119
Effi. $Net_{Ep.250}$	N/A	Yes	0.643	0.159	0.318	0.281	0.403	0.760	9	1119
Effi. $Net_{Ep.500}$	N/A	Yes	0.625	0.159	0.303	0.290	0.407	0.760	9	1119

F_1 scores are recorded for all DR classes
Effi. Net: EfficientNet; CW: Class Weights; Ep: Epoch number to generate synthetic images for augmenting dataset; Mod. NPDR: moderate NPDR; Min: minutes; Ref: Reference work; Reimp: Reimplemented for this work; Tr Tm: Training Time

4.3 Assessment of Synthetic Imagery Using Classification Scores

Table 8 indicates the classification scores of the CNN and EfficientNet classifiers using F_1 score and AUC score when trained on both the original and augmented datasets. Training the CNN was computationally expensive, taking several hours to train each iteration on the whole original dataset. The AUC scores of CNN and EfficientNet for the augmented dataset are improved compared to the original dataset as indicated in Table 8. F_1 scores of the EfficientNet classifier for the PDR class are also improved with the augmented datasets compared to the original dataset. However, there is no significant difference in F_1 and AUC scores of the EfficientNet classifier for augmented datasets with synthetic PDR images of different epochs as indicated in Table 8.

5 Conclusion

This work contributes an empirical interpretation to the selection of synthetic PDR imagery for data augmentation. The contribution of this work is three-fold. First, the selection of suitable evaluation metrics for assessing the similarity and correlation of DR images, representative of their classes and alternate classes. This enabled an effective correlation analysis of PDR images compared to alternate DR images. Second, the selection of suitable evaluation metrics, indicative of their capacity to assess the quality and diversity of DCGAN-based synthetic PDR images and their correlation with classifier performance, is critically assessed. This enabled a quantitative selection of synthetic imagery and an informed augmentation strategy. Third, the selection of synthetic imagery based on the best quality and diversity scores. The efficacy of synthetic images is also evaluated by using them to augment the imbalanced dataset and improve the classification performance of classifiers.

The results demonstrate that MS-SSIM and FID are better at assessing if synthetic imagery belongs to the correct class. The quality of synthetic images is assessed by the FID scores, while diversity is assessed by the MS-SSIM and CD scores. The results indicate the efficacy of synthetic images to augment the imbalanced dataset and improve the F_1 score for the PDR class and the AUC score of the EfficientNet classifier.

This work concludes that evaluation metrics such as MS-SSIM, CD, and FID have a significant impact on assessing the quality and diversity of synthetic images in the biomedical imagery domain. It is important to analyze the impact of different image resolutions, more training epochs, and the lower and upper bound of these metric values for synthetic biomedical imagery, which will be explored as part of future work.

References

1. Cavan, D., Makaroff, L., da Rocha Fernandes, J., Sylvanowicz, M., Ackland, P., Conlon, J., Chaney, D., Malhi, A., Barratt, J.: The diabetic retinopathy barometer study: global perspectives on access to and experiences of diabetic retinopathy screening and treatment. Diabetes Res. and Clin. Pract. **129**, 16–24 (2017). https://doi.org/10.1016/j.diabres.2017.03.023, https://www.sciencedirect.com/science/article/pii/S0168822717304370
2. Wilkinson, C.P., Ferris III, F.L., Klein, R.E., Lee, P.P., Agardh, C.D., Davis, M., Dills, D., Kampik, A., Pararajasegaram, R., Verdaguer, J.T., et al.: Proposed international clinical diabetic retinopathy and diabetic macular edema disease severity scales. Ophthalmology **110**(9), 1677–1682 (2003). https://doi.org/10.1016/S0161-6420(03)00475-5, https://www.sciencedirect.com/science/article/pii/S016164200300475
3. Arora, M., Pandey, M.: Deep neural network for diabetic retinopathy detection. In: 2019 Int. Conf. Mach. Learn., Big Data, Cloud and Parallel Comput. (COMITCon). pp. 189–193. https://doi.org/10.1109/COMITCon.2019.8862217
4. Ghosh, R., Ghosh, K., Maitra, S.: Automatic detection and classification of diabetic retinopathy stages using CNN. In: 2017 4th Int. Conf. Signal Process. and Integr. Netw. (SPIN). pp. 550–554. https://doi.org/10.1109/SPIN.2017.8050011

5. Ni, J., Chen, Q., Liu, C., Wang, H., Cao, Y., Liu, B.: An effective CNN approach for diabetic retinopathy stage classification with dual inputs and selective data sampling. In: 2019 18th IEEE Int. Conf. Mach. Learn. And Appl. (ICMLA). pp. 1578–1584. https://doi.org/10.1109/ICMLA.2019.00260
6. Ali, H., Shah, Z., et al.: Combating covid-19 using generative adversarial networks and artificial intelligence for medical images: Scoping review. JMIR Medical Informatics **10**(6), e37365 (2022)
7. Chen, Y., Yang, X.H., Wei, Z., Heidari, A.A., Zheng, N., Li, Z., Chen, H., Hu, H., Zhou, Q., Guan, Q.: Generative adversarial networks in medical image augmentation: a review. Computers in Biology and Medicine p. 105382 (2022)
8. Saad, M.M., Rehmani, M.H., O'Reilly, R.: Addressing the intra-class mode collapse problem using adaptive input image normalization in GAN-based X-ray images. In: 2022 44th Annual International Conference of the IEEE Engineering in Medicine & Biology Society (EMBC). pp. 2049–2052. IEEE (2022)
9. Rahman, M.M., Davis, D.N.: Addressing the class imbalance problem in medical datasets. Int. J. of Mach. Learn. and Comput. **3**(2), 224–228 (2013)
10. Shorten, C., Khoshgoftaar, T.M.: A survey on image data augmentation for deep learning. Journal of big data **6**(1), 1–48 (2019)
11. Saini, M., Susan, S.: Deep transfer with minority data augmentation for imbalanced breast cancer dataset. Applied Soft Computing **97**, 106759 (2020)
12. Cuadros, J., Bresnick, G.: Eyepacs: an adaptable telemedicine system for diabetic retinopathy screening. J. of Diabetes Sci. and Technol. **3**(3), 509–516 (2009). https://doi.org/10.1177/193229680900300315
13. APTOS 2019 blindness detection | Kaggle, kaggle.com. Available: https://www.kaggle.com/c/aptos2019-blindness-detection (accessed Mar. 03, 2022)
14. Zhou, Y., Wang, B., Huang, L., Cui, S., Shao, L.: A benchmark for studying diabetic retinopathy: Segmentation, grading, and transferability. IEEE Transactions on Medical Imaging **40**(3), 818–828 (2021). https://doi.org/10.1109/TMI.2020.3037771
15. Decencière, E., Zhang, X., Cazuguel, G., Lay, B., Cochener, B., Trone, C., Gain, P., Ordonez, R., Massin, P., Erginay, A., et al.: Feedback on a publicly distributed image database: the Messidor database. Image Anal. & Stereology **33**(3), 231–234 (2014). https://doi.org/10.5566/ias.1155, https://www.ias-iss.org/ojs/IAS/article/view/1155
16. Abràmoff, M.D., Folk, J.C., Han, D.P., Walker, J.D., Williams, D.F., Russell, S.R., Massin, P., Cochener, B., Gain, P., Tang, L., et al.: Automated analysis of retinal images for detection of referable diabetic retinopathy. JAMA Ophthalmology **131**(3), 351–357 (2013). https://doi.org/10.1001/jamaophthalmol.2013.1743
17. Porwal, P., Pachade, S., Kamble, R., Kokare, M., Deshmukh, G., Sahasrabuddhe, V., Meriaudeau, F.: Indian diabetic retinopathy image dataset (idrid) (2018). https://doi.org/10.21227/H25W98, distributed by IEEE Dataport
18. Pires, R., Jelinek, H.F., Wainer, J., Valle, E., Rocha, A.: Advancing bag-of-visual-words representations for lesion classification in retinal images. PloS one **9**(6) (2014)
19. Cen, L.P., Ji, J., Lin, J.W., Ju, S.T., Lin, H.J., Li, T.P., Wang, Y., Yang, J.F., Liu, Y.F., Tan, S., et al.: Automatic detection of 39 fundus diseases and conditions in retinal photographs using deep neural networks. Nature communications **12**(1), 1–13 (2021)
20. Hoover, A., Kouznetsova, V., Goldbaum, M.: Locating blood vessels in retinal images by piecewise threshold probing of a matched filter response. IEEE Trans. on Med. Imag. **19**(3), 203–210 (2000). https://doi.org/10.1109/42.845178
21. Odstrcilik, J., Kolar, R., Budai, A., Hornegger, J., Jan, J., Gazarek, J., Kubena, T., Cernosek, P., Svoboda, O., Angelopoulou, E.: Retinal vessel segmentation by improved matched filtering: evaluation on a new high-resolution fundus image database. IET Image Process. **7**(4), 373–383 (Jun 2013), https://digital-library.theiet.org/content/journals/10.1049/iet-ipr.2012.0455
22. Oza, P., Sharma, P., Patel, S., Adedoyin, F., Bruno, A.: Image augmentation techniques for mammogram analysis. Journal of Imaging **8**(5), 141 (2022)

23. Sengupta, S., Athwale, A., Gulati, T., Zelek, J., Lakshminarayanan, V.: FunSyn-Net: enhanced residual variational auto-encoder and image-to-image translation network for fundus image synthesis. In: Medical Imaging 2020: Image Processing. vol. 11313, pp. 665–671. SPIE (2020)
24. Shi, J., Zhang, P., Zhang, N., Ghazzai, H., Massoud, Y.: Dissolving is amplifying: Towards fine-grained anomaly detection. arXiv preprint arXiv:2302.14696 (2023)
25. Zhou, Y., Wang, B., He, X., Cui, S., Shao, L.: DR-GAN: conditional generative adversarial network for fine-grained lesion synthesis on diabetic retinopathy images. IEEE J. of Biomed. and Health Inform. **26**(1), 56–66 (2022). https://doi.org/10.1109/JBHI.2020.3045475
26. Kebaili, A., Lapuyade-Lahorgue, J., Ruan, S.: Deep learning approaches for data augmentation in medical imaging: A review. Journal of Imaging **9**(4), 81 (2023)
27. Costa, P., Galdran, A., Meyer, M.I., Niemeijer, M., Abràmoff, M., Mendonça, A.M., Campilho, A.: End-to-end adversarial retinal image synthesis. IEEE Trans. on Med. Imag. **37**(3), 781–791 (2018). https://doi.org/10.1109/TMI.2017.2759102
28. Yu, Z., Xiang, Q., Meng, J., Kou, C., Ren, Q., Lu, Y.: Retinal image synthesis from multiple-landmarks input with generative adversarial networks. BioMed. Eng. OnLine **18** (May 2019)
29. Thung, K.H., Raveendran, P.: A survey of image quality measures. In: 2009 Int. Conf. for Knowl. Tech. Postgraduates (TECHPOS). pp. 1–4. https://doi.org/10.1109/TECHPOS.2009.5412098
30. Shmelkov, K., Schmid, C., Alahari, K.: How good is my GAN? In: Proc. of the Eur. Conf. Comput. Vision (ECCV) (Sep 2018)
31. Borji, A.: Pros and cons of GAN evaluation measures. Comput. Vision and Image Understanding **179**, 41–65 (2019). https://doi.org/10.1016/j.cviu.2018.10.009, https://www.sciencedirect.com/science/article/pii/S1077314218304272
32. Wang, Z., Simoncelli, E.P., Bovik, A.C.: Multiscale structural similarity for image quality assessment. In: The Thirty-Seventh Asilomar Conference on Signals, Systems & Computers, 2003. vol. 2, pp. 1398–1402. IEEE (2003)
33. Odena, A., Olah, C., Shlens, J.: Conditional Image Synthesis with Auxiliary Classifier GANs. In: International conference on machine learning. pp. 2642–2651. PMLR (2017)
34. Salimans, T., Zhang, H., Radford, A., Metaxas, D.: Improving GANs using optimal transport. In: International Conference on Learning Representations (2018), https://openreview.net/forum?id=rkQkBnJAb
35. Heusel, M., Ramsauer, H., Unterthiner, T., Nessler, B., Hochreiter, S.: GANs trained by a two time-scale update rule converge to a local Nash equilibrium. Advances in neural information processing systems **30** (2017)
36. Goodfellow, I., Pouget-Abadie, J., Mirza, M., Xu, B., Warde-Farley, D., Ozair, S., Courville, A., Bengio, Y.: Generative adversarial nets advances in neural information processing systems. arXiv preprint arXiv:1406.2661 (2014)
37. Denton, E.L., Chintala, S., Fergus, R., et al.: Deep generative image models using a Laplacian pyramid of adversarial networks. Advances in neural information processing systems **28** (2015)
38. Snell, J., Ridgeway, K., Liao, R., Roads, B.D., Mozer, M.C., Zemel, R.S.: Learning to generate images with perceptual similarity metrics. In: 2017 IEEE International Conference on Image Processing (ICIP). pp. 4277–4281. IEEE (2017)
39. Balasubramanian, R., Sowmya, V., Gopalakrishnan, E.A., Menon, V.K., Sajith Variyar, V.V., Soman, K.P.: Analysis of adversarial based augmentation for diabetic retinopathy disease grading. In: 2020 11th Int. Conf. Comput., Commun. and Netw. Technol. (ICCCNT). pp. 1–5. https://doi.org/10.1109/ICCCNT49239.2020.9225684
40. Lim, G., Thombre, P., Lee, M.L., Hsu, W.: Generative data augmentation for diabetic retinopathy classification. In: 2020 IEEE 32nd Int. Conf. Tools with Artif. Intell. (ICTAI). pp. 1096–1103. https://doi.org/10.1109/ICTAI50040.2020.00167
41. Burlina, P.M., Joshi, N., Pacheco, K.D., Liu, T.A., Bressler, N.M.: Assessment of deep generative models for high-resolution synthetic retinal image generation of age-related macular degeneration. JAMA Ophthalmology **137**(3), 258–264 (2019). https://doi.org/10.1001/jamaophthalmol.2018.6156

42. HaoQi, G., Ogawara, K.: CGAN-based synthetic medical image augmentation between retinal fundus images and vessel segmented images. In: 2020 5th Int. Conf. Control and Robot. Eng. (ICCRE). pp. 218–223. https://doi.org/10.1109/ICCRE49379.2020.9096438
43. Staal, J., Abràmoff, M.D., Niemeijer, M., Viergever, M.A., Van Ginneken, B.: Ridge-based vessel segmentation in color images of the retina. IEEE transactions on medical imaging **23**(4), 501–509 (2004)
44. Sivaswamy, J., Krishnadas, S., Chakravarty, A., Joshi, G., Tabish, A.S., et al.: A comprehensive retinal image dataset for the assessment of glaucoma from the optic nerve head analysis. JSM Biomedical Imaging Data Papers **2**(1), 1004 (2015)
45. Diaz-Pinto, A., Colomer, A., Naranjo, V., Morales, S., Xu, Y., Frangi, A.F.: Retinal image synthesis and semi-supervised learning for glaucoma assessment. IEEE Trans. on Med. Imag. **38**(9), 2211–2218 (2019). https://doi.org/10.1109/TMI.2019.2903434
46. Chen, H., Cao, P.: Deep learning based data augmentation and classification for limited medical data learning. In: 2019 IEEE Int. Conf. Power, Intell. Comput. and Syst. (ICPICS). pp. 300–303. https://doi.org/10.1109/ICPICS47731.2019.8942411
47. Islam, J., Zhang, Y.: GAN-based synthetic brain PET image generation. Brain informatics **7**, 1–12 (2020)
48. Frid-Adar, M., Klang, E., Amitai, M., Goldberger, J., Greenspan, H.: Synthetic data augmentation using GAN for improved liver lesion classification. In: 2018 IEEE 15th Int. Symp. Biomed. Imag. (ISBI). pp. 289–293. https://doi.org/10.1109/ISBI.2018.8363576
49. Han, C., Murao, K., Noguchi, T., Kawata, Y., Uchiyama, F., Rundo, L., Nakayama, H., Satoh, S.: Learning more with less: conditional pggan-based data augmentation for brain metastases detection using highly-rough annotation on mr images. In: Proc. of the 28th ACM Int. Conf. Inf. and Knowl. Manage. p. 119-127. CIKM '19 (Nov.). https://doi.org/10.1145/3357384.3357890
50. Redmon, J., Farhadi, A.: YoloV3: an incremental improvement. arXiv:1804.02767 (2018)
51. Han, C., Rundo, L., Araki, R., Nagano, Y., Furukawa, Y., Mauri, G., Nakayama, H., Hayashi, H.: Combining noise-to-image and image-to-image GANs: brain MR image augmentation for tumor detection. IEEE Access **7**, 156966–156977 (2019). https://doi.org/10.1109/ACCESS.2019.2947606
52. Pei, W., Xue, B., Shang, L., Zhang, M.: A threshold-free classification mechanism in genetic programming for high-dimensional unbalanced classification. In: 2020 IEEE Congr. Evol. Comput. (CEC). pp. 1–8. https://doi.org/10.1109/CEC48606.2020.9185503
53. Kotsiantis, S., Kanellopoulos, D., Pintelas, P.: Handling imbalanced datasets: a review. GESTS Int. Trans. on Comput. Sci. and Eng. **30** (2006)
54. Gayathri, S., Gopi, V.P., Palanisamy, P.: A lightweight CNN for diabetic retinopathy classification from fundus images. Biomed. Signal Process. and Control **62** (2020). https://doi.org/10.1016/j.bspc.2020.102115, https://www.sciencedirect.com/science/article/pii/S1746809420302676
55. Sayres, R., Taly, A., Rahimy, E., Blumer, K., Coz, D., Hammel, N., Krause, J., Narayanaswamy, A., Rastegar, Z., Wu, D., et al.: Using a deep learning algorithm and integrated gradients explanation to assist grading for diabetic retinopathy. Ophthalmology **126**(4), 552–564 (2019). https://doi.org/10.1016/j.ophtha.2018.11.016, https://www.sciencedirect.com/science/article/pii/S0161642018315756
56. Zeng, X., Chen, H., Luo, Y., Ye, W.: Automated diabetic retinopathy detection based on binocular Siamese-like convolutional neural network. IEEE Access **7**, 30744–30753 (2019). https://doi.org/10.1109/ACCESS.2019.2903171
57. Qummar, S., Khan, F.G., Shah, S., Khan, A., Shamshirband, S., Rehman, Z.U., Khan, I.A., Jadoon, W.: A deep learning ensemble approach for diabetic retinopathy detection. IEEE Access **7**, 150530–150539 (2019). https://doi.org/10.1109/ACCESS.2019.2947484
58. Kwasigroch, A., Jarzembinski, B., Grochowski, M.: Deep CNN based decision support system for detection and assessing the stage of diabetic retinopathy. In: 2018 Int. Interdisciplinary PhD Workshop (IIPhDW). pp. 111–116. https://doi.org/10.1109/IIPHDW.2018.8388337
59. Pratt, H., Coenen, F., Broadbent, D.M., Harding, S.P., Zheng, Y.: Convolutional neural networks for diabetic retinopathy. Procedia Comput. Sci. **90**, 200–205 (2016). https://doi.org/10.1016/j.procs.2016.07.014, https://www.sciencedirect.com/science/article/pii/S1877050916311929

60. Sokolova, M., Lapalme, G.: A systematic analysis of performance measures for classification tasks. Inf. Process. & Manage. **45**(4), 427–437 (2009)
61. Zhang, Z., Xue, J., Zhang, J., Yang, M., Meng, B., Tan, Y., Ren, S.: A deep learning automatic classification method for clogging pervious pavement. Construction and Building Mater. **309** (2021). https://doi.org/10.1016/j.conbuildmat.2021.125195, https://www.sciencedirect.com/science/article/pii/S0950061821029391
62. Xu, K., Feng, D., Mi, H.: Deep convolutional neural network-based early automated detection of diabetic retinopathy using fundus image. Molecules **22**(12) (2017). https://doi.org/10.3390/molecules22122054, https://www.mdpi.com/1420-3049/22/12/2054
63. Li, X., Pang, T., Xiong, B., Liu, W., Liang, P., Wang, T.: Convolutional neural networks based transfer learning for diabetic retinopathy fundus image classification. In: 2017 10th Int. Congr. Image and Signal Process., BioMed. Eng. and Inform. (CISP-BMEI). pp. 1–11. https://doi.org/10.1109/CISP-BMEI.2017.8301998
64. Li, D.C., Liu, C.W., Hu, S.C.: A learning method for the class imbalance problem with medical data sets. Comput. in Biol. and Medicine **40**(5), 509–518 (2010). https://doi.org/10.1016/j.compbiomed.2010.03.005, https://www.sciencedirect.com/science/article/pii/S0010482510000405
65. Szegedy, C., Vanhoucke, V., Ioffe, S., Shlens, J., Wojna, Z.: Rethinking the inception architecture for computer vision. In: Proceedings of the IEEE conference on computer vision and pattern recognition. pp. 2818–2826 (2016)
66. Deng, J., Dong, W., Socher, R., Li, L.J., Li, K., Fei-Fei, L.: ImageNet: A large-scale hierarchical image database. In: 2009 IEEE Conference on Computer Vision and Pattern Recognition. pp. 248–255 (2009). https://doi.org/10.1109/CVPR.2009.5206848
67. Wang, Z., She, Q., Ward, T.E.: Generative adversarial networks in computer vision: A survey and taxonomy. ACM Computing Surveys (CSUR) **54**(2), 1–38 (2021)
68. Radford, A., Metz, L., Chintala, S.: Unsupervised representation learning with deep convolutional generative adversarial networks. arXiv:1511.06434v2 (2016)
69. Huang, G., Jafari, A.H.: Enhanced balancing GAN: Minority-class image generation. Neural Computing and Applications. pp. 1–10 (2021)
70. Kurach, K., Lučić, M., Zhai, X., Michalski, M., Gelly, S.: A large-scale study on regularization and normalization in GANs. In: International conference on machine learning. pp. 3581–3590. PMLR (2019)
71. Cristianini, N., Shawe-Taylor, J., et al.: An introduction to support vector machines and other kernel-based learning methods. Cambridge University Press (2000)
72. Tan, M., Le, Q.: EfficientNet: Rethinking model scaling for convolutional neural networks. In: International conference on machine learning. pp. 6105–6114. PMLR (2019)
73. Classification on imbalanced data | TensorFlow Core, tensorflow.org. Available: https://www.tensorflow.org/tutorials/structured_data/imbalanced_data#calculate_class_weights (accessed Feb. 1, 2022)
74. sklearn.ensemble.RandomForestClassifier scikit-learn 1.0.2 documentation, scikit-learn.org. Available: https://scikit-learn.org/stable/modules/generated/sklearn.ensemble.RandomForestClassifier.html (accessed Feb. 1, 2022)
75. Provost, F., Domingos, P.: Well-trained pets: improving probability estimation trees. CeDER Working Paper IS-00-04, Stern School of Business, New York University, New York, NY, USA (2000)

Deep Learning Approaches for End-to-End Modeling of Medical Spatiotemporal Data

Jacqueline K. Harris and Russell Greiner

Abstract For many medical applications, a single, stationary image may not be sufficient for detecting subtle pathology. Advancements in fields such as computer vision have produced robust deep learning (DL) techniques able to effectively learn complex interactions between space and time for prediction. This chapter presents an overview of different medical applications of spatiotemporal DL for prognostic and diagnostic predictive tasks, and how they built on important advancements in DL from other domains. Although many of the current approaches draw heavily from previous works in other fields, adaptation to the medical domain brings unique challenges, which will be discussed, along with techniques being used to address them. Although the use of spatiotemporal DL in medical applications is still relatively new, and lags behind the progress seen from still images, it provides unique opportunities to incorporate information about functional dynamics into prediction, which could be vital in many medical applications. Current medical applications of spatiotemporal DL have demonstrated the potential of these models, and recent advancements make this space poised to produce state-of-the-art models for many medical applications.

Keywords fMRI · Echocardiogram · ECG · EEG · CT Perfusion · Angiography

1 Introduction

Imaging is an important tool for clinicians in diagnosis and prognosis. Various medical imaging modalities enable a view of anatomy not visible to the naked eye and provide information relevant for diagnosis and/or prognosis. Early utilization of medical images for machine learning (ML) largely relied on extracting hand-crafted

J. K. Harris (✉) · R. Greiner
Department of Computing Science, Alberta Machine Intelligence Institute, University of Alberta, Edmonton, AB, Canada
e-mail: jkh@ualberta.ca

R. Greiner
e-mail: rgreiner@ualberta.ca

H. Ali et al. (eds.), *Advances in Deep Generative Models for Medical Artificial Intelligence*, Studies in Computational Intelligence 1124,
https://doi.org/10.1007/978-3-031-46341-9_5

features from the images of an individual that were subsequently fed into a MLed model, which predicted a diagnostic or prognostic value for that individual. These approaches, however, restrict predictive models to information retained in the engineered features, which may not be optimal.

Deep learning (DL) models have demonstrated considerable improvements in performance for many predictive tasks by learning how to transform inputs for prediction. Convolutional neural networks (CNNs), for example, have been widely adopted in computer vision tasks, and have removed the need to first extract human-engineered (but perhaps not useful) features from images before learning a model. In general, utilizing the original image data in a single end-to-end predictive model has been shown to substantially improve performance in many diverse applications and data types [1]. Since medical images share the same structure as any other image data, models developed for computer vision can be (and have been) used in medical applications with little to no modification and achieve similarly impressive results.

In many cases, however, a single, stationary image does not capture all information necessary for accurate prediction. By providing a sequence of still, spatial images, over time (resulting in a temporal dimension), *spatiotemporal data* is able to capture how spatial structures change and evolve. Early development of DL architectures to model spatiotemporal data, or spatiotemporal architectures, centered around tasks such as recognizing actions, which are better captured over a period of time. Similarly, a number of clinical applications also benefit from considering temporal information that can be used to assess functionality. This has long been recognized in fields such as cardiology, where considerable efforts have been made to characterize the dynamics of the heart's motion. Spatiotemporal imaging may also play an important role in early detection of many conditions where any structural indications that would be detectable in still images, if present at all, may only be detectable after prolonged abnormal functioning.

In this chapter, we will provide an overview of clinical applications of spatiotemporal imaging and DL approaches that have been used. Following the trend already observed in more generic imaging tasks, we anticipate that DL models utilizing spatiotemporal data will be able to surpass the performance of models based on still images in many clinical applications. To date, however, clinical utilization of spatiotemporal imaging has been somewhat limited due to the increased resources required for acquisition, and more challenging interpretation. That being said, with advancements in imaging technology, data storage, and computing, these data types will likely become more accessible in the future and drive state-of-the-art model development in various applications.

The scope of this article will be limited to discussing models making a single, or small number of predictions, based on an entire spatiotemporal instance. This means it will *not* cover tasks involving voxel level predictions such as segmentation, or predictions made on each individual frame, such as object tracking. Segmentation, for example, has been a very successful application of DL, largely owing to the fact that each pixel in the training set is given the "true" label, meaning each training image corresponds to many (often tens-of-thousands of) labeled instances - which means fewer training images are needed. This means these tasks have different modeling considerations, and so different approaches may be more appropriate here.

Furthermore, clinical applications of pixel-, or frame-level predictions are often the basis of intermediate measures, such as volume, that are subsequently used to guide downstream clinical decision making such as diagnosis or treatment selection. As discussed in the context of engineered features, producing these intermediate measures disconnects the ultimate predictive label from the raw data, preventing the model from learning what information is of relevance. This is why we suggest many medical applications would be better served by focusing on more direct, actionable labels that are directly predicted from the raw imaging data, leading us to focus on these more end-to-end models in this chapter.

For simplicity, we also limit the scope of this paper to discussion of single session spatiotemporal data; that is, spatiotemporal data that is collected at a single imaging session, rather than a temporal sequence of images collected over many different sessions, usually on different days. In doing this, we can assume that data is collected in a more controlled manner, with a single and consistent imaging device, in the same environment, and with consistent temporal spacing. Further, we will cover only applications using a stationary imaging device, precluding discussion of topics such as endoscopic imaging. We will also limit discussion to modeling data from a single modality, and exclude optical imaging data that is often not considered a medical imaging modality, although it may have clinical applications. Most applications outside of this scope can be modeled using similar methods to those presented in this work, however, they may require adjustments to accommodate additional complexities.

This chapter is organized into three main sections. Section 2 focuses on the background of spatiotemporal DL in a context more general than *medical* imaging, providing a more foundational understanding of the approaches that have since been applied to the clinical domain. Section 3 will provide an overview of selected clinical applications of spatiotemporal DL; N.B., we will not be able to provide a comprehensive review of all works in this area given the broad scope and the growing popularity of DL. Finally, before concluding, Sect. 4 will discuss the challenge of small sample sizes in clinical applications of spatiotemporal DL, and techniques that have been employed to mitigate this problem.

2 Spatial Temporal Deep Learning Background

While this chapter aims to provide an overview of spatiotemporal DL models used in *medical imaging*, it is important to acknowledge that many of the approaches that have been used stem from advancements in fields such as computer vision, and even natural language processing (NLP). Unlike medical data, text and natural image data is much easier to compile since it is freely shared and easily acquired, enabling multiple large scale benchmark datasets to be created for tasks in these spaces. The release of ImageNet [2], for example, fuelled the development of DL architectures for image data capable of surpassing human performance. Recognizing that innovation in DL often requires large, curated datasets, a number of datasets were developed for prediction tasks based on video data, such as action recognition, that propelled the creation of many successful spatiotemporal architectures [3–5].

Working from the success of CNNs for image data, most spatiotemporal modeling approaches focused on how to adjust these spatial models to incorporate temporal information. Since video data is fundamentally a set of still images, naive approaches make a prediction based on each individual frame, and average the predictions over all frames to generate the final prediction for the video. This approach, and others like it, that make predictions based on individual frames, make the assumption that all frames are independent of each other, and ignore important dynamic information encoded in the sequence.

Similar to early approaches modeling imaging data before the development of CNNs, a number of engineered features were developed for spatiotemporal data that attempted to capture information relevant to the predictive task. Many built upon the bag of visual words (BoVW; also referred to as a "bag of features" [6]) representations of images, where images were reduced to a set of visual features that were clustered together and used to form a histogram summarizing the image contents. By tracking the motion of these features through the sequence of images, often using optical flow (OF), a set of spatiotemporal features could be generated [7]. Later approaches improved on BoVW features by densely sampling points [8, 9], rather than using sparse feature interest points over each frame. Generating these engineered features, however, requires substantial computational resources, which becomes prohibitive for larger datasets; and, as we have already mentioned, today's end-to-end models using the raw data now consistently outperform systems based on hand-engineered features.

This section will introduce the DL techniques and models that current medical applications draw from, or directly utilize; these encompass a broad range of work related to spatial and sequence modeling from a number of different fields. While this summary does not intend to present a comprehensive summary of all relevant works, it should, however, provide the context for understanding the use of these models, and similar architectures, in medical applications.

2.1 Convolutional Neural Networks

CNNs have become the default modeling approach for image data. Traditional feed-forward neural networks require the pixel data to be vectorized and treat each pixel as an individual feature. CNNs, however, are able to use the original image structure, can identify and exploit spatial dependencies between pixels, and are able to easily identify objects that are at arbitrary locations within the image [10, 11]. Networks such as AlexNet [12] achieved unprecedented levels of performance in image classification and localization challenges and have since been heavily used for medical image processing for a variety of tasks.

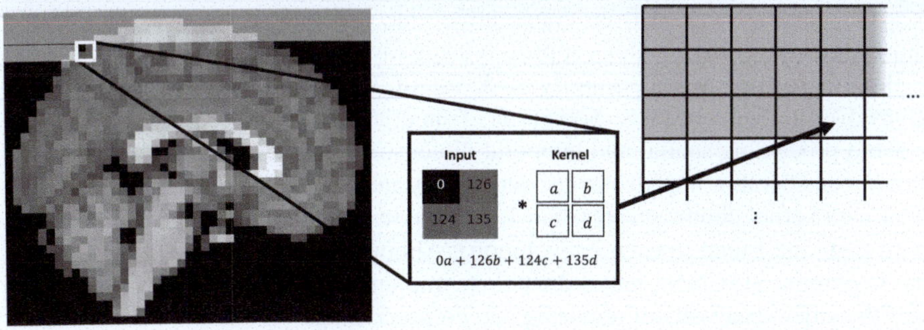

Fig. 1 Diagram demonstrating the use of a convolutional kernel on a 2D image. As the kernel slides over the image, the output of each convolution operation populates the output activation map, which therefore also has a grid structure. Here, the kernel has both a length and width of size 2. Also, the place-holder parameters a, b, c, and d would be numerical values, that are learned through the training process

In general, CNNs are neural networks with at least one convolutional layer, which are designed to work with data in a grid-like structure. Here, the system learns a *convolutional kernel*, which is used rather than the standard matrix multiplication operation performed in vanilla neural networks. Figure 1 shows such a kernel sliding over the input grid, to generate another data grid, often called an activation (or feature) map. Since the dimensionality of the kernel is much smaller than that of the input, convolutional layers are more efficient and require substantially fewer parameters to be learned than a feed forward neural network; this can be an important feature for large, or high resolution images with many pixels. In addition, since the parameters for a given kernel are shared for all locations in the image, the result is location-invariant—i.e., the network can detect objects or spatial features regardless of their relative location in the data grid.

It is natural to progress from still images to videos, as they are simply a sequence of still images; this, however, requires devising a way to incorporate temporal information into these already successful models. Karpathy et al. [4] were one of the first to attempt to both model video data using CNNs in an end-to-end approach, and at the same time compile a benchmark dataset for classifying video content. This team tested different approaches to fusing spatial information over the temporal domain and proposed a multiresolution approach to analyzing images to reduce computational demands. Comparing these spatiotemporal models to a neural network trained with engineered features, they saw a substantial increase in performance. However, the improvement compared to predictions from a CNN using a single frame of the video (or still image) was very modest; bringing into question the value of spatiotemporal models given the added complexity and increase in computational demands.

Soon after, Simonyan and Zisserman [13] proposed a two-stream model for video data, where spatial and temporal information are processed in two separate streams that are fused near the end of the architecture. In this implementation, both streams were implemented using almost identical CNNs architectures, however, the spatial stream accepts individual frames of the video as input, and the temporal stream uses OF fields generated from consecutive video frames. This approach showed improvement over the previous approach using raw stacked frames [4].

Both these approaches primarily made use of 2D convolution and pooling operations over the video frames. Soon after, Tran et al. [14] proposed using 3D CNNs to avoid processing spatial and temporal dimensions independently, which demonstrated considerable improvement over other state-of-the-art models and improvement with kernel depths greater than 1 over the temporal dimension (i.e., including more than one frame in each convolution). Although Tran et al. [14] were not the first to propose 3D CNNs, they were able to implement an approach to work directly with the video data without requiring any preprocessing.

During this time, there were also improvements to CNN architectures for still images. While it was recognized that deeper networks tended to result in better performance, training these networks presented non-trivial challenges. To address these challenges, He et al. [15] introduced a deep residual learning framework (ResNet) that incorporated skip connections between non-adjacent layers in the network that enabled them to train one of the deepest networks at the time, with 152 layers, and set accuracy records on a number of benchmark datasets.

Subsequently, Qui et al. [16] revisited 3D CNNs, questioning if trained 2D CNN architectures for still image tasks could be repurposed for video data, avoiding the need to train 3D CNNs from scratch (which can be very computationally demanding). They proposed a Pseudo-3D ResNet (P3D ResNet) architecture, where the convolutional blocks of the 3D CNN would be replaced by a combination of 2D spatial, and 1D temporal convolutional filters, with the spatial filters initialized from pre-learnt 2D CNNs. This proposed P3D ResNet showed substantial improvement over C3D, the 3D CNN previously proposed by Tran et al. [14]. Notably, Qui et al. [16] also showed that the ResNet-152 architecture [15], using only single frames, also outperformed C3D in many tasks, highlighting the power of deeper architectures.

Later, Tran et al. [17] also revisited their 3D CNN architecture, similarly choosing a ResNet framework with spatial and temporally decomposed 3D convolutional filters, which they named R(2 + 1)D. Using the proposed architecture, Tran et al. [17] demonstrated further improvements in performance on a number of action recognition benchmarks. The R(2 + 1)D model proposed by Tran et al. [17] makes slight, but impactful, modifications to P3D [16], using a single type of spatiotemporal residual block through the depth of the network, and not including bottlenecks.

2.1.1 Learning Long-Range Dependencies

A major drawback of approaches using CNN architectures for spatiotemporal data is that they require temporal sequences to have a fixed length; meaning imaging data of different lengths needs to be preprocessed to a set length, or smaller sequences within the full video can be used separately to generate predictions that are averaged together to generate a video-level prediction. Of course, this might not be problematic in many medical applications, where imaging protocols are often tightly controlled.

More problematically, however, most architectures proposed support only *short* video sequences (aka clips), typically only a few frames long, due to the added computational complexity of 3D architectures. In the context of action recognition, many hypothesized these short clips were not long enough to adequately capture human motion and contributed to the generally underwhelming performance of many spatiotemporal models compared to still images. This fueled investigation into modeling approaches that could better capture long-range temporal information in CNN architectures.

Building on the two-stream architectures, Wang et al. [18] propose the temporal segment model (TSM) for incorporating longer-range temporal information. Noting that consecutive frames are often highly redundant, they propose a sparse temporal sampling scheme, selecting a set of short snippets evenly spaced across the temporal domain. Once the snippets have been selected, RGB (Red Green Blue) images are used in the spatial CNN stream, and each segment is used to calculate OF (or other temporal feature images), which are then used as input into the temporal CNN stream. Finally, action recognition predictions are made based on consensus scores from all snippets, and fused across both streams.

Varol, Laptev, and Schmid [19] propose an approach to extend the C3D architecture [14] to accommodate longer video clips. To better support long-term temporal information, the authors proposed using *Long-term Temporal Convolutions* extending out to 60 frames. Due to the computational complexity, however, they substantially reduce the spatial resolution. Nonetheless, their inclusion of more video frames achieved state-of-the-art performance on action recognition benchmark datasets.

2.2 Recurrent Neural Networks

While 3D CNNs were being developed for spatiotemporal data, alternative approaches were being explored that utilized recurrent neural networks (RNNs) [20]. RNNs had long been known as an approach for modeling sequential data, with many applications in speech and language processing. In contrast to CNN architectures, which were designed to work on data with a grid-like structure, which can include spatiotemporal data of a fixed length, RNNs are able to handle sequences of variable length.

In the RNN architecture, shown in Fig. 2, information about the sequence is stored in a hidden state, h, that summarizes the sequence up to the current time step t. As the sequence progresses, the hidden state is updated such that the value of the hidden state at a given time $h^{(t)}$ is a function of the previous hidden state $h^{(t-1)}$ and the input $x^{(t)}$. Using the same transition function to move from one hidden state to the next the model is able to share a set of parameters across all time steps. Once the end of the sequence has been reached, the final hidden state can be used to generate the prediction. The general RNN architecture can be conceptually broken into 3 modules for (1) generating the hidden state from the input, (2) the transition between hidden states, and (3) generating the output from a hidden state. Each one of these

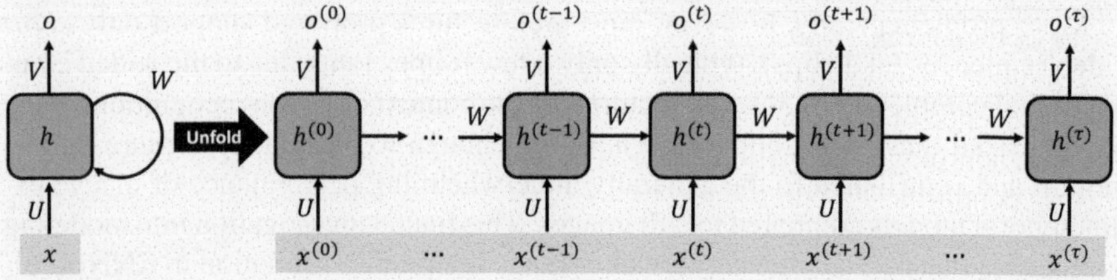

Fig. 2 Diagram of a recurrent neural network (RNN). On the left is the compact representation depicting how the network shares parameters across time-steps by using the same weight matrices: U incorporates information from the input x into the hidden state h; W encodes the transition from one hidden state to the next; and V encodes how to to generate the output o from the hidden state. The right side shows how this RNN unfolds to process an input sequence $x^{(0)} \ldots x^{(\tau)}$. Here, this RNN is generating an output $o^{(t)}$ at each time-step; note other possible RNNs can generate only a single output $o^{(\tau)}$ from the terminal hidden state $h^{(\tau)}$, which is based on the entire sequence. This is the goal of many applications in medical imaging—such as diagnosis

modules is composed of a neural network of varying depth, each with a set of trainable parameters.

In some applications, it may also be important to consider not only what information preceded the current state, but also what information lies in the future. To incorporate information from future timepoints into prediction, bidirectional RNN architectures, shown in Fig. 3, have two separate networks, one that runs in the forward direction, as previously described, and a second running from the end of the sequence moving in reverse. This second network works in the same way, producing a hidden state at each time-step, $g^{(t)}$, except $g^{(t)}$ is a function of $g^{(t+1)}$, summarizing information from all future timepoints, and the input $x^{(t)}$. The two sub-networks do not interact with one another, but both hidden states, $h^{(t)}$ and $g^{(t)}$, are used to generate the prediction at time t.

While RNNs can theoretically handle sequences of variable length, in their most basic form, it was quickly discovered that they struggle to learn long-term dependencies due to vanishing and exploding gradients [21]; a problem also observed in other deep networks when the gradient needs to propagate through many layers. This typically means that longer-term interactions are given much smaller weight than shorter-term ones. Many approaches were suggested for managing this problem that allow the model to operate on multiple timescales.

Most modern architectures now utilize gating to control information flow, allowing the network to possibly forget information from previous time-steps that is no longer needed. An early implementation called long short-term memory (LSTM) [22] remains a popular model to date. This implementation introduced an internal cell state $c^{(t)}$ with a self-loop allowing information to flow for long durations, and included gating on input and output streams to control flow of irrelevant information. By including a learned weight on the self-loop, the model can also learn to forget longer-scale information no longer needed [23], making the network able to dynamically adjust time scale, and capable of modeling long-term dependencies.

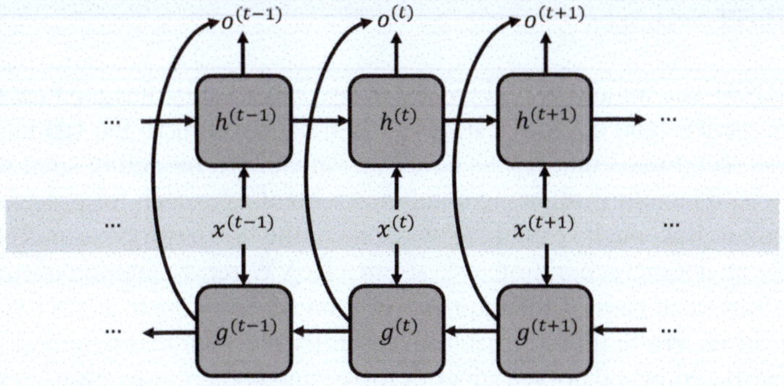

Fig. 3 While the standard recurrent neural network (RNN) architecture goes in only one direction (typically from the start time to the end time), *bidirectional RNNs* introduce a second RNN passing information from the end of the sequence, backwards. Output generated from the bidirectional RNN at a given time-step, $o^{(t)}$, is the function of both the hidden states $h^{(t)}$ from the forward passing RNN, and $g^{(t)}$ from the backward passing RNN; thus, incorporating information from the sequences both before and after the current time-step in the prediction

More recently, Cho et al. [24] introduced a similar gated recurrent unit (GRU), which makes minor updates to the LSTM unit, primarily, replacing forget and input gates of the LSTM with a single update gate (see Fig. 4). In practice, however, neither architecture demonstrates a clear dominance over the other in all applications [25].

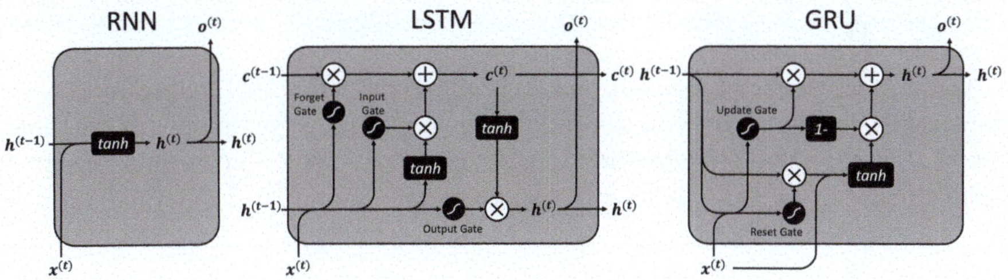

Fig. 4 Cells of RNN (left), LSTM (center), and GRU (right). Both LSTM and GRU cells include gate functions, each with its own set of learned parameters to control the flow of information based on context provided by the hidden state from the previous time-step $h^{(t-1)}$ and the current input $x^{(t)}$. The LSTM cell has three gates: forget, input, and output. Each LSTM cell also has an internal cell state, $c^{(t)}$, which allows information to flow more effectively over long periods of time. Retention of information in the internal cell state is controlled by the forget gate, integration of the current input into the cell state is controlled by the input gate, and the updated cell state interacts with the output gate to generate the updated hidden state $h^{(t)}$. In contrast, GRU cells have only two gates, update and reset, and do not make use of an internal cell state. Similar to the LSTM's forget gate, the GRU's update gate controls what information from the previous time-step should be retained and, in addition, controls what new information is integrated into the updated hidden state $h^{(t)}$. The reset gate controls how much of the previous hidden state $h^{(t-1)}$ is used to generate the updated hidden state $h^{(t)}$

2.2.1 Hybrid Networks

Although RNNs can handle spatial data, they are specifically designed for handling temporal sequences and so do not necessarily translate well to the spatial domain. While it was recognized that RNNs could be valuable in modeling spatiotemporal data, they would benefit from being combined with an approach for processing spatial information. Baccouche et al. [26] were one of the first to propose an RNN based approach for an action recognition task, using a BoVW representation to summarize each video frame and passing the sequence of frame descriptors to an LSTM network for classification. While this approach successfully incorporated temporal information into classification and proved superior to averaged predictions from single frame models, it relied on engineered feature representations. An attractive alternative to this involves combining RNN and CNN architectures into a single hybrid network, leveraging the respective strengths of each model in temporal and spatial domains.

Specifically motivated by the short duration of clips used in most 3D CNN architectures at the time (due to their high computational demand), Ng et al. [27] proposed feeding each video frame through a CNN that directly feeds into an LSTM model - in effect modeling the sequence of CNN activations; an approach also proposed by Donahue et al. [28]. In addition to working from the raw data, Ng et al. [27] also included a separate CNN/LSTM stream for OF data and fused the output of the two models for prediction. They also proposed a temporal feature pooling architecture, similar to Karpathy et al. [4], where the outputs of CNN applied to each frame are pooled over different durations for prediction. Both approaches performed very similarly to one another, achieving state-of-the-art performance on action recognition benchmarks (exceeding Karpathy et al. [4]) and demonstrating the value of longer-range temporal information.

As discussed previously, advancements in spatiotemporal CNN architectures soon enabled CNN architectures to accommodate longer-range temporal information; however, these CNN/RNN hybrids remain a popular choice in medical imaging applications.

2.3 *Attention*

In the field of NLP, machine translation involves taking one or more sentences in the source language, and returning one or more sentences in a destination language, which retains the intended meaning; note this can be a very challenging task, even for humans. Many implementations of machine translation models use an encoder-decoder model, where the input sequence (decreased to a fixed length vector) is used to generate the output sequence by the decoder; which can be implemented by two RNN networks. In these RNN encoder-decoder networks, each element in the input sequence is fed through the encoder RNN, and the sequence of hidden states of the entire word sequence is used to generate a context vector. The decoder network is then used to generate words, one at a time—predicting the next word in the sequence using the content vector from the encoder, the hidden state of the decoder, and the last word that was predicted in the output sequence.

In these approaches, information passed to the decoder about the input sequence is stored in the content vector that has a fixed length regardless of the length of the input. This creates a bottleneck, limiting what information can be passed to the decoder, especially as the input sequence grows in length. To get around this, Bahdanau et al. [29] proposed the first implementation of an *attention mechanism*, where a context vector would be generated for each word in the output sequence. Each context vector is essentially computed as a weighted sum of the encoder hidden states (from a bidirectional RNN), where the weights are based on how well each position in the input sequence matches the current position in the output sequence. By considering alignment between the input and output sequences, this approach proved to perform much better on longer sequences, allowing the model to focus on relevant information from the input sequence when making predictions.

More generally, attention mechanisms learn what words, or tokens, are most relevant to one another. During translation, a representation for each token in the input sequence is generated by the encoder. This representation, or query, is scored against the learned keys of all possible tokens in the database to generate a weighting for each token. Attention is then, again, calculated as the weighted sum of all tokens stored as value vectors. Learning the encoder, keys, and value vectors, the attention mechanism is able to learn what tokens are relevant to the token being predicted, and place more emphasis on those relevant tokens.

2.3.1 Transformers

Building on the success of attention networks, Vaswani et al. [30] proposed a related architecture, transformers, built around self-attention mechanisms. Like the previous architectures, the transformer is composed of an encoder and decoder, however, to enable more parallelization and computational efficiency it replaces the RNN networks with an architecture made of multiple layers, each composed of multi-head self-attention and feed forward networks. By implementing these changes, transformers are able to reduce computational complexity and achieve state-of-the-art performance on translation tasks.

Since their conception, transformers have grown in popularity—in particular, making huge progress in NLP. Recently, Devlin et al. [31] proposed a transformer-based architecture, "Bidirectional Encoder Representations from Transformers" (BERT), which has become a widely used tool for many language tasks. One of the major contributions of this work, however, was the use of unsupervised pre-training (see Sect. 4.1.2) that enabled the model to first learn general language properties on large amounts of unlabelled text data, before being fine-tuned for specific down-stream tasks. This implementation used two pre-training tasks: (1) *Masked Language Model*—where random words are masked in the input sequence that the model learns to predict, and (2) *Next Sentence Prediction*—where the model is given two sentences as input and tasked with predicting if the second sentence follows the first in the original document, or is a random sentence from the corpus. BERT is one of the first in a class of models, now called *Large Language Models*, that currently have millions, to billions, of trainable parameters, and learn general language properties from enormous text datasets; all of these models are based around transformers that enable efficient training of these massive models.

The successes of transformers, however, have not been limited to NLP tasks. Unlike text data, which is composed of a set of discrete tokens, imaging data is continuous, and applying the self-attention mechanism to every pixel in the image would be prohibitively expensive. Making minimal changes to the original transformer, Dosovitskiy et al. [32] proposed a *Vision Transformer*, where images are divided into a smaller number of image patches that are embedded to form the 1D input sequence. Although they were not the first to purpose transformer-based models for imaging data, Dosovitskiy et al. [32] show that, with sufficiently large pre-training datasets (14M–300M images), their model surpasses CNN architectures, demonstrating that with enough data the transformer models make up any advantage gained by the additional inductive biases of CNNs.

The computational efficiency of transformers has enabled models with billions of parameters to be trained using massive datasets. State-of-the-art models in various fields continue to employ transformers as the basis of their models, showing that with larger models, and more training data, performance continues to improve. As more data continues to become available, and computational hardware becomes more efficient, these models will likely continue to grow in size and become even more accurate.

3 Medical Imaging Applications

While the approaches described in the previous section can be readily translated to medical data, each specific modality may require different considerations and accommodations. In many proposals, raw imaging data is preprocessed or reformatted to match the input structure of pre-developed models. This approach enables off-the-shelf use of existing models that may have already been trained on another task and can simply be fine-tuned for the current application. We will discuss this technique, called "transfer learning", in Sect. 4.1.1. While this approach can expedite model development, avoiding time spent on developing and training a new architecture, pre-existing models, especially from other fields, may not be optimal for applications using medical imaging data.

A major obstacle when using medical imaging data is that it often has much higher resolution, or longer sequence lengths, than the data used for developing the previously mentioned spatiotemporal models [33]. Spatiotemporal medical imaging data also regularly captures 3D spatial information to cover anatomical structures, rather than a representative slice, resulting in 4D data that is not compatible with most previously discussed architectures. Given that computational complexity was already a concern, these factors can further increase the time and resources needed to train these models for medical applications. These factors are further exacerbated by the relatively limited number of available training instances for clinical applications; see Sect. 4.

This section will introduce a number of medical imaging modalities, and clinical applications of spatiotemporal DL models used to date. Currently, proposed methods have focused heavily on neurological and cardiovascular applications, however, these models have more widespread applicability given the dynamic nature of the body. In particular, the following sections will show that proposed works tend to cluster around certain applications, largely a result of the release of datasets in those areas that are large enough for training these complex models. We will specifically focus on biopotential imaging modalities, cardiac imaging, angiography/perfusion imaging, and functional magnetic resonance imaging (fMRI)—giving a brief overview of each modality and data structure, as well as touching on clinical applications. Given the broad range of current and potential clinical applications of spatiotemporal DL, the scope of this review will cover only a small subset of current applications but should provide a high-level overview of the space.

3.1 Biopotential Imaging

Biopotential imaging can be used for a wide range of clinical applications, broadly encompassing modalities such as electroencephalogram (EEG) for probing neurological function, and electrocardiogram (ECG) to measure electrical function of the heart. Generally, biopotential imaging involves measuring electrical signals using sensors, or electrodes, placed on the skin's surface. Unlike many of the other modalities that will be discussed, this type of data does not resemble an anatomical image, as the spatial components of the data are not directly encoded. Instead, two or more electrodes are used to generate a temporal signal of electrical activity from the underlying tissue. As a result, the data has largely been thought of as a set of temporal signals that can be stacked to form a 2D matrix.

Since the data is stored in a 2D matrix, without intrinsically encoding the original spatial information, biopotential imaging modalities may arguably be outside the scope of this chapter; however, they benefit from many of the same modeling approaches as the other modalities discussed in subsequent sections. In particular, they are conceptually quite similar to data from fMRI, and often used in similar applications. The following sections will discuss some current applications of biopotential imaging and how they are being modeled using novel DL approaches; specifically focusing on applications of EEG, ECG, and models for human-machine interaction.

3.1.1 Electroencephalogram

The brain functions by passing electrical signals through different cells. Using an EEG, fluctuations in these electrical signals can be measured. Typically, data collection is performed by placing electrodes positioned in a standard arrangement on the participant's scalp. The electrodes are used to measure electrical signals generated by the underlying neuronal tissue, providing a way to monitor brain activity. Rather than directly using the measurements from individual electrodes, the temporal signals generated by an EEG system, referred to as channels, are generated by passing the signals from two electrodes through a differential amplifier. Depending on the specific EEG configuration being used, each channel may result from two individual electrodes, or by comparing each electrode to a shared reference.

Compared to many other modalities, EEG, and other biopotential imaging modalities have very high *temporal* resolution, capable of recording activity at sub-millisecond resolution. This, however, comes at the cost of *spatial* resolution, as EEG typically involves collecting from a small number of electrodes spread across the scalp; for example, the widely used 10–20 system [34] for EEG electrode placement involves only 21 electrodes, and hence only 21 signals, from the surface of the brain. In addition, because measurements are made from the scalp, the signals cannot be directly linked to specific neuroanatomical regions. Typically, there exists a trade-off between spatial resolution, temporal resolution, and signal-to-noise ratio in imaging modalities. For example, fMRI (another modality for imaging neuronal function) can provide much higher spatial resolution with full 3D brain coverage typically on the order of a few millimeters, but with only a single image acquired every few seconds.

A number of studies have investigated using EEG-based DL architectures to detect human emotions. While this task has obvious applications to human-computer interaction, it may also be useful in psychiatric conditions such as major depression. Salama et al. [35] attempted to model EEG data from the DEAP [36] benchmark dataset for emotion recognition using a 3D CNN architecture. To work in this architecture, they first reformatted the EEG data into 3-dimensions by segmenting the temporal sequence into a set of frames with a set width (number of temporal samples per frame), creating a set of 2D frames with dimensions equal to the number of EEG channels and the width of the frame. Finally, a small number of frames are stacked to create 3D volumes, where the label is determined by majority vote over all frames in the volume. Using this 3D CNN, they are able to demonstrate improved performance over other models using engineered features.

When using the raw channel data, as many have proposed, little to no information about the actual spatial location of the electrodes will be incorporated into the model. In many cases, however, EEG electrodes are arranged in a standardized pattern on the scalp, making it possible to reconstruct the spatial organization of the raw channel signals. To reconstruct the EEG spatial domain, Cho and Hwang [37] proposed mapping the electrodes to the appropriate coordinates in a sparse 2D matrix and using a radial basis function (RBF) to interpolate values in-between electrodes. This spatial reconstruction creates a 2D frame for each timepoint, allowing a 3D volume to be constructed by stacking consecutive frames. They then modeled this data using C3D [14] (a 3D CNN architecture) and R(2 + 1)D [17], with an adjustment to the kernel size, extending it from 3 to 7 along the temporal domain to better accommodate the EEG signal. Using the same DEAP dataset [36] for emotion recognition, they are able to outperform the previous 3D CNN from Salama et al. [35] that worked with the raw signal data. This work suggests that, while the spatial locations of the electrodes are not inherently captured in EEG data, it may be relevant, and worth reincorporating.

Although CNN architectures are a popular modeling approach for biopotential imaging data, they are not necessarily good for incorporating longer-range temporal interactions. Song et al. [38] proposed a transformer-based architecture, S3T (Spatial-Temporal Tiny Transformer), that allows interactions across multiple timescales to be considered during prediction. This architecture has two attention mechanisms: (1) a feature–channel attention mechanism, used to focus attention on more relevant electrode channels; and (2) a temporal transformer, used to determine temporal dependencies in the signal. This approach was able to outperform other DL approaches, including CNN and various hybrid architectures, on the BCI (brain computer interface) competition dataset [39] for identifying a number of body movements. Performing an ablation study, where different portions of the full S3T model are removed, they are able to show that the temporal transformer has the greatest impact on overall performance.

Beyond the studies described above, EEG data have been proposed for a number of other clinical applications. Early identification and classification of epileptic seizures can help determine which preventative treatments to use to stop, or minimize, the episode. A number of studies have identified and explored this as an application of EEG based DL models [40]. EEG is also an important modality for investigating psychiatric disorders that present without obvious lesions, nor other anatomical markers. As mentioned previously, emotion recognition could be used for clinical applications involving psychiatric disorders such as major depressive disorder (MDD), however, a number of studies have also attempted more directly predicting diagnosis and treatment outcome prediction tasks [41, 42].

Sleep is another application that has been investigated using EEG data, where different sleep stages have been shown to have specific characteristic waveform patterns. Using EEG collected during sleep, a number of sleep disorders can be identified, however, reviewing hours of EEG signals can be a tedious and time-consuming task for sleep experts. As a result, a number of automated approaches have sought to classify sleep data based on EEG recordings. Mousavi, Afghan, and Acharya [43], for example, propose a CNN/BiLSTM to successfully classify sleep stages.

3.1.2 Electrocardiogram

As part of regular function, the heart's pumping action is generated by a controlled sequence of electrical stimuli dictating when specific muscles should contract. This pumping action is a critical bodily function and is responsible for moving blood (along with oxygen, nutrients, and other important substances) around the body. As a result, it is imperative that the heart maintains a regular and consistent rhythm of electrical stimuli, which can be measured by an ECG. During an ECG exam, a

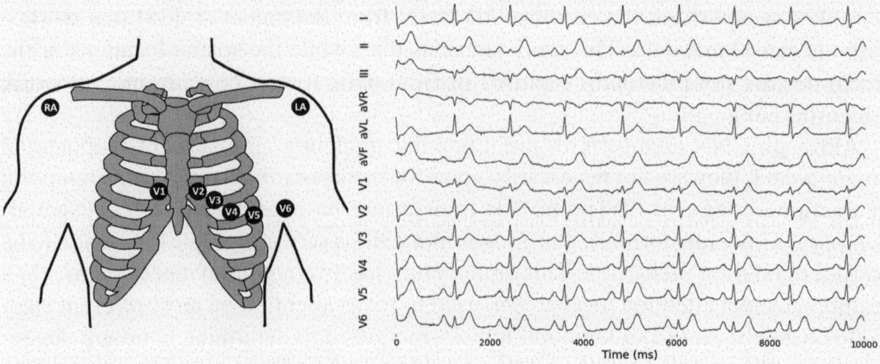

Fig. 5 Diagram of the standard 12-lead ECG configuration consisting of six precordial electrodes, V1–V6, placed across the chest (primarily on the patient's left side) as well as four limb electrodes placed respectively on the right arm (RA), left arm (LA), right leg (RL) and left leg (LL) (RL and LL electrode placement not shown). From these 10 electrodes, 12 signals (called "leads") are calculated, each providing a slightly different view of the heart's activity. Each lead is captured simultaneously during the recording period and represented as a waveform, an example of which is shown on the right

number of electrodes are placed in specific configurations at locations across the chest, back, and extremities (Fig. 5). The final temporal signals, referred to as leads in this context, are generated from the recordings of two or more electrodes. Similar to other biophysical imaging modalities, ECG is a relatively low cost, and effective tool for assessing functionality, and as a result, is regularly used as part of routine clinical practice to assess heart function [44]. Newer technology has also made it possible to incorporate ECG into personal wearable devices, such as smartwatches [45].

This imaging modality is a very valuable tool for assessing heart health and can be used to identify many cardiac conditions (and some non-cardiac conditions [46]). Like the other biophysical imaging modalities, the temporal component of ECG is often considered of greater importance than the spatial dimension. Since the beating of the heart involves a cyclic pattern of electrical activity, looking at the signals collected from the heart over a number of beat cycles can be effective for identifying irregularities. Arrhythmia, or the general presence of irregular heart rhythms, can be assessed using ECG data, and can be important to identify before more serious, and potentially life-threatening, conditions develop.

Spatial information in ECG, however, is not disregarded during assessment. While arrhythmia refers to the general presence of heart rhythm irregularities, the underlying etiology can be a number of different conditions. The placement of electrodes couples the signals with specific underlying anatomy, which can be important for localizing underlying abnormalities. For example, left bundle branch block (LBBB) occurs when there is a disruption of the electrical conduction pathway to the left ventricle, causing delayed contraction and inefficient blood ejection. To diagnose a LBBB, specific wave abnormalities are identified from electrodes placed on the lateral left chest.

The use of automated approaches for the identification of different arrhythmias is particularly attractive as arrhythmias may only arise during certain activities such as sleep or exercise. To identify these conditions an ambulatory ECG can be used, where signals are collected for long durations of time (i.e., days) while performing regular activities. As a result, large amounts of data can be accumulated while waiting for a cardiac event to occur. Given the spatiotemporal characterization of these different conditions on ECG, significant interest has been placed on developing automated DL models for arrhythmia classification based on ECG signals.

Yao et al. [47] propose a model for differentially diagnosing eight types of arrhythmias based on 12-lead ECG data using a hybrid CNN/LSTM with attention module. In this approach, a CNN is applied to the raw ECG data to extract spatial information from the different leads, which is then fed into an LSTM network and a subsequent attention mechanism then used to incorporate temporal information. Class prediction is made directly from the attention module, without incorporating fully connected layers, which allows the model the flexibility to work with sequences of different lengths. The performance of the proposed architecture was compared to 2D CNN networks using inputs with varying temporal length, and an architecture similar to theirs but without the attention mechanism. Results show that their proposed architecture consistently outperformed the comparison models across the different prediction classes.

Using the same dataset for arrhythmia classification, Che et al. [48] propose using a CNN with embedded transformer network. Here, the ECG signal is divided along the temporal dimension into a sequence of smaller windows of fixed length. Each window is passed through a 2D CNN, and the sequence of outputs from all windows are used by a transformer to capture additional temporal information before classification. When compared to other state-of-the-art models, the proposed architecture has the highest classification accuracy for most arrhythmia classes. Che et al. [48] also performed an ablation study to test the value of different components of their model; however, they demonstrate no consistent results when considering modifications such as swapping the transformer for bi-directional LSTM or using an attention module. Although not directly compared in the study, these results are consistent with the reported results from the previously discussed CNN/LSTM/Attention network proposed by Yao et al. [47], which indicate no model consistently performs better across all classes.

While spatiotemporal DL models based on ECG have been enthusiastically studied for predictive tasks relating to arrhythmia, similar approaches can be used for other cardiovascular disorders. A number of additional studies have used ECG DL models for diagnosing conditions such as valvulopathy, cardiomyopathy, and ischemia (see [49] for a review).

3.1.3 Human–Machine Interaction

An advantage of biopotential imaging is that these systems are considerably cheaper and more transportable than many of the modalities described later. As a result, many applications of human–machine interaction, where a human interfaces or communicates with a machine, have been proposed using biopotential imaging. These applications can be very impactful for individuals with amputations or conditions that reduce mobility. As mentioned in Sect. 3.1.1, EEG has been explored for BCI applications such as identifying neural signatures of bodily movements.

Another biopotential modality, electromyogram (EMG), which measures electrical signals from skeletal muscle, has become an attractive modality for controlling prosthetic limbs in amputees; given that the electrodes can be easily and comfortably worn on the skin while the limb is in use. To facilitate the development of EMG based control systems, datasets such as the Ninapore database [50] have been released. Since then, a number of DL architectures have been proposed to perform tasks such as gesture recognition.

Park and Lee [51], for example, use a CNN on signals extracted from a sliding window to classify hand movements. To better adapt the architecture for individual users, they propose a user-adaptive decoder that is fine-tuned using a small amount of data for a new user. Comparing the proposed CNN to another study using a more traditional support vector machine (SVM) model [52], they show improved performance, especially when using the user-adaptive approach.

In a more comprehensive study of potential modeling approaches and the value of transfer learning, Côté-Allard et al. [53] test a number of different CNN architectures with different configurations. In addition to the raw EMG signals, Côté-Allard et al. [53] also test two additional input features derived from EMG data: (1) Fourier transform-based spectrogram, and (2) Continuous Wavelet Transform (CWT). Generating each of these derived features results in a 3D matrix that the authors model using a CNN model with temporal fusion, similar to Karpathy et al. [4], whereas the raw data is only 2D and instead modeled using a more conventional 2D CNN architecture. Further, they test the value of pre-training the network on a large dataset from many individuals and fine-tuning the network for a specific user. For all input types, the authors show the use of transfer learning improves performance and, out of the three input types, the raw EMG performed best: marginally outperforming the other CNN models and showing an even larger margin of improvement over other engineered feature types used in more traditional classifiers such as SVM.

Similarly, in motor neuron diseases, the neurons that control skeletal muscle gradually degenerate and die, making it progressively more difficult for patients to walk, eat, and breathe. As the motor neurons begin to degrade, the use of EMG, as described previously, becomes less feasible, as the skeletal muscles no longer receive nerve activation. To assist patients with amyotrophic lateral sclerosis (ALS), the most common motor neuron disease, Ravichandran et al. [54] proposed an electrooculogram (EOG) based classification system that could classify eye movements. For ALS patients who lose the ability to walk, these eye movements can be used to drive a wheelchair. Requiring only 4 sensors placed around the eye, the use of EOG data for this application is ideal because it is not overly cumbersome for patients to wear and relatively low cost. Their study tested CNN and LSTM networks for classification, demonstrating impressive results by all proposed models, but marginally better performance by the CNN.

3.2 *Cardiac Imaging*

Composed of the heart and blood vessels, the cardiovascular system is responsible for transporting blood, and its components, to all parts of the body. Compared to other organ systems, cardiovascular functionality is tightly coupled to mechanical motion, as the heart constantly pumps blood around the body using contractile force. As cardiac function involves such robust movement, modeling approaches originally developed for motion-based tasks, such as action recognition, are relatively easy to transfer to applications in cardiology.

Echocardiogram, which uses ultrasound (US) imaging to image the heart, is routinely used to assess cardiac health. Like biopotential imaging, US is relatively inexpensive, portable, and non-invasive, leading to its wide use. Unlike biopotential imaging, however, echocardiograms do generate a spatial image of the heart, allowing clinicians to examine anatomical structures such as the atria, and ventricles. Typically, this data is collected as a 3D volume, capturing a 2D slice through the heart over time. Although there are many attractive qualities of echocardiogram, the images can be challenging to interpret as they are very noisy, and acquisition is performed using a hand-held probe that can create substantial variability in the image acquisition plane. Together, these factors make it challenging for practitioners to assess complex spatial and temporal dynamics by visual inspection only.

This has motivated a number of clinical measures used to summarize relevant characteristics of cardiac motion from echocardiogram images. Since these measures have become the basis for diagnosis of many cardiac conditions, many DL applications have focused on automatically generating these engineered measures, rather than more directly predicting diagnosis or prognosis. For example, DL models have been used to segment different cardiac structures, track motion, and perform strain analysis (see [55] for review).

Automated indexing of end-systole (ES) and end-diastole (ED) frames in echocardiogram videos has been an application of particular interest, as these frames are used for generating important clinical measurements such as left-ventricular (LV) ejection fraction (EF). A number of earlier papers propose similar hybrid architectures for predicting ED and/or ES frame indices by first extracting image features with a CNN that are subsequently fed into a RNN to model temporal dependencies [56–58].

In a more direct approach, Ouyang et al. [59] use the R(2 + 1)D architecture [17] to generate predictions of LVEF directly from echocardiogram videos. Ultimately, however, their final model (EchoNet-Dynamic) works in conjunction with a frame-level CNN for LV segmentation, used to identify the start and end of beat-cycles in the sequence. To generate the final LVEF prediction for a single echocardiogram, they average five beat-level LVEF predictions. They then diagnose cardiomyopathy by applying a common threshold to the predicted LVEF. Importantly, that team also publicly released the large training dataset that was used to develop the model, which included over 10K echocardiograms collected during routine clinical practice and annotated by clinical experts.

Rather than making beat-level predictions, Reynaud et al. [60] used the full-length video to predict ES/ED frame locations, as well as LVEF, using transformers. Their model included three modules: (1) A residual autoencoder (AE) to reduce dimensionality; (2) a BERT-based model for spatiotemporal reasoning; and (3) regressors for prediction. After training the AE separately, the encoder portion is used to generate compressed representations of spatial frames that are stacked into clips to be fed into the BERT module, where the full architecture (all three modules) is trained end-to-end. This approach did not perform as well as the EchoNet-Dynamic model from Ouyang et al. [59]; however, they did outperform single-beat predictions made by the EchoNet-Dynamic base architectures, suggesting EchoNet-Dynamic's superior performance may arise from post-processing steps external to the DL architecture.

The utility of LVEF as a prognostic marker, however, has long been in question, and may not be an ideal choice for many patients, as it often fails to identify early (subclinical) cardiac impairment [61]. A recognized challenge in calculating LVEF is measurement variability, which can be even more difficult in the presence of ectopic beats, and can result in substantial differences in LVEF measurements from one beat to another. Ouyang et al. [59] address this challenge by averaging predicted LVEF from five separate heartbeats, a practice also recommended by clinical guidelines for manual evaluation of LVEF, showing lower error measurements compared to single beat predictions. While this seems advantageous, it disregards heartbeat variability as a meaningful factor in prognosis, despite having demonstrated utility conditions such as heart failure [62], where utilizing the entire video, or at least multiple heartbeats, in predictive models may prove to be more valuable.

Shad et al. [63] recently learned a model that could use preoperative echocardiograms to predict postoperative right ventricular failure in patients implanted with a left ventricular assist device (LVAD); allowing clinicians to use aggressive treatment in those predicted to be at high risk. The proposed model applied a two-stream approach - one for grayscale images, and a second for OF - using a 3D CNN [14] with residual blocks [15]. The proposed network uses 32 frame clips from the original sequence to generate a prediction, but the final prediction is generated by randomly sampling, and averaging the predictions from 5 different clips. Shad et al. [63] demonstrated that their spatiotemporal DL model performed better than standard clinical risk scores and clinical experts with access to the same images, suggesting the importance of end-to-end prediction.

In another approach, Hwang et al. [64] proposed an end-to-end CNN-LSTM hybrid architecture for differential diagnosis of LV hypertrophy (LVH) from echocardiogram videos. To limit computational load, the model makes predictions based on 12 frames sampled at regular intervals from a single cardiac cycle. In the proposed architecture, five separate CNN-LSTM streams, one for each of the five standard cardiac views, are trained in parallel, and the outputs from each are concatenated together to form the input for a fully connected NN that ultimately makes the classification prediction; outperforming clinical experts and demonstrating the value of including multiple cardiac views in predictions.

Similarly, Zaman et al. [65] used a hybrid CNN-LSTM architecture, along with 2D and 3D CNN architectures, to differentially diagnose Takotsubo syndrome; a disorder that can be easily misdiagnosed by ECG and lead to potentially dangerous treatment interventions. Using echocardiogram data as input, the spatiotemporal DL architectures outperformed clinical experts, with the 3D CNN architecture performing better than the 2D (still-frame) CNN models.

While most spatiotemporal DL models currently use echocardiogram data, many studies have shown that many cardiac conditions are better assessed by cardiac CT or MRI [66]. This is likely (at least) in part due to the widespread clinical use of echocardiograms, which are comparatively low cost, making it highly accessible and a first-line choice in assessing cardiovascular health. As a result, large echocardiogram datasets originating from routine clinical use have become available for training these data-hungry models. While these datasets drive development, they may also limit applications to specific use cases and labels [67]. Focusing on predicting current clinical metrics derived from imaging data may not be an ideal use of spatiotemporal data, which often oversimplify complex dynamic information that may be meaningful in appropriate diagnosis and prognosis, leaving the potential of these complex models largely still untapped in this space.

3.3 Angiography and Perfusion Imaging

Computed Tomography Perfusion (CTP) has become an important modality for imaging ischemic strokes, where blood flow to the brain is cut off, or reduced, by a clot in an arterial vessel. Here, a contrast agent is injected intravenously, and a series of images are acquired as the contrast agent passes through the brain's blood vessels. Voxel intensity values in each frame indicate the concentration of the contrast agent at that location over the course of time, which can be used to quantify dynamics of vascular flow, and so indicate where blood flow may be restricted, and to what extent, which helps determine the appropriate treatment. The calculation of these measures from the CTP images can depend on a number of patient-specific factors. Moreover, after images have been acquired, if the vessels remain blocked, tissue damage will worsen and spread as time goes on—which may change highly time-sensitive treatment decisions. Thus, it is incredibly important to be able to both identify the location and size of the ischemia from these images and also predict how the stroke will progress over time.

Mittermeier et al. [68] proposed a spatiotemporal model to predict the size of the ischemic core (either small or large) in stroke patients based on their CTP images, which can be used to help decide if a patient would be a good candidate for reperfusion therapy. Their proposed architecture consisted of two identical streams, each using video data from one of two selected image slices covering the middle cerebral artery territory. Each stream uses a 2D CNN architecture, specifically VGG19 [69], to extract spatial features from each image frame. The extracted features are then concatenated and fed into a temporal feature extraction module with two pathways, local and global, applying convolutional filters of different depths to capture multi-resolution temporal dynamics. The authors use an ablation study, comparing the full model to variations with only one of the two temporal pathways, to demonstrate the value of using both streams together, which supports the understood importance of both short- (spiking) and long-term (wash-out) tracer dynamics in prediction.

This work is presented as a proof-of-concept study, demonstrating the capacity of the DL model to learn meaningful relationships between CTP data and tissue properties without the need to derive tracer-kinetic measures. They acknowledge that the predicted labels are a simplified target, suggesting, however, that with the appropriate data for training this approach could be used for more meaningful prognostic labels, such as predicting future impairment. Note that the authors made a conscious decision when developing their model to use only two image slices, citing limited availability of 3D CTP at stroke centers.

In another application, Hu et al. [70] propose a spatiotemporal model that uses a similar vascular imaging modality, digital subtraction angiography (DSA), to diagnose moyamoya disease, which causes restricted blood flow to major cerebral arteries. For input, 10 images from each DSA sequence are extracted and used to generate 2 sets of OF images (transverse and longitudinal). Each image type is then fed into an independent architecture, each composed of the sequence: 2D CNN, Bidirectional Convolutional GRU, and 3D CNN. The outputs from each input stream are ultimately fused and fed into a fully connected NN for classification. The authors argue here that each component of the full architecture has a quality that should improve overall performance, specifically, that 3D CNNs are better for shorter-term temporal dynamics, and GRUs are better for longer-term temporal dynamics, both of which may be relevant for prediction. When the authors compare their proposed architecture to more simplistic variations of their architecture, where they omitted the 3D CNN, and/or replaced the bi-directional GRU with a unidirectional GRU, however, the difference in performance was less than 3%, and no model had lower than 95% accuracy; which was also consistent when comparing with more basic spatiotemporal models such as C3D [14].

Choosing the appropriate course of treatment of acute ischemic stroke (AIS) can be challenging. Mechanical thrombectomy (MT), a procedure where blood clots are removed from vessels, can be highly effective for some individuals. To assess who will be a good candidate for MT, an ordinal Thrombectomy in Cerebral Infarction (TICI) score is generated based on DSA images. A major problem with this measurement, however, is that it can be highly variable depending on the imaging center and specific grader. To generate more objective and consistent scores, Nielsen et al. [71] propose a GRU-based DL architecture for predicting TICI based on DSA. Their approach uses two DSA orientations, frontal and lateral, that are modeled in two GRU arms with shared weights [72]. In this proof-of-concept study, they demonstrate promising results predicting TICI, that could be extended to a wider population.

3.4 Functional Magnetic Resonance Imaging

Functional magnetic resonance imaging (fMRI), like EEG, measures functional activity of the brain. Instead of measuring electrical signals, however, fMRI is able to detect subtle changes in blood flow, indirectly measuring neuronal activity as a temporal sequence of 3D images over the brain volume. This, and other modalities that measure neurological function, have been particularly useful for investigating psychiatric conditions that present without obvious lesions or structural changes visible in anatomical images.

Since the brain's functionality is not coupled with motion, it is assumed that a given voxel corresponds to the same anatomical position for the duration of the scan. As a result, the 4D fMRI dataset can be viewed as a time-series from each voxel, or region (Fig. 6). This format of data is far more analogous to EEG and other physiological signal data than cardiac imaging, where functionality is tightly linked to motion. This is why most engineered features for spatiotemporal data from early computer vision, which focused on action recognition and similar tasks (using approaches such as OF), do not translate well to fMRI.

As discussed in Sect. 3.1.1, EEG has poor spatial resolution, limited to electrical signals measured at the scalp. Alternatively, fMRI provides full brain coverage, at the expense of lower temporal resolution. Although this makes fMRI useful for investigating specific spatial activations in the brain, it drastically increases dimensionality. As a result, ML pipelines rarely work with the raw, pixel-level data, and instead exploit parcellation approaches as part of data preprocessing; where voxels are grouped together into a smaller number of regions of interest (ROIs) based on either anatomical or functional characteristics, and the signal for each ROI is

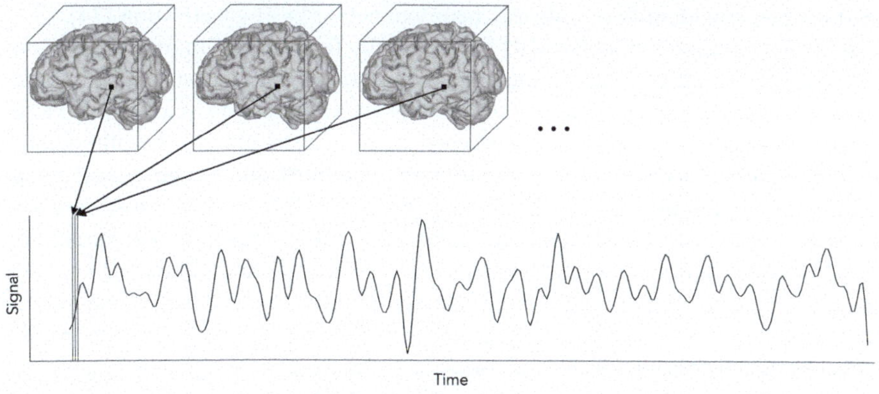

Fig. 6 Functional magnetic resonance imaging (fMRI) data is typically 4D, consisting of a sequence of 3D images acquired at regular time intervals. Since the brain is a stationary structure within the skull, each voxel is assumed to correspond to the same anatomical location in each image volume. As a result, the signal intensities from a single voxel over the duration of the scan forms a time-series representing the fluctuating neuronal activity in that region

generated based on some function, often the mean, of the underlying signals from individual constituent voxels. Though straightforward, parcellation can have a substantial impact on dimensionality, and the choice of parcellation scheme can have considerable implications on downstream predictive performance. In future, it would be preferable to omit this step, preventing any possible information loss when combining voxel level signals to generate the combined ROI time-series. However, with today's limited data, it is often necessary and almost universally used.

fMRI data is typically categorized as either task-based or resting state; each involves its own acquisition paradigms and analysis techniques, even though the data itself shares the same format. Task-based fMRI, as the name suggests, involves having participants engage in some task during imaging (e.g., watch a sequence of images, or making a sequence of decisions) to elicit a specific mental response. The imaging sequence is coupled with a corresponding sequence of temporal labels indicating what specific task the participant was engaging in when each 3D volume was collected [73]. The use of task-based fMRI in clinical applications can be complicated by the process of task design, which is often application specific. Further, because of the number of different tasks, and specific designs, it can be difficult to accumulate large amounts of consistent, labeled data. This approach, however, can make image analysis more straightforward as neuronal activity can be directly tied to specific stimuli. Typically, this can be done by segmenting the sequence by stimuli and comparing neuronal activation under different conditions.

In contrast, resting state fMRI (rs-fMRI) is acquired while the participant remains at rest in the MRI scanner, not actively engaging in any specified activity or thought process. Since rs-fMRI does not have any temporal labels, the entire scan needs to be considered as a whole, without any additional information to help guide how it is analyzed. As a result, most rs-fMRI analysis is based on engineered feature extraction or unsupervised learning approaches, where patterns within the data are uncovered; most focusing on identifying intrinsic neuronal networks of coactivation [74].

Extracted measures from rs-fMRI have typically focused on summarizing temporal activation patterns. Notably, functional connectivity (FC) measures the pairwise correlation between the time-series of different spatial locations as a means to infer which regions are communicating with each other. Investigating FC has illuminated numerous alterations associated with different conditions, and has been used extensively, and with some success, as input features for ML models. More recently, however, the use of FC has come into question, as it ignores temporal variability, condensing the entire temporal dimension into a single measure. While that has been useful in reducing dimensionality, it ignores how connectivity patterns may fluctuate over time, which may be an important consideration in many applications. As such, considerable efforts have been made to better model and understand temporal variability, which may benefit from spatiotemporal DL.

Although rs-fMRI data is conceptually more challenging to analyze and interpret, it has also proven to be an important modality for investigating numerous disorders and represents an important component of neuronal functioning. Moreover, because there is far less variability in resting state paradigms as compared to task-based images, resting state scans are an almost ubiquitous component of fMRI protocols, making it much easier to accumulate large amounts of data and combine data across studies.

The 4D structure of fMRI data can be challenging to use, having an additional dimension beyond even the more conventional 3D spatiotemporal data that early models used. In 2018, Li et al. [75] noted that many previous attempts to model fMRI data largely ignored the 3D spatial structure of the data, focusing more heavily on temporal signals. To address this, and retain more of the original data structure, they proposed using a 3D CNN architecture on data from temporal sliding windows to diagnose autism spectrum disorder (ASD). Their approach moved a sliding window across the temporal axis, creating smaller temporal sequences over the duration of the scan. For each sliding window, they calculated the mean and standard deviation of the time-series for each voxel, then generated a 3D mean and standard deviation image for each window. Using a modified version of the previously discussed 3D CNN model C3D [14], they treat the mean and standard deviation images as separate channels in the model, making a prediction based on every window, then combining these predictions, using a majority vote, over the duration of the scan to make a prediction for each subject.

Interestingly, Li et al. [75] choose to treat the entire session as a contiguous sequence, sliding the window along the entire length of the session using a consistent stride; however, the imaging data being used was actually task-based fMRI of block design, where stimuli are presented for 24 s at a time, and no attempt is made to incorporate the task design into the model. They do, however, note that utilizing the raw fMRI data did not work well, and instead use the residual signals after modeling out task data with a GLM. While the authors do note that window lengths between 3–5 frames perform better than shorter windows, this averaging approach over windows is only a minor step away from standard frame-based prediction models and still largely ignores important temporal dynamics.

Building on their previous work, Riaz et al. [76] propose an end-to-end model centered around a CNN architecture to predict FC between two time-series. Rather than using learned FC features as input to a more traditional machine learning model as they had done previously [77], they instead trained the feature extractor and FC network in an end-to-end model for predicting attention-deficit/hyperactivity disorder (ADHD) diagnosis. Their full model contained 3 modules: (1) a feature extractor network that accepts time-series data from 90 parcellation ROIs. In the proposed architecture each ROI has its own CNN network, although weights are shared between all streams. (2) a functional connectivity network that operates on the outputs from the CNN streams, measuring the similarity between pairs of regions. The measures between all pairs of regions are then mapped together and passed to (3) a classification network. Interestingly, the use of CNNs in this implementation is not for spatial information, but instead uses only 1D kernels along the time dimension of regional time-series. In effect, this model largely disregards the 3D spatial structure of the fMRI data.

Zhang et al. [78] similarly propose an architecture where individual ROI time series are fed through a CNN network with shared parameters, called a separated channel (SC) CNN. They then test passing the learned CNN representations along to either a dense, LSTM, or attention network. Results show that the CNN-attention network outperforms the other network variants, as well as other results on the ADHD-200 dataset, including the FC based architecture from Riaz et al. [76] described in the previous paragraph.

Li et al. [79] also propose a CNN/LSTM hybrid, called C3d-LSTM, for differential diagnosis of Alzheimer's disease (AD) and mild cognitive impairment (MCI). Unlike the previous two approaches, however, this approach uses 3D CNN modules, without shared parameters, directly on the 3D image volumes from the preprocessed fMRI sequence. The spatial representations learned from these CNN modules are concatenated and passed through the LSTM for prediction, demonstrating improved performance over 3D and 2D CNN architectures.

Taking a different approach to a hybrid CNN/LSTM architecture, Wang et al. [80] directly incorporated convolutions into an LSTM model during the state-to-state transition, and input networks. This allows the network to learn temporal dynamics while directly considering spatial information. This work was not carried out on a clinical task, focusing instead on individual subject identification, but the authors demonstrate improvement over RNN-only architectures in this novel approach to hybrid models for fMRI.

To more directly model both spatial and temporal dimensions, Mao et al. [81] attempt using 4D convolutions to predict ADHD diagnosis from rs-fMRI. Similar to the P3D [16] and R(2 + 1)D [17] architectures, Mao et al. [81] propose to decompose the convolutional filter into spatial and temporal components, except in this implementation the spatial dimension is 3D. They also compare this approach to a single frame 3D CNN, temporal pooling model, and CNN/LSTM hybrid models. As previously discussed in the context of 3D CNN architectures, adding another dimension to the CNN architecture significantly increases the computation complexity. To address this, the authors base predictions off relatively short clips (16 frames) sampled from the full scan. Results from this study show a modest improvement of the 4D CNN and CNN/LSTM architectures compared to the other architectures tested and previous results on the ADHD-200 dataset.

Taking a different approach to modeling the full spatiotemporal fMRI sequence using a CNN architecture, Xie et al. [82] converted the 4D image data into 3D volumes by reshaping the signal from all ROIs at a given timepoint into a 2D matrix, then concatenating the matrices from each time point along the third dimension. The authors suggest this approach is better than the more straightforward 2D representation of concatenated ROIs time-series, as it allows more ROIs to be included in a single convolution and formats the data to be compatible with other pre-trained architectures. This data is fed through a CNN network applying $1 \times 1 \times t$ (where t the size of the temporal dimension) convolutional filter to the 3D volume, ultimately generating a new 3D volume with depth 3 that is passed to the ResNet34 pre-trained CNN architecture [15]. On data from individual sites, this CNN based approach performs quite similarly to both the DeepFMRI model from Riaz et al. [76] and SC-CNN attention network from Zhang et al. [78], with no single model performing best for all sites in the ADHD-200 dataset.

While these previous works do demonstrate improvement over models using still images, or extracted (engineered) features, the results are modest, and leave much room for improvement. Despite using some of the largest fMRI datasets available for a single task, these are still substantially smaller than the video, or text, datasets that were used for developing the models described in Sect. 2. In addition, fMRI data have much higher resolution, and overall larger size compared to more generic videos, further increasing the need for more training data.

A more recent study from Thomas et al. [83] proposed using the same strategy as many of the successful *large language models*: leveraging the large banks of open fMRI data resources, the authors pre-train transformer-based models including an autoencoder, causal sequence model (CSM), and BERT architectures inspired by advances in NLP. To use these models, the authors reformat the 4D fMRI data into a 2D matrix of time-series derived from a functional parcellation. In this format, each timepoint in the scan can be represented as a vector of the intensity values from each region in the parcellation, similar to the word embedding structure used in NLP. When used for mental-decoding tasks, the pre-trained models significantly outperformed baseline models, with the CSM performing the best. The results from the pre-trained models were especially impressive when using small amounts of task-specific fine-tuning. The CSM, for example, was able to exceed 80% accuracy on two different datasets with fine-tuning data from only 3 participants, compared to the best results from the baseline models on the two datasets of 54% and 75%. While mental state decoding is not a clinical application, this stream of work investigating approaches to leverage pre-training could be valuable and potentially applied to medical tasks.

3.4.1 Graph Neural Networks

Another class of DL architecture, called graph neural networks (GNNs), have also garnered significant attention for modeling fMRI data. It has long been recognized that fMRI data may be represented as a graph structure, where spatial regions are represented as nodes, and an edge between two such nodes is labeled with the similarity between the time-series of the two regions associated with those nodes. While GNNs are specifically designed to work with and leverage the unique properties of graphs, to use these models, in most cases, it is required that fMRI data is first formatted into a graph structure, rather than working with the raw fMRI signals.

Most often, this is accomplished by generating FC matrices for the data, that can be either static (over the full scan) or dynamic (generated from sliding windows). Kong et al. [84], for example, used a dynamic GNN to diagnose MDD and predict treatment response using thresholded FC matrices generated from sliding windows. They proposed a spatiotemporal graph convolutional network (STGCN) that learns graph features from each window and performs temporal fusion using LSTM. This approach yielded impressive results of $\sim$84% diagnostic accuracy, and as high as 89% accuracy for predicting treatment response.

Contrarily, a more recent benchmark analysis of different GNN models for fMRI data [85], tested on large fMRI datasets for MDD diagnosis, ASD diagnosis, and sex classification, found relatively poor performance of GNN architectures when compared to non-graphical baseline models, including a SVM with radial basis function kernel using static FC features. These results were also significantly lower than what had been reported by Kong et al. [84] for MDD diagnosis, reaching only $\sim$58% balanced accuracy, despite considering a similar STGCN architecture (among others). Ultimately, the authors argue that the excitement around GNNs currently is not matched by their results.

4 Learning from Small Samples

When spatiotemporal models were first being explored in computer vision, Karpathy et al. [4] noted the lack of video datasets of size and variety comparable to the image datasets driving the development of CNN architectures. Following the release of their benchmark action recognition dataset, and others like it, however, substantial and rapid progress was made in spatiotemporal DL. In much the same way, current medical imaging applications of spatiotemporal DL have been hindered by the lack of available training datasets. While substantial progress has been made in releasing benchmark datasets in the medical imaging domain, they still lag behind natural image datasets.

In addition to the added challenges of compiling video datasets for DL, medical imaging data is highly controlled due to privacy and sharing restrictions, making the public release of these data more difficult. Annotation for supervised learning in medical applications can also be more challenging on the scale required for DL as it often requires specialized training or medical expertise. Moreover, routine clinical practice does not always lead clinicians to collect many of the spatiotemporal modalities discussed, nor other emerging imaging technologies. fMRI, for example, is only routinely used as part of presurgical planning for conditions such as epilepsy or brain tumors [86], despite considerable interest in the modality for applications such as psychiatry. As a result, these data are typically only collected as part of research studies, which typically have limited budgets and resources.

Spatiotemporal DL has great potential to produce more accurate predictive models in medicine, however, the potential cannot be fully explored without adequate amounts of data. This creates a kind of negative feedback loop, where without sufficient data, DL models cannot be developed, and without models, or tools to make sense of that data, many spatiotemporal imaging modalities will remain out of the clinical workflow.

Although medical imaging may pose additional challenges when creating datasets, small sample size has been a problem in many applications of DL and has been a focus of considerable research. The remainder of this section will describe several techniques that have been proposed for improving performance in DL models when data resources are limited. Given the breadth of research in this field, we will limit discussion to specific spatiotemporal implementations of select techniques, and considerations that should be made when applying them in medical imaging applications.

4.1 *Network Pre-training*

While medical spatiotemporal data can be difficult to accumulate, it is often more challenging to have sufficient amounts of data *labeled for a particular task*. Data from clinical research studies have protocols dictating strict inclusion and exclusion criteria, limiting the sample to a specific clinical population of interest. In addition, study protocols will strictly dictate what information is collected from patients, making it difficult to use data from one study for a different application, even if the populations of interest do overlap. Similarly, data collected in a clinical setting can be difficult to work with because only information relevant to patient treatment will be collected, and is often poorly annotated. Furthermore, records for a given patient may be kept in disjoint databases. Clinical data may also have poor population coverage, introducing substantial biases and limiting the capacity of models to generalize and work effectively when used in their target clinical setting.

Recognizing data sharing as a means to accelerate scientific research, many open clinical datasets have been released. These datasets may be annotated for a specific clinical task, and/or more openly combine images with various demographic and clinical variables. As these datasets may be collected for different tasks, they may have different types of labels, and so cannot be combined for any specific classification task. However, the rs-fMRI data collected for one study, is still rs-fMRI. Is it possible to use the rs-fMRI data collected for (say) MDD prediction, to help a study related to ADHD? As we do not know the ADHD-status of those MDD study subjects, those instances will be unlabeled. But there may still be ways to use that unlabelled data to improve the performance of an ADHD prediction model. (Of course, our use of rs-fMRI, MDD, ADHD is just for illustration; this could apply to an arbitrary imaging modality, and different study goals.)

Network pre-training approaches involve first training a model to perform a predictive task that is not the one of ultimate interest, and subsequently fine-tuning the same network on the smaller set of labeled data. The intuition behind these approaches is that the network first learns to perform a task on a large amount of available data, and then can transfer what has been learned to perform the task of interest. An important consideration in these approaches is what to use as a pre-training task, as it should enable the model to learn information that will ultimately aid in performing the final predictive task. In the subsequent sections we will discuss two popular techniques for model pre-training: (1) transfer learning, and (2) self-supervised learning (SSL), which differ in the type of task that is used to pre-train the network.

4.1.1 Transfer Learning

In the context of network pre-training, transfer learning involves learning a task from one dataset, and using the learned model as the basis for prediction on a different dataset - e.g., first learning a MDD model, then tweaking this to be an ADHD model. If an appropriate pre-training task is chosen, the learned representations should transfer to the new task to help improve generalization. Early adoption of transfer learning in imaging involved pre-training on large image datasets (such as ImageNet [2]) and fine-tuning on smaller datasets for the desired task; an approach that resulted in state-of-the-art performance on many tasks. The use of pre-trained 2D image data was also successfully used as the basis of many spatiotemporal models. As previously discussed, the pseudo-3D CNN architecture P3D ResNet [16] used pre-trained 2D CNN weights to initialize spatial filters. Many hypothesized that with sufficiently large datasets more general image features could be learnt and used for nearly every computer vision task.

Expectations have since been significantly dampened. He, Girshick, and Dollár [87] were one of the first to question whether blanket use of pre-training on massive image datasets provided as much benefit as many believed. Ultimately, they found that the same performance could be achieved by training models from random initialization, and pre-training on these massive datasets did not learn more "universal" features that would "solve" computer vision; for some tasks, these pre-trained models actually performed worse than models trained from scratch.

The same approach has been applied in medical imaging; directly utilizing off-the-shelf models from computer vision for medical applications. However, concerns have been raised about the use of natural image datasets for pre-training in medical applications [88], noting fundamental differences between the image types [33]. When comparing the performance of pre-trained models to those trained from scratch in various medical applications, Raghu et al. [88] found very little difference, but did note many pre-trained architectures were over-parameterized and could be replaced by much smaller architectures. These results, along with those from He, Girshick, and Dollár [87], were, however, based on still image prediction, and may not necessarily translate directly to spatiotemporal models.

In the clinical applications previously mentioned, a number of studies employed transfer learning techniques as part of development; many specifically using models trained on natural imaging data [59, 63, 68]. In a different approach, Côté-Allard et al. [53] use an inter-subject dataset to pre-train their gesture recognition model, and later fine-tune for individual users. Rather than simply using the pre-trained weights for initialization, they employ a number of techniques to avoid catastrophic forgetting [89].

The use of transfer learning, however, does not guarantee better model performance. For example, Thomas et al. [83] found pre-training their popular NLP models on text datasets provided no added benefit when working with fMRI data. Interestingly, Shad et al. [63] were able to effectively use an action recognition dataset to pre-train their model, but found that using another echocardiogram dataset did not improve performance.

Despite these findings, many agree that the use of transfer learning for tasks with especially small datasets is still valuable. As the size of medical imaging datasets continue to grow, however, this approach may become less useful.

4.1.2 Self-supervised Learning

In contrast to transfer learning, which involves learning from another annotated dataset, SSL approaches formulate learning tasks for *unlabelled* data—an idea we first introduced in Sect. 2.3.1 in the context of BERT [31] and large language models. Training the model to re-identify masked words and predict if different sentences originally belonged together in text, using massive, unlabelled text corpora, BERT was able to achieve impressive results—inspiring these approaches to be used in subsequent, larger NLP models.

As previously mentioned, Thomas et al. [83] were able to use similar SSL approaches to pre-train their NLP inspired models for fMRI data by asking the models to predict masked timepoints and determine if one sequence follows another. Since these tasks do not involve any information about the imaged subject, or their health status, they were able to leverage large amounts of fMRI data from different studies and open databases for pre-training.

One of the most popular approaches to SSL, also used by Thomas et al. [83], is *autoencoders*. Here, a NN is tasked with reconstructing the original input data, however, the data must pass through a bottleneck with lower dimensionality than the input, thus forcing the model to learn a compressed representation of the data. The encoder portion of the network, that transforms the original data to the compressed representation, can then be used as a component of a different supervised model.

To implement an autoencoder for fMRI data, Thomas et al. [83] used a bi-directional LSTM for their encoder, whose output, after pre-training, is fed to a decoding head for the downstream prediction task. Using this approach, they found very little difference in performance compared to models pre-trained with the NLP-inspired SSL tasks described previously, and again, substantially better than models without pre-training. Reynaud et al. [60] also used an autoencoder as part of their architecture, however, they use it to reduce spatial dimensionality; applying a 3D CNN ResNet autoencoder to every ultrasound frame before feeding the output into the spatiotemporal architecture.

The task of annotating datasets at the scale required for DL is extremely labor intensive, and in medical applications that require some degree of expertise, it may simply be infeasible. The value of SSL has already been demonstrated in the success of large language models, and as medical image data continues to be shared more openly, SSL approaches will likely become even more attractive for training DL models.

4.2 Regularization

Working with large, complex models, and relatively small amounts of training data, overfitting is a major concern: here, during training, models will appear to perform well on validation sets, but not generalize well on test data. Encompassing a large number of approaches to mitigate this, *regularization* refers to any modification made to model learning that should improve generalization error [90].

Many approaches involve expressing preferences for certain qualities of learned models. The classic examples being *L1-regularization* and *L2-regularization*, that each add an additional term to the cost function penalizing the use of larger weights. In effect, these models express a preference towards models utilizing fewer input features for prediction. Other approaches have been proposed more specifically for avoiding overfitting in DL architectures, such as dropout [91]. Here, however, we will limit discussion to more specific approaches used for spatiotemporal models, and considerations for applications using medical imaging. In particular, focusing on data augmentation approaches for spatiotemporal images, and multi-task learning.

4.2.1 Data Augmentation

Data augmentation approaches work to directly address limited training data by artificially inflating the number of training instances. A number of different approaches can be used to do this, from very simple random perturbations to more complex generative DL models. Given the ease with which simple approaches can be used, data augmentation of some form has become a nearly ubiquitous component of training DL architectures.

Many of the standard approaches used to augment image datasets can also be used for video data, with the stipulation that transformations, such as rotations, cropping, and translation are applied consistently to all frames in the temporal sequence. Many of these approaches were used in the applications discussed previously, including random rotations [63, 68], window cropping [13, 19, 27, 59], translation [59, 68], flipping [68], intensity perturbation [63], and noise injection [35]. While most of these approaches can be used in medical applications, special care should be taken to choose appropriate methods. The use of random horizontal flips, for example, may not be advisable for fMRI data where there may be unique unilateral functional properties. (In general, each of these transformations is applicable only in situations where the label does not depend on that transformation - e.g., if a certain shape at one location is a lesion, then that shape at a different location is also a lesion, etc.)

In addition to these spatial augmentation approaches, the temporal domain can also be used to generate additional training data. Like spatial cropping, temporal cropping can be applied to generate a number of clips of a fixed length from the full video sequence by randomly selecting different starting frames [13, 19, 27]. Mao et al. [81] took a slightly different approach: generating short clips by randomly sampling a small number of frames at fixed intervals in the temporal dimension. These approaches can be particularly well-suited to CNN architectures that require a fixed length input. Using short clips can also help to reduce computational complexity but may result in the loss of important long-range temporal information if the clip length is too short. Another spatial processing approach, cutout [92], involves occluding random image patches, simulating object occlusion and forcing the model to use more of the image when making predictions. Yao et al. [47] adapted this approach for temporal signals by randomly masking short temporal segments with zeros.

Again, the use of temporal augmentation approaches need to be thoughtfully considered in medical applications. When developing an echocardiogram-based approach for estimating LVEF, Reynaud et al. [60] note that, while most videos contain at least three cardiac cycles, the ground truth segmentations are only provided for the ES and ED frames from a single, representative cycle in each video. To avoid training the model with unlabelled ES/ED frames, they devise a guided random sampling approach where labeled frames are sampled, along with varying distances on either side that are small enough to guarantee no unlabelled ES/ED frames are included in the clip. They also use a mirroring approach where, instead of including a random number of frames on either side of the labeled frame, the transition frames either before or after the labeled frame are mirrored on the other side.

Beyond these simple techniques discussed here, more sophisticated models can be learned to generate new training examples. Most notably among these, generative adversarial networks (GANs) [93] can be used to generate realistic image data. GANs, and other generative models, are able to generate new, realistic data instances by learning a distribution from the training dataset, and then sampling from it. Although these approaches have had considerable success generating image data, extending these models to spatiotemporal data is not necessarily a straightforward task. In a recent report, Liu et al. [94] propose a conditional GAN (cGAN) [95] architecture for generating paired fMRI and structural MRI data, which were then added to the training set. The accuracy of the resulting learned model was only slightly ($<5\%$) better in diagnosing different psychiatric disorders than models trained on data from simpler augmentation approaches, or including no augmentation at all. In addition, these models can be very complex, computationally expensive, and also require substantial amounts of training data.

4.2.2 Multi-task Learning

Training on more than one label can constrain the model to learn more general representations that perform well on different tasks. While the idea of multi-task learning (MTL) [96] is similar to transfer learning and SSL (discussed in Sect. 4.1), there is a slight distinction. In network pre-raining approaches the networks are pre-trained and fine-tuned in two separate steps, whereas MTL involves co-learning the desired task and representations at the same time. In doing this, an inductive bias is imposed such that the model learns to perform well on all tasks simultaneously.

In the context of medical applications, there are often readily available labels that can be used for these purposes. In one of the first applications of MTL, Caruana et al. [97] use the results of future clinical tests (e.g., blood work, blood pressure) as additional training labels to improve patient risk assessment; showing an upwards of 10% improvement in error rate in some cases. More specifically, for medical imaging applications, auxiliary labels may include segmentations, anatomical localization, and parameter quantification (see [98] for a review).

Xue et al. [99] for example, use MTL to simultaneously quantify many indices of the LV since they are often highly correlated, along with cardiac phase identification.

Using a CNN/LSTM hybrid, where the frames from a cardiac MRI are passed through a shared CNN, and the representations are then used by two parallel RNN streams, one for LV quantification indices, and the second for cardiac phase identification, they demonstrate improved performance using MTL. In another example, Jahren et al. [58] include an auxiliary modality prediction task in their echocardiogram phase indexing model.

5 Conclusion

The improvements in accuracy observed moving from static images to video-based prediction highlights the importance of considering full spatiotemporal data in DL models. Given the importance of functionality in many clinical conditions, predictive models may need to incorporate temporal information to be sufficiently accurate for many clinical applications.

This chapter has provided an overview of advancements in spatiotemporal DL that form the basis of the architectures used in current medical imaging applications. As discussed, many proposed models for clinical applications draw heavily from, if not directly utilize, architectures proposed in other domains, such as C3D [14], R(2 + 1)D [17], hybrid CNN-LSTM, and BERT [31]. While these models have demonstrated the potential of spatiotemporal DL in medical imaging, architectures more specifically designed for the unique attributes of medical imaging data may yield further improvements [33]. (There are yet other directions to consider - e.g., incorporating multi-modality, and longitudinal data - which are beyond the scope of this article.)

Although the value of spatiotemporal DL in medical applications has been recognized, the development of these models has been significantly hindered by the lack of appropriate training datasets. As discussed, medical imaging data has strict privacy regulations controlling how the data is shared, and acquisition of these images is often expensive and typically limited to clinical and research settings. The task of curating a dataset of the size and variety needed for training these large and complex models requires significant time and resources, so it is not surprising that once a dataset is released, many models will be proposed using said data. As a result, clinical applications tend to cluster around available data resources.

While these large datasets are imperative for the continued development of DL models, they also push development disproportionately towards specific applications with available data [67], often constraining applications to focus on predetermined labels that may not be optimal. Limited availability of data is currently one of the greatest barriers to developing state-of-the-art DL models for medical imaging data, and significant future efforts should focus on increasing open data sharing initiatives; especially in light of the successful SSL approaches capable of learning from large, unlabelled datasets.

In the future, the demand for data will only continue to grow. As Dosovitskiy et al. [32] demonstrated in their work, with large enough pre-training datasets, a more general transformer architecture can outperform the inductive bias of CNNs for static image data. In our review of current clinical applications of spatiotemporal DL, there has also been an apparent shift towards more attention- and transformer-based architectures. From the success of ResNet [15] in increasing network depth, to the massive number of parameters in state-of-the-art large language models, model complexity has been consistently demonstrated as a way to improve performance.

Following the trend observed in computer vision, spatiotemporal DL in medical imaging has been able to demonstrate superior performance to models using static images in many applications. Advances in imaging technologies, data storage, computer hardware, and modeling approaches will enable the continued development of larger, and more complex models. While still in its infancy, the adoption of spatiotemporal DL into the medical domain has already produced impressive results and will likely become more routinely used as the performance of these models continues to improve.

References

1. LeCun Y, Bengio Y, Hinton G (2015) Deep learning. Nat 521:436–444
2. Deng J, Dong W, Socher R et al (2009) ImageNet: A large-scale hierarchical image database. In: 2009 IEEE Conf on Comput Vis and Pattern Recognit (pp. 248–255)
3. Soomro K, Zamir AR, Shah M (2012) UCF101: A dataset of 101 human actions classes from videos in the wild. arXiv preprint arXiv:1212.0402
4. Karpathy A, Toderici G, Shetty S et al (2014) Large-Scale Video Classification with Convolutional Neural Networks. In: 2014 IEEE Conf on Comput Vis and Pattern Recognit, (pp. 1725–1732)
5. Kay W, Carreira J, Simonyan K et al (2017) The kinetics human action video dataset. arXiv preprint arXiv:1705.06950.
6. Willamowski J, Arregui D, Csurka G et al (2004) Categorizing nine visual classes using local appearance descriptors. Illum 17(21)
7. Laptev I, Marszalek M, Schmid C et al (2008) Learning realistic human actions from movies. In: 2008 IEEE Conf on Comput Vis and Pattern Recognit (pp. 1–8)
8. Wang H, Kläser A, Schmid C et al (2013) Dense Trajectories and Motion Boundary Descriptors for Action Recognition. Int J Comput Vis 103:60–79
9. Wang H, Schmid C (2013) Action Recognition with Improved Trajectories. In: 2013 IEEE Int Conf on Comput Vis (pp. 3551–3558)
10. Lecun Y, Bottou L, Bengio Y et al (1998) Gradient-based learning applied to document recognition. In: Proc of the IEEE (pp. 2278–2324)
11. LeCun Y, Huang FJ, Bottou L (2004) Learning methods for generic object recognition with invariance to pose and lighting. In: Proc of the 2004 IEEE Comput Society Conf on Comput Vis and Pattern Recognit (pp. II–104)
12. Krizhevsky Alex, Sutskever I, Hinton G (2012) ImageNet Classification with Deep Convolutional Neural Networks. In: Adv in Neural Inf Process Syst
13. Simonyan K, Zisserman A (2014) Two-stream convolutional networks for action recognition in videos. In: Adv in Neural Inf Process Syst 27 (2014)
14. Tran D, Bourdev L, Fergus R et al (2014) Learning Spatiotemporal Features with 3D Convolutional Networks. In: Proc of the IEEE Int Conf on Comput Vis (pp. 4489–4497).
15. He K, Zhang X, Ren S et al (2016) Identity mappings in deep residual networks. In: Proc of the Comput Vis-ECCV 2016: 14th Eur Conf (pp. 630–645)

16. Qiu Z, Yao T, Mei T (2017) Learning Spatio-Temporal Representation with Pseudo-3D Residual Networks. In: Proc of the IEEE Int Conf on Comput Vis(pp. 5533–5541)
17. Tran D, Wang H, Torresani L et al (2018). A Closer Look at Spatiotemporal Convolutions for Action Recognition. In: Proc of the IEEE Conf on Comput Vis and Pattern Recognit (pp. 6450–6459)
18. Wang L, Xiong Y, Wang Z et al (2016) Temporal Segment Networks: Towards Good Practices for Deep Action Recognition. Temporal segment networks: Towards good practices for deep action recognition. In: Eur Conf on Comput Vis (pp. 20–36)
19. Varol G, Laptev I, Schmid C (2017) Long-term temporal convolutions for action recognition. IEEE Trans on Pattern Anal and Mach Intell 40(6):1510–1517
20. Rumelhart DE, Hinton GE, Williams RJ (1986) Learning representations by back-propagating errors. Nat 323(6088):533–536
21. Bengio Y, Simard P, Frasconi P (1994) Learning long-term dependencies with gradient descent is difficult. IEEE Trans on Neural Netw 5(2):157–166, 1994
22. Hochreiter S, Schmidhuber J (1997) Long Short-Term Memory. Neural Comput 9(8):1735–1780
23. Gers FA, Schmidhuber J, Cummins F (2000) Learning to Forget: Continual Prediction with LSTM. Neural Comput 12(10):2451–2471
24. Cho K, Merriënboer B, Bahdanau D, Bengio Y (2014) On the Properties of Neural Machine Translation: Encoder-decoder Approaches. In: Proc of SSST-8, Eighth Workshop on Syntax, Semant and Struct in Stat Transl
25. Chung J, Gulcehre C, Cho K, Bengio Y (2014) Empirical Evaluation of Gated Recurrent Neural Networks on Sequence Modeling. arXiv preprint, arXiv:1412.3555
26. Baccouche M, Mamalet F, Wolf C et al (2010) Action classification in soccer videos with long short-term memory recurrent neural networks. In: Proc ICANN(2)
27. Ng JYH, Hausknecht M, Vijayanarasimhan S et al (2015) Beyond Short Snippets: Deep Networks for Video Classification. In: Proc of the IEEE Conf on Comput Vis and Pattern Recognit (CVPR)
28. Donahue J, Anne Hendricks, L., Guadarrama S, Rohrbach M et al (2015) Long-term recurrent convolutional networks for visual recognition and description. In: Proc of the IEEE Conf on Comput Vis and Pattern Recognit (pp. 2625–2634)
29. Bahdanau D, Cho K, Yoshua B (2014) Neural Machine Translation by Jointly Learning to Align and Translate. arXiv preprint arXiv:1409.0473
30. Vaswani A, Shazeer N, Parmar N, Uszkoreit J, Jones L, Gomez AN, Kaiser L, Polosukhin I (2017) Attention Is All You Need. In: Proc of the 31st Int Conf on Neural Inf Process Syst
31. Devlin J, Chang MW, Lee K et al (2018) Bert: Pre-training of deep bidirectional transformers for language understanding. arXiv preprint arXiv:1810.04805.
32. Dosovitskiy A, Beyer L, Kolesnikov A, Weissenborn D, Zhai X, Unterthiner T, Dehghani M, Minderer M, Heigold G Gelly S, Uszkoreit J, Houlsby N (2020) An Image is Worth 16x16 Words: Transformers for Image Recognition at Scale. arXiv preprint arXiv:2010.11929
33. Langlotz CP, Allen B, Erickson BJ, et al (2019) A roadmap for foundational research on artificial intelligence in medical imaging: from the 2018 NIH/RSNA/ACR/The Academy Workshop. Radiol 291(3):781–791
34. Klem GH, Lüders HO, Jasper HH, et al (1999) The ten-twenty electrode system of the International Federation. The Int Fed of Clin Neurophysiol. Electroencephalogr Clin Neurophysiol Suppl 52:3–6
35. Salama ES, El-Khoribi RA, Shoman ME et al (2018) EEG-Based Emotion Recognition using 3D Convolutional Neural Networks. Int J of Adv Comput Sci and Appl 9(8)
36. Koelstra S, Muhl C, Soleymani M (2012) DEAP: A database for emotion analysis using physiological signals. IEEE Trans on Affect Comput 3(1):18–31
37. Cho J, Hwang H (2020) Spatio-temporal representation of an electoencephalogram for emotion recognition using a three-dimensional convolutional neural network. Sensors 20(12)
38. Song Y, Jia X, Yang L (2021) Transformer-based Spatial-Temporal Feature Learning for EEG Decoding. arXiv preprint arXiv:2106.11170

39. Brunner C, Leeb R, Muller-Putz GR et al (2008) BCI Competition 2008-Graz data set A. Inst for Knowl Discov (Laboratory of Brain-Computer Interfaces), Graz Univ of Technol, 16, 1–6
40. Aslam MH, Usman SM, Khalid S et al (2022) Classification of EEG Signals for Prediction of Epileptic Seizures. Appl Sci 12(14):7251
41. Bardeci M, Ip CT, Olbrich S (2021) Deep learning applied to electroencephalogram data in mental disorders: A systematic review. Biological Psychol 162:108–117
42. Liu Y, Pu C, Xia S et al (2022) Machine learning approaches for diagnosing depression using EEG: A review. Transl Neurosci 13(1):224–235
43. Mousavi S, Afghah F, Acharya UR (2019) SleepEEGNet: Automated sleep stage scoring with sequence to sequence deep learning approach. PLOS ONE 14(5)
44. Rafie N, Kashou AH, Noseworthy PA (2021) ECG Interpretation: Clinical Relevance, Challenges, and Advances. Hearts 2(4):505–513
45. Pantelopoulos A, Bourbakis NG (2010) A Survey on Wearable Sensor-Based Systems for Health Monitoring and Prognosis. IEEE Transact on Syst, Man, and Cybern, Part C (Appl and Rev). 40(1):1–12
46. Sun W, Kalmady SV, Salimi A et al (2022) ECG for high-throughput screening of multiple diseases: Proof-of-concept using multi-diagnosis deep learning from population-based datasets. arXiv preprint arXiv:2210.06291
47. Yao Q, Wang R, Fan X et al (2020) Multi-class Arrhythmia detection from 12-lead varied-length ECG using Attention-based Time-Incremental Convolutional Neural Network. Inf Fusion 53:174–182
48. Che C, Zhang P, Zhu M et al (2021) Constrained transformer network for ECG signal processing and arrhythmia classification. BMC Med Inform Decis Mak 21(184)
49. Somani S, Russak AJ, Richter F et al (2021) Deep learning and the electrocardiogram: review of the current state-of-the-art. EP Europace 23(8):1179–1191
50. Atzori M, Gijsberts A, Kuzborskij I et al (2015) Characterization of a benchmark database for myoelectric movement classification. IEEE Transact on Neural Syst and Rehabilitation Eng 23(1):73–83
51. Park KH, Lee SW (2016) Movement intention decoding based on deep learning for multiuser myoelectric interfaces. In: 4th Int Winter Conf on Brain-Comput Interface
52. Tommasi T, Orabona F, Castellini C et al (2013) Improving Control of Dexterous Hand Prostheses Using Adaptive Learning. IEEE Transact on Robotics 29(1):207–219
53. Côté-Allard U, Fall CL, Drouin A et al (2019) Deep Learning for Electromyographic Hand Gesture Signal Classification Using Transfer Learning. IEEE Transact on Neural Syst and Rehabilitation Eng 27(4):760–771
54. Ravichandran T, Kamel N, Al-Ezzi AA et al (2021) Electrooculography-based Eye Movement Classification using Deep Learning Models. In: 2020 IEEE-EMBS Conf on Biomedical Eng and Sci (IECBES) (pp. 57–61)
55. Hernandez KAL, Rienmüller T, Baumgartner D et al (2021) Deep learning in spatiotemporal cardiac imaging: A review of methodologies and clinical usability. Comput in Biology and Medicine 130
56. Fiorito AM, Østvik A, Smistad E et al (2018) Detection of cardiac events in echocardiography using 3D convolutional recurrent neural networks. In: 2018 IEEE Int Ultrasonics Symp (IUS) (pp. 1–4)
57. Dezaki TF, Liao Z, Luong C et al (2019) Cardiac phase detection in echocardiograms with densely gated recurrent neural networks and global extrema loss. IEEE Trans Med Imag 38(8):1821–1832
58. Jahren TS, Steen EN, Aase SA et al (2020) Estimation of End-Diastole in Cardiac Spectral Doppler Using Deep Learning. IEEE Trans on Ultrason, Ferroelectr, and Freq Control 67(12):2605–2614
59. Ouyang D, He B, Ghorbani A et al (2020) Video-based AI for beat-to-beat assessment of cardiac function. Nat 580:252–256
60. Reynaud H, Vlontzos A, Hou B et al (2021) Ultrasound Video Transformers for Cardiac Ejection Fraction Estimation. In: Proc of Med Image Comput and Comput Assist Interv-MICCAI 2021, Part VI 24 (pp. 495–505)

61. Kalam K, Otahal P, Marwick TH (2014) Prognostic implications of global LV dysfunction: a systematic review and meta-analysis of global longitudinal strain and ejection fraction. Heart. 100(21):1673–80
62. Tsai CH, Ma HP, Lin YT et al (2020) Usefulness of heart rhythm complexity in heart failure detection and diagnosis. Sci Rep 10(1):14916
63. Shad R, Quach N, Fong R et al (2021) Predicting post-operative right ventricular failure using video-based deep learning. Nat Commun 12:5192
64. Hwang IC, Choi D, Choi YJ et al (2022) Differential diagnosis of common etiologies of left ventricular hypertrophy using a hybrid CNN-LSTM model. Sci Rep 12:20998
65. Zaman F, Ponnapureddy R, Wang YG et al (2021) Spatio-temporal Hybrid Neural Networks Reduce Erroneous Human "Judgment Calls" in the Diagnosis of Takotsubo Syndrome. EClinicalMedicine 40:101115
66. Kwong RY, Yucel EK (2003) Computed Tomography Scan and Magnetic Resonance Imaging. Circ 108(15):e104–e106
67. Varoquaux G, Cheplygina V (2022) Machine learning for medical imaging: methodological failures and recommendations for the future. NPJ Digit. Med. 5(1):48
68. Mittermeier A, Reidler P, Fabritius MP et al (2022) End-to-End Deep Learning Approach for Perfusion Data: A Proof-of-Concept Study to Classify Core Volume in Stroke CT. Diagn 12(5):1142
69. Simonyan K, Zisserman A (2014) Very deep convolutional networks for large-scale image recognition. arXiv preprint arXiv:1409.1556
70. Hu T, Lei Y, Su J et al (2021) Learning spatiotemporal features of DSA using 3D CNN and BiConvGRU for ischemic moyamoya disease detection. Int J of Neurosci 1–11
71. Nielsen M, WaldmannM, Frölich AM et al (2021) Deep Learning-Based Automated Thrombolysis in Cerebral Infarction Scoring: A Timely Proof-of-Principle Study. Stroke 52:3497–3504
72. Tan M, Le QV (2019) EfficientNet: Rethinking model scaling for convolutional neural networks. In: Int Conf on Machine Learn (pp. 6105–6114)
73. Ashby FG (2015) An introduction to fMRI. In: Forstmann BU, Wagenmakers E-J (ed) An introduction to model-based cognitive neuroscience, 91–112. Springer International Publishing
74. Damoiseaux JS, Rombouts SARB, Barkhof F et al (2006) Consistent resting-state networks across healthy subjects. Proc Natl Acad Sci USA 103(37):13848–13853
75. Li X, Dvornek NC, Papademetris X, et al (2018) 2-Channel convolutional 3D deep neural network (2CC3D) for fMRI analysis: ASD classification and feature learning. In: IEEE Int Symp on Biomed Imaging (pp. 1252–1255)
76. Riaz A, Asad M ,Alsano E et al (2020) DeepFMRI: End-to-end deep learning for functional connectivity and classification of ADHD using fMRI. J Neurosci Methods 335:0165–0270
77. Riaz A, Asad M, Al-Arid SMMR, et al (2017) Fcnet: a convolutional neural network for calculating functional connectivity from functional mri. In: Proc Int Workshop on Connectomics in NeuroImaging (pp. 70–78)
78. Zhang T, Li C, Li P et al (2020) Separated Channel Attention Convolutional Neural Network (SC-CNN-Attention) to Identify ADHD in Multi-Site Rs-fMRI Dataset. Entropy 22(8):893
79. Li W, Lin X, Chen X (2020) Detecting Alzheimer's disease Based on 4D fMRI: An exploration under deep learning framework. Neurocomputing 388:280–287
80. Wang L, Li K, Chen X et al (2019) Application of convolutional recurrent neural network for individual recognition based on resting state fMRI data. Front in Neurosci 13:434
81. Mao Z, Su Y, Xu G, et al (2019) Spatio-temporal deep learning method for ADHD fMRI classification. Inf Sci 499:1–11
82. Xie J, Huo Z, Liu X et al (2022) An fMRI Sequence Representation Learning Framework for Attention Deficit Hyperactivity Disorder Classification. Appl Sci 12(12):6211
83. Thomas AW, Ré C, Poldrack RA (2022) Self-supervised learning of brain dynamics from broad neuroimaging data. arXiv preprint arXiv:2206.11417
84. Kong Y, Gao S, Yue Y et al (2021) Spatio-temporal graph convolutional network for diagnosis and treatment response prediction of major depressive disorder from functional connectivity. Hum Brain Mapp 42(12):3922–3933

85. El Gazzar A, Thomas R, Van Wingen G (2022) Benchmarking Graph Neural Networks for FMRI analysis. arXiv preprint arXiv:2211.08927
86. Specht K (2020) Current challenges in translational and clinical fMRI and future directions. Front Psychiatry 10:924
87. He K, Girshick R, Dollár P (2018) Rethinking ImageNet Pre-training. In: Procof the IEEE/CVF Int Conf on Comput Vis (pp. 4918–4927)
88. Raghu M, Zhang C, Kleinberg J et al (2019) Transfusion: Understanding Transfer Learning for Medical Imaging. Adv in Neural Inf Process Syst 32
89. Rusu AA, Rabinowitz NC, Desjardins G et al (2016) Progressive neural networks. arXiv preprint arXiv:1606.04671.
90. Goodfellow I, Bengion Y, Courville A (2016) Deep Learning. MIT Press
91. Srivastava N, Hinton G, Krizhevsky A et al (2014) Dropout: A Simple Way to Prevent Neural Networks from Overfitting. J of Mach Learn Res 15(56):1929–1958
92. DeVries T, Taylor GW (2017) Improved regularization of convolutional neural networks with cutout, arXiv preprint arXiv:1708.04552.
93. Goodfellow IJ, Pouget-Abadie J, Mirza M et al (2014) Generative Adversarial Networks. Commun ACM 63(11):139–144.
94. Liu R, Huang ZA, Hu Y et al (2022) Attention-Like Multimodality Fusion With Data Augmentation for Diagnosis of Mental Disorders Using MRI. In: IEEE Trans on Neural Netw and Learn Syst
95. Mirza M, Osindero S (2014) Conditional Generative Adversarial Nets. arXiv preprint arXiv:1411.1784
96. Caruana R (1993) Multitask learning: A knowledge-based source of inductive bias1. In: Proc of the Tenth Int Conf on Mach Learn (pp. 41–48)
97. Caruana R, Baluja S, Mitchell T (1995) Using the future to "sort out" the present: Rankprop and multitask learning for medical risk evaluation. In: Adv in Neural Inf Process Syst 8
98. Zhao Y, Wang X, Che T et al (2023) Multi-task deep learning for medical image computing and analysis: A review. Comput Biol Med 153:106496
99. Xue W, Brahm G, Pandey S et al (2017) Full left ventricle quantification via deep multitask relationships learning. Med Image Anal43:54–65

Skin Cancer Classification with Convolutional Deep Neural Networks and Vision Transformers Using Transfer Learning

Muniba Ashfaq and Asif Ahmad

Abstract The deadliest type of skin cancer is melanoma. Melanocytes are the cells where cancerous growths take place. The cells create melanin pigment, which gives skin its color. Sun exposure to bodily parts is the primary cause of cancer. The formation of a new pigment, changes to an existing mole, or unusual growth on the skin are all indicators of malignancy. A patient with melanoma who receives early detection and treatment has a 99% probability of surviving five years. A melanoma patient who has had malignant (cancerous) tissue removed can recover when the disease is still in its early stages. Malignant (non-cancerous) tumors frequently form in melanocytes. These benign tumors resemble melanoma in many ways and take the shape of moles (nevi). It might be challenging for doctors to distinguish benign tumors from melanoma. Various deep neural networks (DNN) have been taken into consideration. Our research compares the results obtained by using traditional Convolutional Neural Networks (CNN) with those obtained using Vision Transformer (ViT) for skin cancer classification. We fine-tuned the pre-trained Vision Transformer (ViT) model on ImageNet 2012, which contains one million images and one thousand classes, at a resolution of 224 × 224. Prior to that, the model was pre-trained on ImageNet-21k, which includes 14 million images and 21,843 classes, also at a resolution of 224 × 224. The results show that EfficientNet-B3 performed best as compared to other CNN models and vision transformer with the same input image resolution of 224 × 224 and top layers configuration.

Keywords Transfer Learning · Neural network · Vision Transformer · Medical images classification

M. Ashfaq (✉)
Department of Computer Systems Engineering, University of Engineering and Technology Peshawar, Peshawar, Pakistan
e-mail: muniba@uetpeshawar.edu.pk

A. Ahmad
Faculty of Engineering Sciences, Ghulam Ishaq Khan Institute of Engineering Sciences and Technology, Topi, Pakistan
e-mail: asif.ahmad@giki.edu.pk

H. Ali et al. (eds.), *Advances in Deep Generative Models for Medical Artificial Intelligence*, Studies in Computational Intelligence 1124,
https://doi.org/10.1007/978-3-031-46341-9_6

1 Introduction

In many regions of the world, skin cancer is more common among individuals with fair skin. There is a significant emergence of public health issues with the increasing ratio of incidence and the rates of morbidity and mortality. Ultra-violet radiation (UVR) is the primary factor that contributes to formation of skin cancers. The DNA damage and genetic mutations brought on by UVR results in its development [1]. World Health Organization reports that skin cancer is one-third of all cancer cases world-wide. The major health concern that impacts people is skin cancer [2]. Non-melanoma skin cancer (NMSC) predominantly consists of basal cell carcinoma (BCC) and squamous cell carcinoma (SCC), which are the most prevalent forms of cancer among people across the globe [3]. Nearly 1% of skin cancer diagnoses in the US are melanoma, yet it is this disease that results in the majority of skin cancer fatalities. Many melanoma patients recover fully from their initial surgery. From the time of initial diagnosis, the 5-year survival rate in melanoma cases is 93% [4].

Globally, the (Asymmetry, Border Irregularity, Color, Diameter, and Evolution) ABCD(E) criteria are used in medical education for assessing pigmented lesions that need to be further analyzed by a dermatologist [5]. In melanocytes, benign (non-cancerous) tumours frequently form. These benign tumours resemble melanoma in appearance and take the shape of moles (nevi). Traditional methods of detection, such as visual inspection by a dermatologist or the use of dermoscopic images, have limited accuracy and are subject to human error. It might be challenging for a dermatologist to distinguish benign tumours from melanoma. It also depends on their expertise and years of experience [6].

To help dermatologists and enable automatic melanoma detection, computer-aided diagnosis systems (CAD) are necessary. In this context, deep learning has revolutionized, particularly in the detection of melanoma, the most deadly form of skin cancer. Deep learning makes use of artificial neural networks and final decision based on learning input images using training. The purpose of these neural networks is to simulate how the human brain processes information, analyze large data and identify patterns that may be too subtle for humans to detect. Moreover, train the deep learning algorithms to analyze skin lesions images and identify the presence of melanoma with high accuracy [7–9].

There are several ways in which deep learning can be used to detect melanoma. One approach is to use deep learning algorithms to analyze images of skin lesions and identify those that are likely to be melanoma. Different techniques can be used, including convolutional neural networks (CNNs) [10], which are well suited to image analysis tasks. Another approach is to use deep learning to analyze data from electronic health records (EHRs) [11] to identify risk factors for melanoma. This can help doctors to identify individuals who may be at higher risk of developing the disease and take preventive measures to reduce that risk.

Moreover, transfer learning is a powerful strategy where the training is initially on a specific classification and then extending it to produce results for some different but related classification using fine-tuning. In order to train a high-performing model, this can lower the requirement of computational resources and the amount of data, making it a particularly useful approach in situations where there is limited data available.

In the context of skin cancer melanoma detection, transfer learning has been used to leverage the large data and computational resources to train models for image classification on the ImageNet [12] dataset. By using a already trained model as an initial point and after that fine-tuning for skin cancer melanoma detection, researchers have been able to achieve high levels of accuracy with relatively small annotated data.

Recent studies have demonstrated the effectiveness of transfer learning using a variety of pre-trained models and fine-tuning strategies. Different CNN architectures are available that include AlexNet [13], VGG Net [14], GoogleNet [15, 16], ResNet [16], ResNeXt [17], inception-V3 [18], Inception-V4 [19] and Inception-ResNet [19], DenseNet [20], and Xception [21]. In particular, for melanoma detection, the authors [22] used five different models that include VGG16, VGG19, ResNet50, DenseNet121, and Inception V3 model. They validated significant improvement in the transfer learning and data augmentation techniques as compared to the baseline method. These studies demonstrate the potential of transfer learning to enable accurate and efficient skin cancer melanoma detection. The transfer learning will likely continue its contribution to the development of effective and practical solutions for multiple real world problems. The detection and treatment of skin cancer, particularly melanoma, have the potential to be completely transformed by deep learning. By harnessing the power of artificial intelligence, we may be able to detect melanoma at an earlier stage and improve the chances of survival for those who are diagnosed with the disease.

Overall, deep learning has the power and capability to revolutionize the way that we detect and treat skin cancer, including melanoma. By harnessing the power of artificial intelligence, we may be able to detect melanoma at an earlier stage and improve the chances of survival for those who are diagnosed with the disease.

2 Related Work

Several studies have depicted the effectiveness of deep learning in skin cancer categorization. Authors [8] used DCNN-SVM where the usefulness of transfer learning is analyzed. In one study [23] pre-trained CNN models (VGG16, VGG19, MobileNet, and NASNet) are used for its classification. Moreover, Sparrow Search Algorithm is used as an optimizer to further improve the results on HAM10K dataset. Similarly, authors [24] used ResNet-50, and EfficientNet-B0 and fine-tuned these models on HAM10K dataset of skin cancers. The modified architecture and fine-tuned ResNet50 are deployed to classify skin cancers [25]. The class-weighted learning strategy allocates different weights to different classes and balances the data. The use of the loss function known as focal loss is an additional approach to get better performance. The ResNet50 model is evaluated against VGG16, MobileNet, and EfficientNet B1 as base models. Furthermore, the classification of skin cancer is performed followed by segmentation [26]. The decorrelation formulation technique is used to preprocess the images. The MASK-RCNN model is used to segment skin lesions and the DenseNet model is used to extract features using average pool and fully connected by employing transfer learning in ISBI2016, ISBI2017, and HAM10000 datasets.

In [27] authors considered a two steps classification using transfer learning and deep learning by dividing the skin cancer class types into two sets. The dataset HAM10K is used for classification purposes. They utilized randomly selected images for training and testing as 80 and 20 in the first place and 20 and 5 in the second place respectively. The modified architecture of pre-trained Xception model [28] is used for skin cancer classification using transfer learning and is accomplished by introducing additional one, two, and one layers of pooling, dense, and dropout respectively. The Fully Connected (FC) layer is transformed to classify seven skin disease classes. To overcome the data misbalancing data augmentation technique is used.

Moreover, the transfer learning method is also used in plain and hierarchical classification models to distinguish between seven classes of moles [29] and data augmentation to balance data. The DenseNet201 network achieved high classification accuracy. The hierarchical model is used to overcome the data preference for the nevi class.

In another study [30], authors used balanced accuracy and precision as performance metrics to evaluate ResNet, Xception, and DenseNet models on the HAM10000 dataset. Here, the Xception models only achieved better performance in the case of balanced accuracy, DenseNet was able to achieve both good balanced accuracy and precision, while ResNet's results were low in all.

Another popular technique called atrous or, dilated convolution using transfer learning is proposed on VGG16, VGG19, MobileNet, and InceptionV3 models [31]. The dilated convolution performed better on as compared to the traditional CNN with the same computational cost.

Moreover, skin image datasets acquired from two different sites (different clinical settings) are used for melanoma detection [32]. They presented the cross-domain skin disease recognition capability of the two-step progressive transfer learning on pre-trained models and suggested adversarial learning to domain adaptation strategy.

These findings suggest that deep learning can greatly be used to get better accuracy and quick detection of melanoma. Recently, the computer vision community has taken an interest in applying Transformer networks [33], which have been successful in natural language processing (NLP), to vision-related problems. For skin cancer classification, a new and improved transformer network called SkinTrans [34] has been proposed, which uses a three-step process. First, the Vision Transformer (ViT) network is utilized, followed by multi-scale and overlapping sliding windows with multi-scale patch embedding used to serialize the images. Finally, to ensure similar skin cancer data is encoded similarly, contrastive learning is used to make the distinct encoding outcomes of data.

Furthermore, a two-step approach is utilized to classify skin cancer using the Medical Vision Transformer (MVT) [35]. The primary stage addresses data unbalancing through data augmentation, while the MVT is employed in the subsequent stage. MVT utilized smaller patches of input image, which are subsequently passed in a sequential pattern and Multi-Layer Perceptron (MLP) at the end is used for classification.

DeepViT [36] is another transformer network utilized and the performance of both ViT and DeepViT is compared to that of VGGNet and ResNet pre-trained models. DeepViT distinguishes itself from ViT by using a re-attention mechanism. However, experimental results have demonstrated that CNN models perform better than ViT and DeepViT, particularly with small medical datasets.

Another study revealed the use of TransSLC [37] for skin cancer classification. The bi-directional encoder representation is used in the transformer model on HAM10K dataset. Other versions of the transformer for skin cancer classification include an enhanced deep bottleneck transformer model [38], swin transformer model [39], MT-TransUNet [40], and fully transformer network [41].

The research study and the techniques presented here related to applying vision transformer is mostly consuming more computational power to execute large deep networks to get trained and then test for unknown skin cancer data. The architectural details of some of the methodologies are also not clear to reproduce the results. Moreover, the classification result of each class of skin cancer is not presented in some of the previous research related to vision transformers. Furthermore, the base model name of the vision transformer is also not mentioned. Mostly, the standard vision transformer has been modified with extended layers and is integrated with other techniques to produce skin based vision transformers. Contrary to the previous research, our main aim is to apply transfer learning to the traditional and most popular pre-trained convolutional neural network models and the vision transformer. For performance comparison purposes, the top layers are replaced by the same common layers to categorize skin cancer. In addition to this, less computational power and memory requirement as compared to the skin based vision transformers is used such that it is easily accessible to the research community through online freely available platforms i.e., Google Colab, and Kaggle. Overall, the usefulness of deep learning in skin cancer detection shows significant promise for enhancing melanoma early detection and care. Further research is needed to optimize the use of these algorithms and to explore their potential for use in other forms of skin cancer detection.

3 Methodology

Four different convolutional neural network-based models and vision transformer are used to categorize skin cancer as melanoma and non-melanoma. DL algorithms' fundamental building blocks are neural networks. They are made up of input, hidden, and output layers. Each node inside each layer is connected to other nodes and has a corresponding weight and threshold. The node is triggered and begins sending data to the following layer if the output exceeds the threshold value. CNNs are extensively used for medical image analysis and diagnosis. Here, huge deep neural networks that have already been trained and optimized are employed in conjunction with transfer learning approaches. The dataset used here is HAM10000 ISIC dataset. In the first step, we configure and initialize the deep neural network models (VGG16, ResNET50, InceptionResnerv2, and EfficientNet-B3) for the detection of melanoma. In the second step, we used pre-trained deep neural networks and apply transfer learning by fine-tuning with the HAM10000 ISIC dataset. We compare the classification results of traditional CNN-based models i.e., VGG16, ResNET50, InceptionResnerv2, and EfficientNet with the powerful vision transformer (ViT). The Vision Transformer (ViT) is an encoder architecture transformer based model that has been trained in a supervised manner using a vast collection of images, particularly the ImageNet-21k dataset. The model has a resolution of 224×224 pixels and was fine-tuned on the ImageNet dataset, which consists of 1 million images and 1,000 categories, also at a resolution of 224×224.

3.1 Dataset

Initially, the skin cancer detection, classification, and segmentation studies were based on limited skin lesion datasets. With the introduction of deep learning models, there was a need for a vast amount of data to train these models for high accuracy. To overcome this issue and to provide the research community with a comprehensive skin cancer classification dataset, the HAM10000 dataset was introduced in 2018 [42]. This dataset consists of 10,015 dermoscopy images of skin lesions, with seven distinct categories of skin cancer as shown in Fig. 1. The dataset includes two malig-

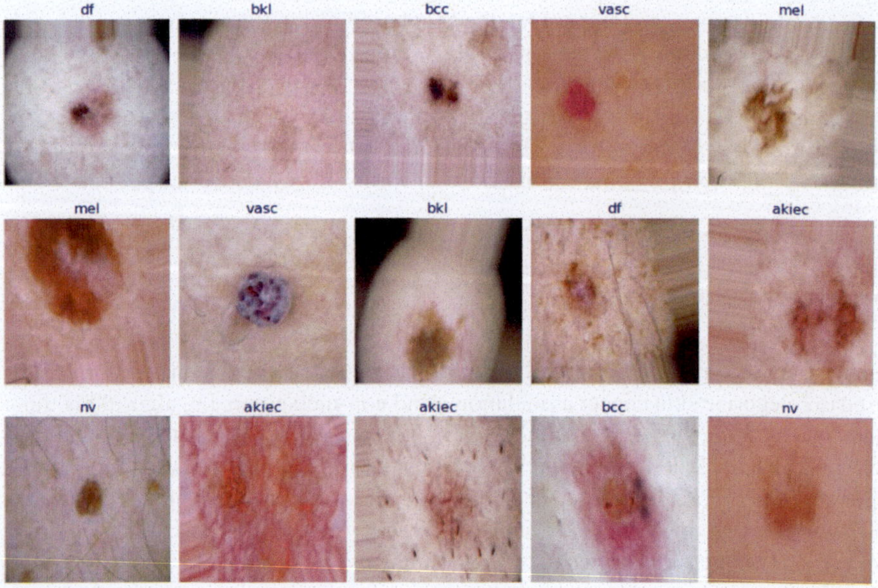

Fig. 1 Skin Cancer Cases (Actinic Kerastoses (akiec), Basal Cell Carninoma (bcc), Benign Keratosis (bkl), Dermatofibroma (df), Melanocytic nervi (nv), Vascular Skin Lesions (vasc), and Melanoma (mel)) from HAM10000 dataset after applying data augmentation technique

Table 1 HAM10000 dataset classes and details

Abbreviation	Class	Value	No. of Samples	Type
akiec	Actinic Kerastoses	0	327	Benign or Malignant
bcc	Basal Cell Carcinoma	1	514	Malignant
bkl	Benign Keratosis	2	1099	Benign
df	Dermatofibroma	3	115	Benign
nv	Melanocytic nervi	4	6705	Benign
vasc	Vascular Skin Lesions	5	142	Benign or Malignant
mel	Melanoma	6	1113	Malignant

nant classes, which are 1113 cases of melanoma (mel) and 514 cases of basal cell carcinoma (bcc). Furthermore, it comprises five benign classes, including 6705 cases of melanocytic nevi (nv), 1099 cases of benign keratosis-like lesion (bkl), 327 cases of Actinic keratoses/ Bowen's disease (akiec), and 142 cases of vascular(vasc). The images used in the study were collected from two sources: the Department of Dermatology at the Medical University of Vienna in Austria, and the skin cancer practice of Cliff Rosendahl in Queensland, Australia. The data was obtained over a period of 20 years and the image labels were confirmed using various methods including histopathology, reflectance confocal microscopy, follow-up, and expert consensus. The pixel resolution of the skin cancer images is 600×450. Despite having 10,015 skin lesion images, an analysis of the metadata reveals that there are only 7470 distinct skin lesions. The remaining images are duplicates taken at various magnifications or perspectives. The dataset is also very unbalanced. As an illustration, the largest class (nv) has 6705 images, whilst the smallest class (df) only has 115. Since there are not an equal amount of images in each class, the model will be heavily biased toward the largest class, which accounts for about 67% of the total data, if training is done using this unequal amount of data for each class. The total samples and abbreviation of each skin cancer class along with the type as benign or malignant is shown in Table 1. Moreover, the abbreviation and corresponding label values are also shown.

3.2 *Preprocessing*

There are collectively seven distinct types of skin cancer in HAM10000 dataset. We separate each class's data and divided it into training, validation, and testing sets. The training set is 70% of the data selected from each class. The validation is 20% and testing is 10% of the dataset of each class. In this way, 10,015 skin images are now divided into 7007 training, 1008 testing, and 2000 validation samples. This dataset has highly imbalanced classes. On one side, one class melanocytic nervi has 6705 samples and on the other hand, dermatofibroma is as low as 115 samples. To deal with the highly imbalanced class effect, data augmentation is performed. We select a threshold of 3000 training samples and 500 validation samples for each class. Only

3000 samples are consumed even for the case where samples are more than 3000. The class that has fewer samples is populated to the 3000 samples using the data augmentation technique. Similar is the case for the validation set with 500 samples for each class. However, the testing set is the same as the result of initial segregation to the testing set and all samples are preserved for this purpose.

The data is augmented to modify the image transformations in any of the image dimensions. The dimensions that we set for modifications include horizontal and vertical flips. Moreover, the rotation is set to randomly select in the range of + 20 to – 20 °C. Images can be shifted horizontally or vertically with the value of horizontal and vertical shift set to 0.2. Besides, the images may undergo zoom in/out and shear with 0.2 factor. The data is normalized per sample by subtracting the mean and dividing by the standard deviation. Furthermore, to guarantee the standardized image resolution, the images are resized to 224×224.

3.3 Pre-trained Model Architectures

3.3.1 VGG16

The VGG16 is a variant of VGGNet released by the University of Oxford Visual Geometry Group (VGG) [14] in 2014. It is trained on ImageNet dataset [43] of 14 million images and contains 1000 classes. The VGG16 model was developed to increase the depth and the convolutional layers to increase the accuracy of image classification problems. It outperforms AlexNet and showed that increasing the performance depth of architecture makes significant improvement as compared to expansion. The VGG16 architecture is extensively used as a benchmark model in computer vision research because it performs well in a variety of image classification tasks.

The VGG16 model is composed of 16 layers, which consist of 3 fully-connected layers and 13 convolutional layers, as well as 5 max pooling layers. The model uses convolutional layers for input image intricate features, while the fully connected layers are employed to classify skin cancer. In comparison to AlexNet (11×11), VGG16 uses smaller convolutional filters (3×3), which helps to increase the model's depth without populating the number of parameters. Max-pooling layers with convolution kernel of size (2×2) and stride of 2, which are used in VGG16, lower the spatial dimension of the feature maps and strengthen the model's translation invariance. AlexNet employs average pooling, which is less efficient. All convolutional layers in VGG16 have the same amount of filters (3×3) and stride 1, simplifying the architecture and improving training efficiency. Three fully connected layers are incorporated in the VGG16 model. A max-pooling layer and a ReLU activation function are added after each convolutional layer. In the VGG16 model, each of the three fully connected layers is followed by a ReLU activation function. A probability distribution over the classes is generated by feeding the output of the final fully connected layer into a softmax activation function, which uses the fully connected layers for classification.

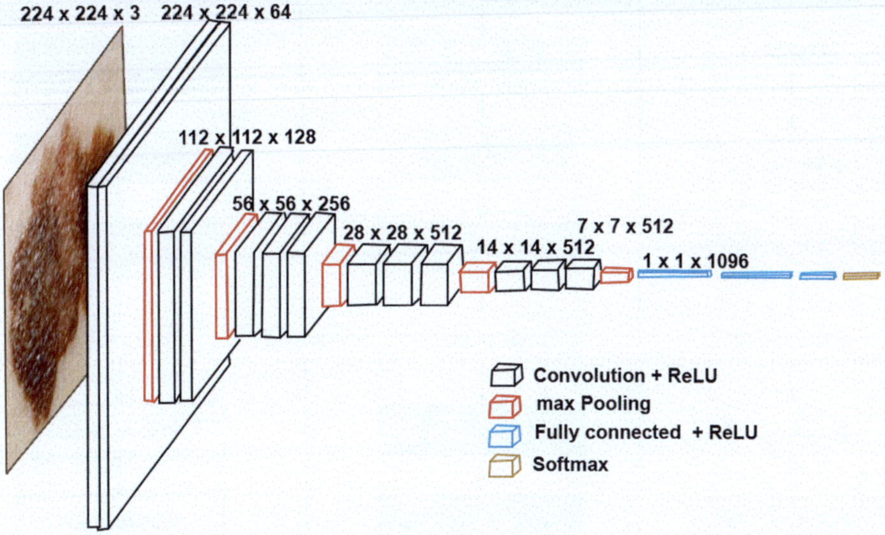

Fig. 2 VGG16 Architecture containing convolution, max pooling, and fully connected layers

The dimension of the input image to the VGG16 model is ($224 \times 224 \times 3$) displayed in Fig. 2. The first convolutional layer, composed of 64 filters, is run over the input image. The consecutive convolutional layers apply 128, 256, and 512 filters. Max pooling layers are placed after each set of convolutional layers. Three fully connected layers are used to further process the output of the final max pooling layer, with the number of neurons in each layer dropping from 4096 to 4096 and 1000, respectively. The network's final output is produced by passing the output of the third fully connected layer through a softmax activation function. Figure 3 displays the architectural details of the VGG16 model.

3.3.2 ResNET50

ResNet50 was trained on the ImageNet dataset and was released by Microsoft Research Asia. This model won the ILSVRC 2015 classification competition [16], indicating its exceptional performance. ResNet50 is an extended version of the ResNet architecture, which stands for "Residual Network". ResNet50 comprises 50 layers in its architecture and was designed to address the problem of vanishing gradients. Vanishing gradients occur due to the increased depth of the network, which can make learning difficult during backpropagation, as the gradient becomes smaller and smaller. To overcome this issue, the authors of ResNet50 introduced the concept of "residual connections", which are short-cut connections that allow gradients to move straight to earlier layers by skipping one or more network layers. This ensures that gradient information is preserved, enabling the network to learn even with a much more complex architecture.

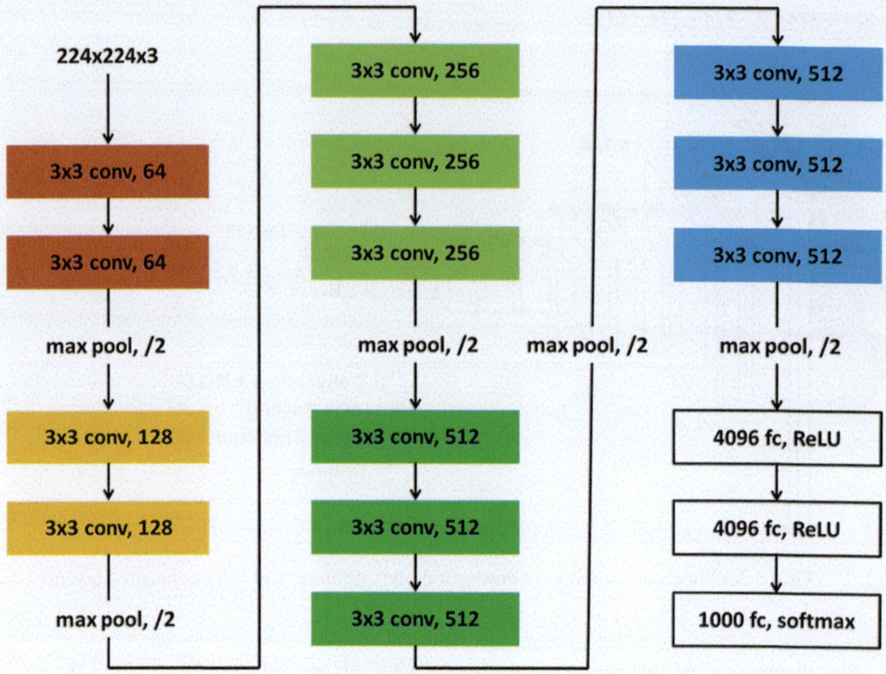

Fig. 3 VGG16 model's details

The ResNet50 architecture takes an image of size $(224 \times 224 \times 3)$ as input. The model uses convolutional and max pooling layers for input image feature extraction. The first convolutional layer employs a 7×7 filter with a stride of 2, and the input is zero-padded to retain the spatial dimensions of the image. A 3×3 max pooling layer follows with a stride of 2. The model also includes four blocks of residual layers, where each block contains several bottleneck layers consisting of a 1×1 followed by 3×3 and another 1×1 convolutional layer. These layers are linked by shortcut connections. The model concludes with a global average pooling layer that transforms the feature maps to a one-dimensional vector after the four blocks of residual layers. Finally, the output of the model is generated by passing this vector through a fully connected layer producing a 1000-dimensional vector that represents the class probabilities. The architectural details of ResNet50 model is shown in the Fig. 4.

ResNet50 is a complex and deep architecture that can effectively extract features from images. Its use of residual connections enables it to train much deeper than previous architectures, resulting in superior performance on image classification tasks.

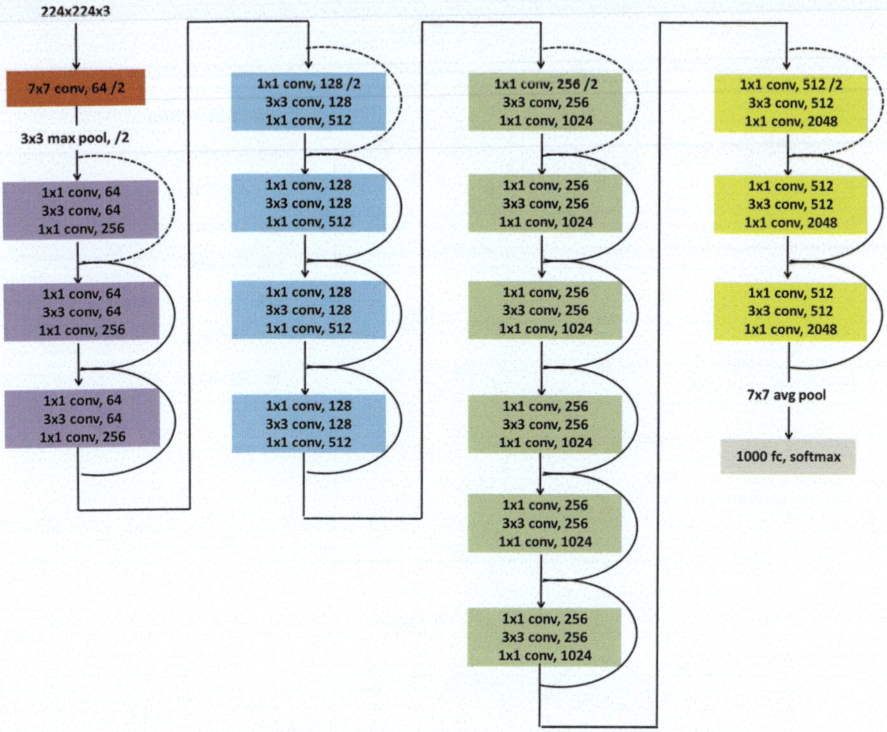

Fig. 4 ResNET50 model's details

3.3.3 Inception-Resnet-v2

The Inception-ResNet v2 model is an improved version of the original Inception-ResNet model with increased accuracy and efficiency, which was designed specifically for image classification tasks [18, 19]. The model utilizes Inception modules, which are multi-layered blocks that extract input features, and residual connections that help to solve the vanishing gradient problem and enhance the network's learning ability.

The architecture of the Inception-ResNet v2 model is composed of different components, starting with the stem which applies convolutional and max-pooling layers to the input image to maximize the amount of feature maps and minimize the spatial resolution. The Inception blocks are the building blocks of the network that extract features from the input image at multiple scales as each block is composed of multiple branches with different convolutional kernel sizes. The reduction blocks are used for the spatial resolution reduction of the feature maps and enhance the computational efficiency of the model. Furthermore, residual connections are used to solve the vanishing gradient issue and improve the network's learning capability. These connections are created by adding the block input to the output, enabling information

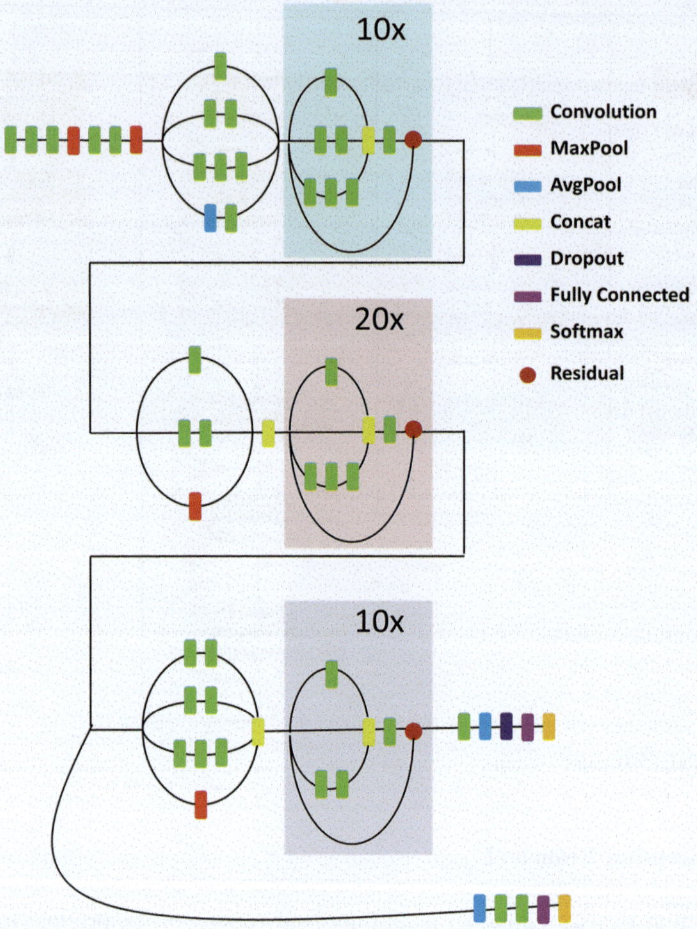

Fig. 5 Inception-Resnet-v2 model's details

to flow directly from the input to the output. Finally, at the end of the model network fully connected layers are followed by a softmax activation function. These layers categorize the input image into predefined classes. The architectural details of the Inception-ResNet v2 is shown in Fig. 5. Overall, the Inception-ResNet v2 employs various advanced techniques to improve performance.

The Inception-ResNet v2 architecture was developed to deal with the shortcomings of the previously existing models such as AlexNet in the field of image classification. The Inception-ResNet v2 model's strength lies in its deep structure, consisting of hundreds of layers that can extract a wider range of features from input images, leading to improved accuracy. Furthermore, the incorporation of residual connections into the architecture helps to address the vanishing gradient problem, enhancing the model's learning capabilities. Additionally, the Inception-ResNet v2 model was trained on a larger dataset of over 2 million images, which increases its robustness and generalization abilities. In contrast, AlexNet only has 8 layers, lacks residual connections, and training was done on 1.2 million images of small dataset.

3.3.4 EfficientNet-B3

EfficientNet is a convolutional neural network and is designed with improved accuracy having less number of parameters. Tan [44] studied the relationship and evidenced that the careful balancing of the width, depth, and resolution for model scaling of the convolutional neural networks can lead to better performance. They designed a new baseline model and scale it up to get a family of seven EfficientNet models namely EfficientNetB0 - EfficientNetB7. These models when applied to ImageNet dataset showed Top-1 accuracy for image classification tasks. The compound scaling method outperformed conventional scaling techniques and uniformly scales each of the three dimensions (width, depth, and resolution) with an exact ratio.

The main building block of the architecture is the mobile inverted bottleneck convolutional (MBConv) block. Besides, the other important components are inverted residual connections and linear bottlenecks. The MBConv idea is based on the MobileNet models while (inverted residual connections and linear bottlenecks) are borrowed from the MobileNet-V2. In the original residual block, layers with wide number of channels (64) have skip connections while it is squeezed to 16 in the inverted residual blocks. In the inverted residual block, the skip connections occur in narrower layers and fewer channels so are called inverted. Moreover, the linear bottlenecks refer to the use of linear activation function in the squeezed layer with less number of channels. The linear activation function in the inverted residual block for the bottleneck layer is better than ReLU. The ReLU activation ignores the values less than zero in the inverted residual block. The architectural details of EfficientNet-B3 is shown in Fig. 6. A new activation function Swish is also used in the EfficientNet model architecture. Mathematically, it is formulated in (1)

$$f_{Swish}(x) = \frac{x}{1 + e^{-\beta x}} \tag{1}$$

where parameter $\beta \geq 0$ is learned during the training stage. For $\beta = 0$, the Swish function becomes a linear activation function and it is similar to ReLU for $\beta \to \infty$ except it is smoother than ReLU and LeakyReLU. Additionally, the squeeze-and-excitation (SE) module in MBConv block further improves the performance. EfficientNet is a promising architecture for deep learning models as it delivers greater accuracy and efficiency than earlier models. It is a useful tool for computer vision researchers and practitioners since the compound scaling method and pre-trained models enable simple adaption to a variety of tasks.

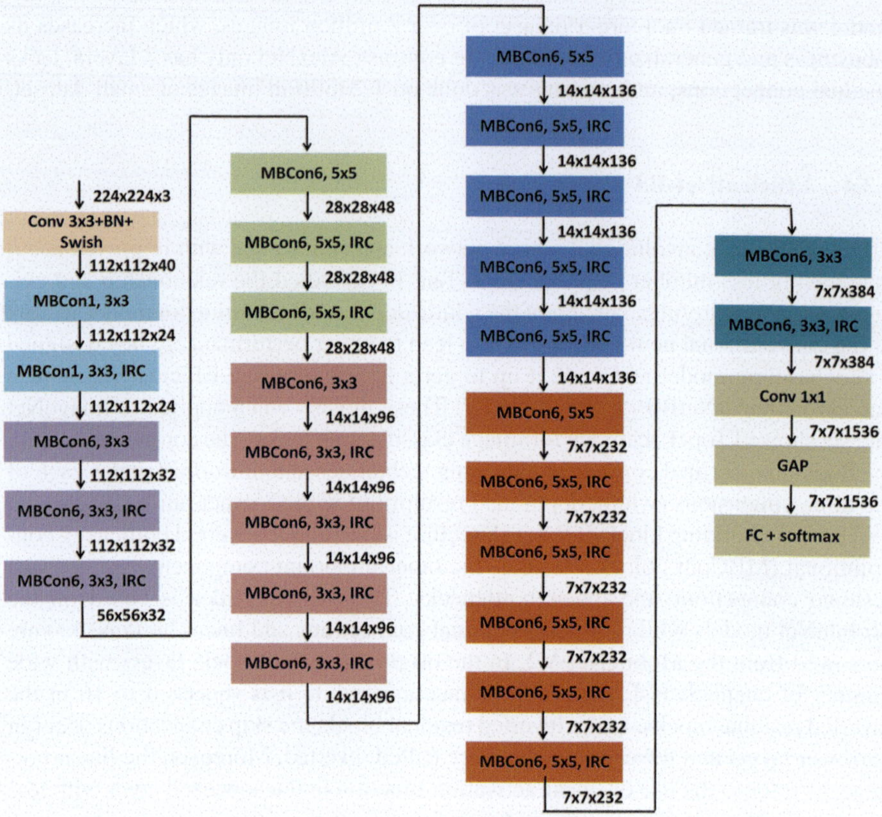

Fig. 6 EfficientNet-B3 model's details

3.3.5 Vision Transformer

The Vision Transformer is a transformer architecture, which was originally designed for natural language processing tasks, to handle image data. This model was proposed by Dosovitskiy [45] and it is an adaptation of the original transformer that is designed to work with sequences of image patches. The input image is first divided into non-overlapping patches and passed through convolutional layers to extract feature maps, which are then reshaped and fed into the transformer architecture. The transformer consists of multiple layers of self-attention and fully connected layers, where the self-attention layers compute attention weights between different regions of the image, enabling the model to learn relationships between them. This is essential for tasks such as object detection and segmentation. The output of the self-attention layers is then passed through a feed-forward neural network composed of fully connected layers. The final output of the network is generated by a linear layer. The Vision Transformer architecture allows for the handling of input images of various sizes

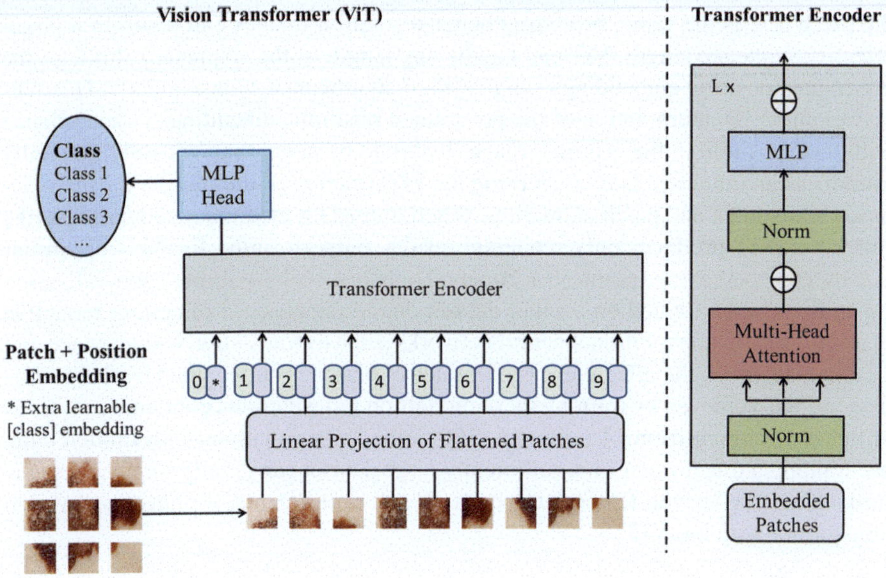

Fig. 7 Vision transformer model's details

and aspect ratios while maintaining high performance. Moreover, the patch-based approach facilitates efficient parallel processing and reduces the memory requirements of the model. An illustration of the architecture of the Vision Transformer is depicted in Fig. 7.

Mathematically, the input 2D image is represented as $x \in \mathbb{R}^{H \times W \times C}$ and transformed into a sequence of flattened 2D image patches $x_p \in \mathbb{R}^{N \times (P^2.C)}$. The resolution of the input 2D image is (H, W) with C channels and that of the individual patch is (P, P). The transformer's sequence length becomes $N = HW/P^2$. The patch embeddings, which are generated by a trainable linear projection, map each vectorized patch to the model dimension D. This is because the transformer architecture employs constant widths in all of its layers. Similar to the [class] token used in BERT, a learnable embedding is applied to the sequence of embedding patches. The image is represented by the state of this embedding. During both the pre-training and fine-tuning phases, the classification heads are attached to networks of the same size. Dosovitskiy investigated various 2D-aware position embedding variations, but none of them produce appreciable improvements over conventional 1D position embeddings. The encoder receives the joint embeddings split as input. It should be noted that ViT only uses the encoder from a standard transformer, whose output comes before an MLP head. For smaller downstream tasks, ViT is typically fine-tuned after pre-training on big datasets. This is accomplished by removing the pre-trained prediction head and attaching a zero-initialized $D \times K$ feed-forward layer, where K is the total number of classes in the downstream classes. It is frequently advantageous to use higher resolutions for fine-tuning than for pre-training. For instance, even though the patch size is the same, providing better-resolution images can result in a larger effective sequence length. ViT can handle any length of the sequence, although the pre-trained position embeddings can lose their significance. Consequently, Dosovitskiy employ 2D interpolation of the pre-trained position embeddings in accordance with their position in the original image. It should be noted that ViT only manually introduces an inductive bias concerning the 2D structure of the images during resolution adjustment and patch extraction. When trained on medium-sized datasets like ImageNet, ViT produces only moderate results, outperforming ResNets of similar size by a few percentage points in accuracy. Transformers have limited generalization capabilities when trained on a small dataset due to the absence of certain inductive biases present in convolutional neural networks, such as translation equivariance and locality. However, the effectiveness of inductive biases is outweighed by the performance gains achieved by training these models on large datasets containing millions of images (ranging from 14 million to 300 million). In situations with limited data, pre-training a transformer on a sufficiently large dataset can greatly improve its performance on tasks with fewer data points. In our experiments, we have used vision transformer with base 32.

4 Results and Discussion

The deep neural network models VGG16, ResNET50, Inception-Resnet-v2, EfficientNet-B3, and Vision Transformer are used for the evaluation of skin cancer classification. The classification results obtained from traditional CNNs are compared with the Vision Transformer. In our study, we replaced the top layers of all the pre-trained models i.e., VGG16, ResNET50, Inception- Resnet-v2, and EfficientNet-B3 with a set of a batch normalization layer, dense layer with 128 units, ReLU activation function, and a dropout layer with 45% rate in the same sequence as shown in Fig. 8. A dense layer then follows all the above layers with 7 units and a softmax activation function for the prediction of the classes. However, for the vision transformer, we replaced the top layers with a flattening layer, batch normalization layer, dense layer with 256 units, ReLU activation function followed by a dense layer with 7 units and a softmax activation function for the prediction of the classes and is shown in Fig. 9.

For training of the CNN pre-trained models, we have used hyperparameters including 100 epochs with early stopping, batch size of 32, Adamx optimization function with 0.0001 learning rate, and categorical cross-entropy loss function. The dataset is divided into 70% of training, 20% of validation, and 10% of testing sets. The input image of resolution 224×224 is fed to both CNN pre-trained models and vision transformer.

Figures 10, 11, 12, and 13 show the best results of training and validation loss are found at epoch 13, 21, 18, 24, and 16 for VGG16, ResNET50, Inception-Resnet-v2, EfficientNet-B3, and Vision Transformer respectively. Comparing EfficientNet-B3's training and validation graph to those of other deep neural networks and vision transformers, Fig. 13 reveals that it is smoother. The over fitting problem is less observable

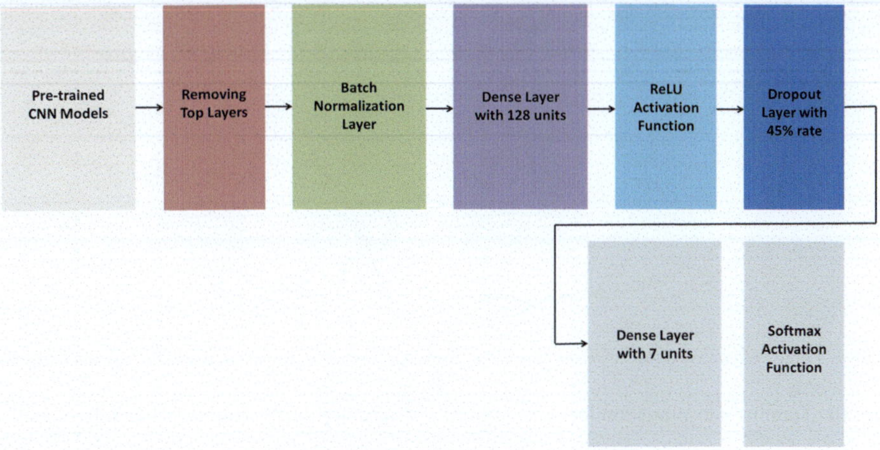

Fig. 8 Pre-trained CNN models and fine tuning using transfer learning

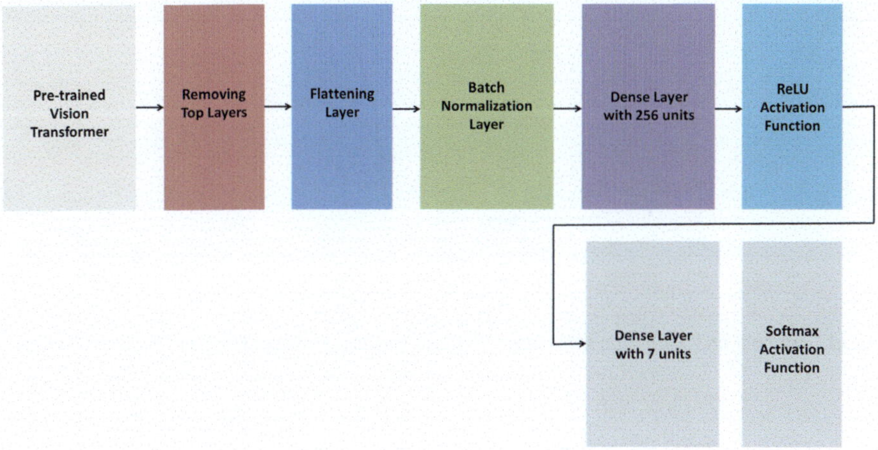

Fig. 9 Pre-trained vision transformer and fine tuning using transfer learning

in VGG-16 and EfficientNet-B3 as compared to ResNet50 and InceptionResnet-v2. Overall the performance of EfficientNet-B3 is best as compared to all other CNN models and vision transformer.

The performance of the ViT is poor as compared to the CNN models in general. The reason is the less available skin cancer data with high data imbalances. The graph of training and validation accuracy as shown in Fig. 14 also show more fluctuations and over-fitting problem. The dropout technique is used to reduce over-fitting problems and to balance cancer classes data augmentation is used. The big problem lies in the huge difference in the number of samples in the highest class samples and the lowest class samples. The threshold of 3000 is taken which cut off some

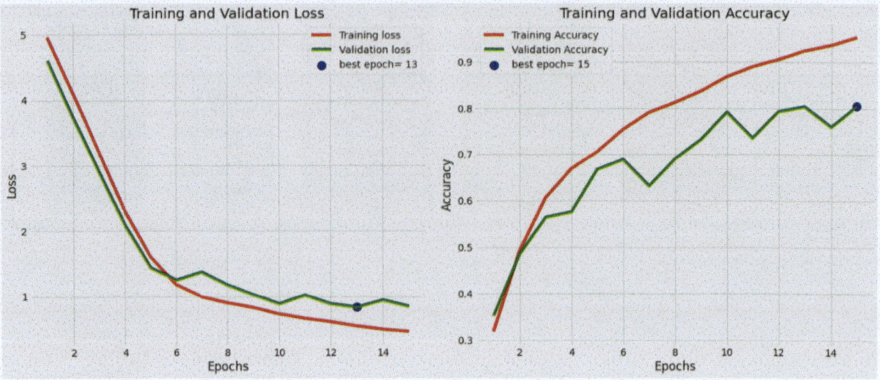

Fig. 10 Training and validation loss curves (left) and accuracy curves (right) of VGG-16 model

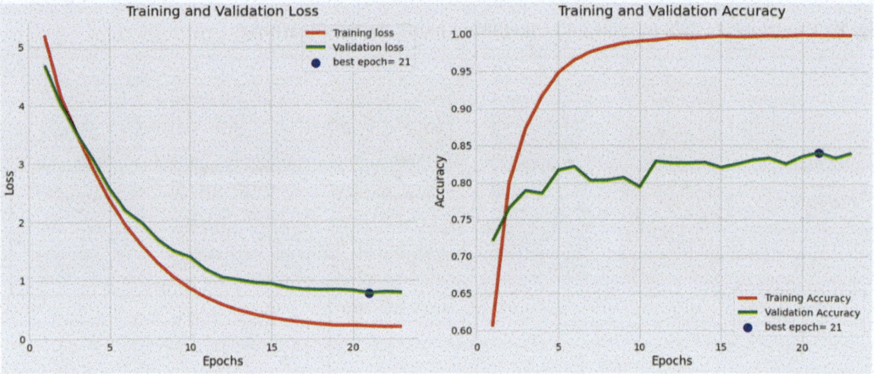

Fig. 11 Training and validation loss curves (left) and accuracy curves (right) of ResNet50 model

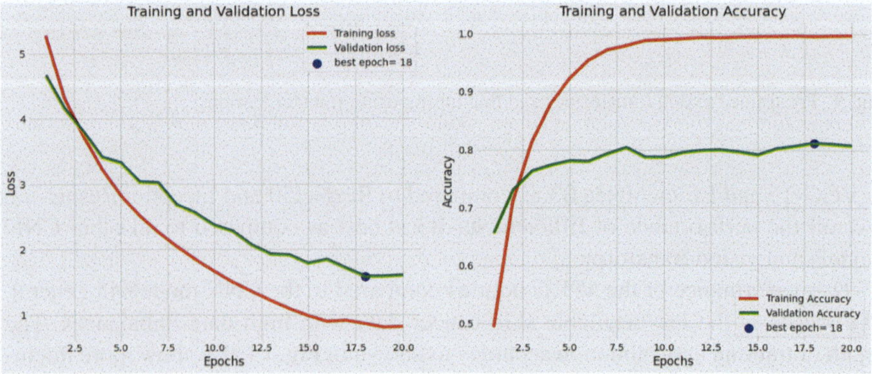

Fig. 12 Training and validation loss curves (left) and accuracy curves (right) of Inception-Resnet-v2 model

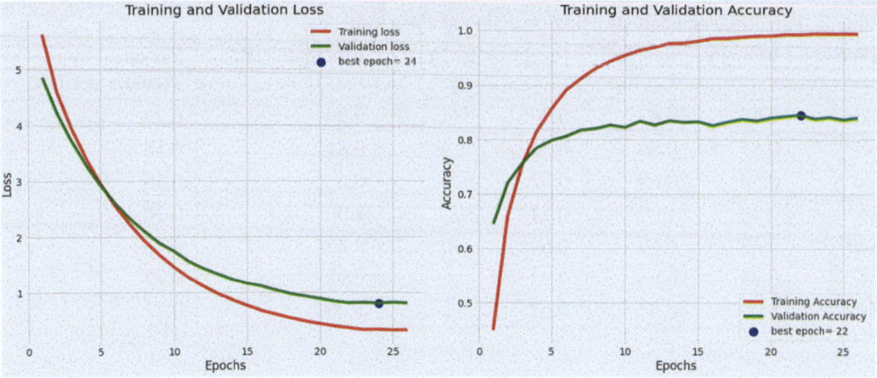

Fig. 13 Training and validation loss curves (left) and accuracy curves (right) of EfficientNet-B3 model

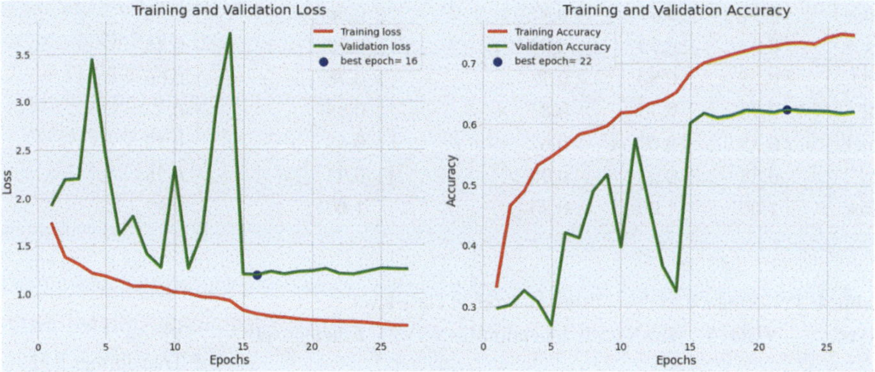

Fig. 14 Training and validation loss curves (left) and accuracy curves (right) of Vision Transformer

samples from the highest class samples and more samples are added to the lowest class samples. The further reduction in the threshold value may result in the loss of important features in the highest class samples. The replication of most of the features can be observed as we try to compensate the lowest class samples and balance them according to the set threshold. Besides this, the vision transformer model did not converge to a good solution within the given number of epochs, resulting in unstable curves which shows its less adaptive nature to new domains though having high transferability. CNN models achieve better results in the given epochs and data for fine tuning to adapt themselves to new domains as compared to vision transformer to achieve better results.

Moreover, Tables 2, 3 and 4 shows the performance analysis of the CNN models i.e., VGG-16, ResNet50, InceptionResNet v2, and EfficientNet-B3 and Vision Transformer. Here, while considering the individual classes Table 2 shows that the precision of akiec, df, nv, and vasc is high as compared to the other models and the precision of bcc, bkl, and mel is high in ResNet50. Table 3 shows that the recall

Table 2 Performance analysis using precision at class level

Type	VGG16	ResNet50	InceptionResNetV2	EfficientNetB3	Vision Transformer B32
akiec	0.45	0.67	0.70	0.90	0.33
bcc	0.65	0.86	0.75	0.84	0.38
bkl	0.60	0.68	0.62	0.6	0.40
df	0.70	1.00	0.77	1.00	0.20
mel	0.67	0.69	0.64	0.64	0.43
nv	0.94	0.93	0.93	0.95	0.92
vasc	1.00	0.94	0.67	1.00	0.72

Table 3 Performance analysis of using recall at class level

Type	VGG16	ResNet50	InceptionResNetV2	EfficientNetB3	Vision Transformer B32
akiec	0.71	0.47	0.47	0.56	0.35
bcc	0.83	0.79	0.83	0.79	0.45
bkl	0.75	0.80	0.73	0.76	0.66
df	0.58	0.75	0.83	0.83	0.33
mel	0.55	0.69	0.62	0.67	0.53
nv	0.88	0.93	0.90	0.93	0.76
vasc	1.00	1.00	0.93	1.00	0.87

Table 4 Performance analysis using f1-score at class level

Type	VGG16	ResNet50	InceptionResNetV2	EfficientNetB3	Vision Transformer B32
akiec	0.55	0.55	0.56	0.69	0.34
bcc	0.73	0.82	0.79	0.82	0.41
bkl	0.66	0.74	0.67	0.67	0.50
df	0.64	0.86	0.80	0.91	0.25
mel	0.60	0.69	0.63	0.66	0.48
nv	0.91	0.93	0.91	0.94	0.84
vasc	1.00	0.97	0.78	1.00	0.79

of df is high in EfficientNetB3 as compared to ResNet50 and that of bkl and mel is high in ResNet50 and comparable results in case of bcc, nv, and vasc in comparison with EfficientNetB3. Table 4 shows the F1-score of akiec, df, nv, and vasc is better in the case of EfficientNet-B3 as compared to ResNet50. The F1-score is highest in ResNet50 for melanoma case. The F1-score for the bcc class is same for both ResNet50 and EfficientNet-B3. The F1-score of only two classes bkl and melanoma is better in ResNet50. The Table 5 shows the accuracy of ResNet50 and EfficientNet-B3 is high as compared to other CNN models and the vision trans-

Table 5 Overall Performance analysis using accuracy, precision, recall, and f1-score

Performance Metrics	VGG16	ResNet50	InceptionResNetV2	EfficientNetB3	Vision Transformer B32
Accuracy	0.82	0.86	0.83	0.86	0.69
Precision (Macro Avg)	0.71	0.82	0.72	0.85	0.49
Recall (Macro Avg)	0.76	0.78	0.76	0.79	0.56
F1-Score (Macro Avg)	0.73	0.79	0.73	0.81	0.52
Precision (Weighted Avg)	0.84	0.87	0.84	0.87	0.75
Recall (Weighted Avg)	0.82	0.86	0.83	0.86	0.69
F1-Score (Weighted Avg)	0.82	0.86	0.83	0.86	0.71

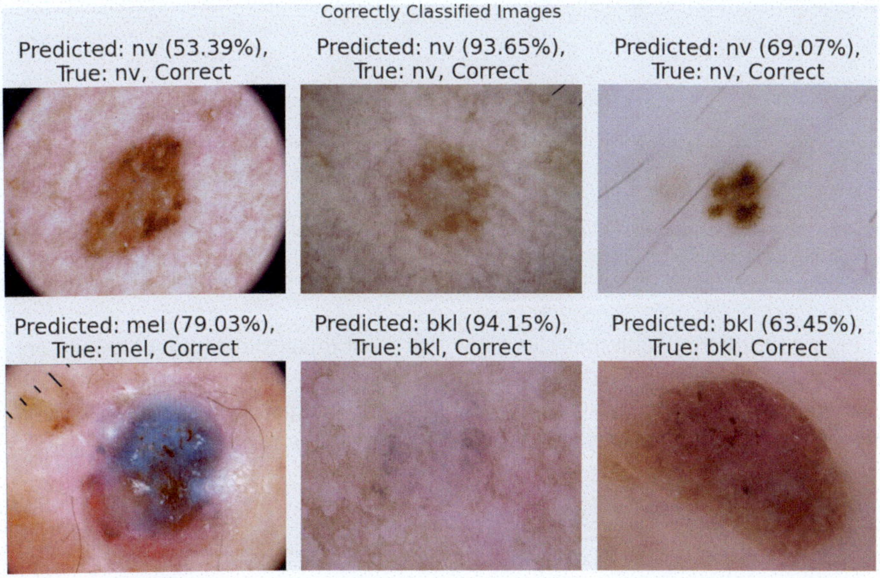

Fig. 15 Correctly classified skin cancer image samples obtained from highly accurate EfficientNetB3 skin cancer CNN classification model

former. The macro average of precision, recall, and f1-score using EfficientNetB3 is highest while in case of weighted average both EfficientNetB3 and ResNet50 have comparable results. The overall performance using accuracy, macro average, and weighted average of EfficientNet-B3 is better as compared to the other models and have comparable results in some cases with ResNet50.

Figures 15 and 16, show correctly and incorrectly classified images of the best accuracy achieved model, EfficientNetB3 respectively. The model correctly classified most of the images from the test data set that have clear and distinctive features, such as shape, color, texture, and border. However, the model also makes some mistakes when the images have similar or vague features, such as overlapping or irregular shapes, varying or mixed colors, noisy or blurred textures, and unclear or fuzzy borders.

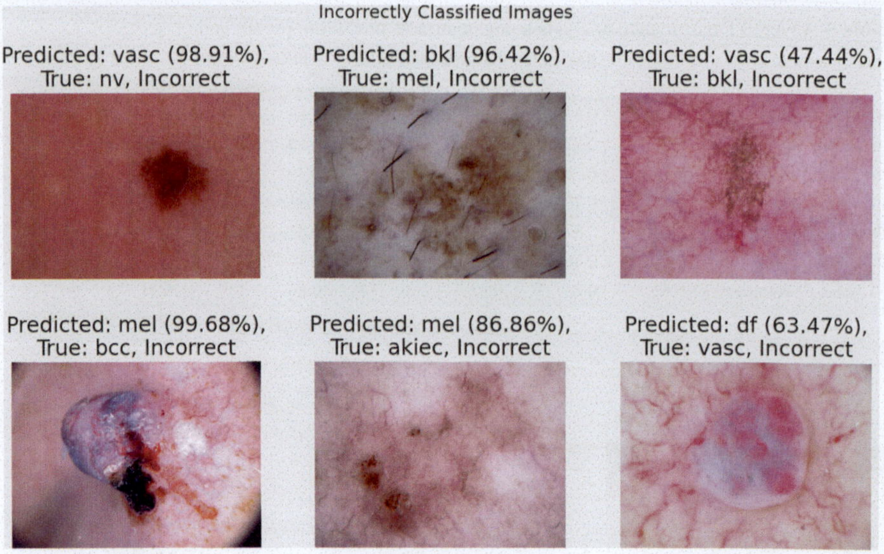

Fig. 16 Incorrectly classified skin cancer image samples obtained from highly accurate EfficientNetB3 skin cancer CNN classification model

Figure 17, of confusion matrices show that most images in nv are classified correctly by the models followed by bkl and mel, and also among the classes, most of the nv are misclassified as mel followed by bkl. Also in comparison to the other classes, most of the mel class images are classified incorrectly as bkl and nv class images.

5 Conclusion

Melanoma is the deadliest skin cancer. The early detection of melanoma can increase the survival rate. The early diagnosis is a difficult task as the melanoma case resembles a non-melanoma. The accurate detection of melanoma cases depends on the year of experience of medical experts. The automatic detection of skin cancer will be helpful for physicians and will assist them. The ongoing research to provide more accurate deep learning-based models is helpful for the categorization of skin cancer, particularly melanoma detection in the initial stages. The dataset used here is HAM10000 ISIC dataset. The CNN models VGG16, ResNET50, Inception-Resnet-v2, and EfficientNet-B3 are used for the classification results. Moreover, these CNN models are compared with the Vision Transformer. The results explore the best-performing deep network model using transfer learning. The EfficientNet-B3 performed well in the case of accuracy and F1- score for individual classes of skin cancer. The performance of vision transformer is low as compared to all CNN models in general. The performance of vision transformer can be improved with the use of more computational resources and use of balanced medical data.

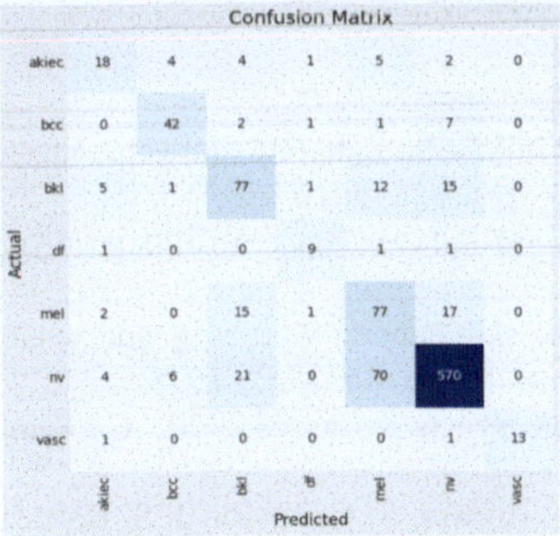

(a) Confusion Matrix of VGG16

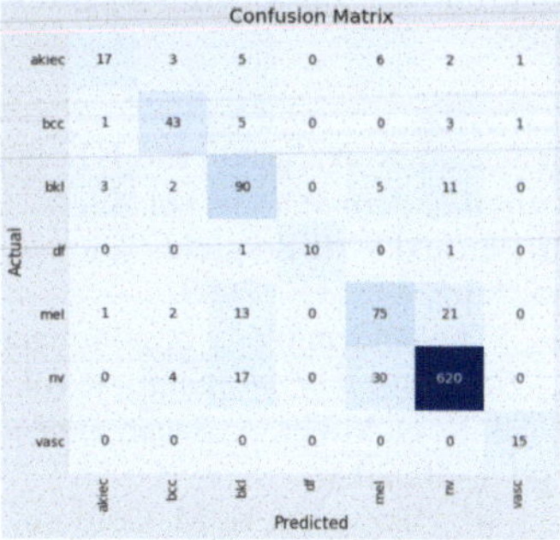

(b) Confusion Matrix of ResNet50

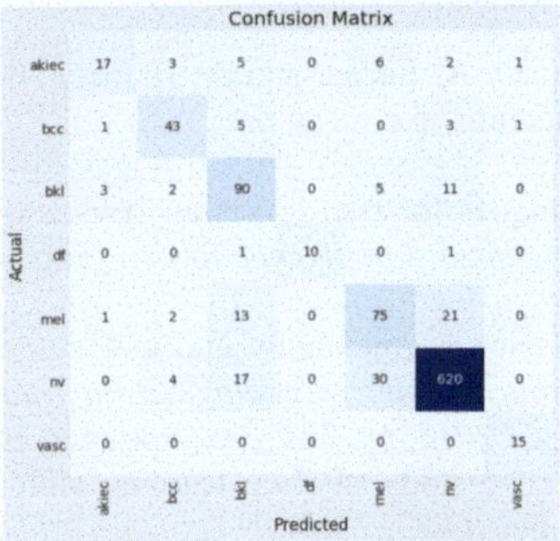

(c) Confusion Matrix of Inception-ResNetV2

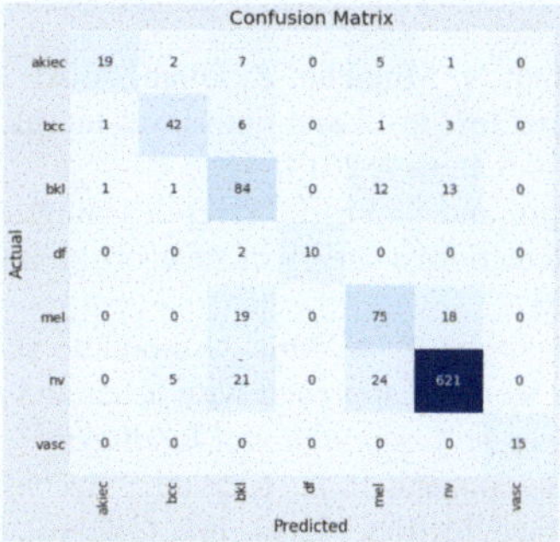

(d) Confusion Matrix of Efficient-NetB3

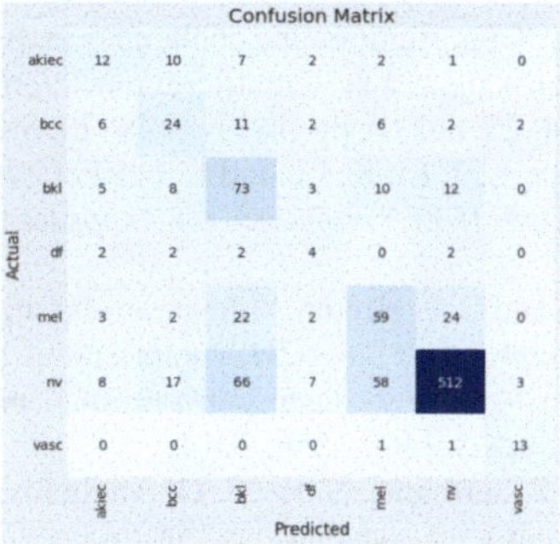

(e) Confusion Matrix of Vision Transformer B32

Fig. 17 Confusion matrices of CNN models and vision transformer

References

1. D. L. Narayanan, R. N. Saladi, and J. L. Fox, "Ultraviolet radiation and skin cancer," *International journal of dermatology*, vol. 49, no. 9, pp. 978–986, 2010.
2. S. C. Harrison and W. F. Bergfeld, "Ultraviolet light and skin cancer in athletes," *Sports health*, vol. 1, no. 4, pp. 335–340, 2009.
3. R. Marks, "The epidemiology of non-melanoma skin cancer: who, why and what can we do about it," *The Journal of dermatology*, vol. 22, no. 11, pp. 853–857, 1995.
4. R. L. Siegel, K. D. Miller, A. Sauer, *et al.*, "Cancer facts & figures 2020," *CA Cancer J. Clin*, vol. 70, pp. 7–30, 2020.
5. H. Tsao, J. M. Olazagasti, K. M. Cordoro, J. D. Brewer, S. C. Taylor, J. S. Bordeaux, M.-M. Chren, A. J. Sober, C. Tegeler, R. Bhushan, *et al.*, "Early detection of melanoma: reviewing the abcdes," *Journal of the American Academy of Dermatology*, vol. 72, no. 4, pp. 717–723, 2015.
6. M. Ashfaq, N. Minallah, Z. Ullah, A. M. Ahmad, A. Saeed, and A. Hafeez, "Performance analysis of low-level and high-level intuitive features for melanoma detection," *Electronics*, vol. 8, no. 6, p. 672, 2019.
7. A. Adegun and S. Viriri, "Deep learning techniques for skin lesion analysis and melanoma cancer detection: a survey of state-of-the-art," *Artificial Intelligence Review*, vol. 54, pp. 811–841, 2021.
8. Z. A. Nazi and T. A. Abir, "Automatic skin lesion segmentation and melanoma detection: Transfer learning approach with u-net and dcnn-svm," in *Proceedings of International Joint Conference on Computational Intelligence: IJCCI 2018*, pp. 371–381, Springer, 2020.
9. S. H. Kassani and P. H. Kassani, "A comparative study of deep learning architectures on melanoma detection," *Tissue and Cell*, vol. 58, pp. 76–83, 2019.
10. A. Esteva, B. Kuprel, R. A. Novoa, J. Ko, S. M. Swetter, H. M. Blau, and S. Thrun, "Dermatologist-level classification of skin cancer with deep neural networks," *nature*, vol. 542, no. 7639, pp. 115–118, 2017.
11. C. Xiao, E. Choi, and J. Sun, "Opportunities and challenges in developing deep learning models using electronic health records data: a systematic review," *Journal of the American Medical Informatics Association*, vol. 25, no. 10, pp. 1419–1428, 2018.
12. J. Deng, W. Dong, R. Socher, L.-J. Li, K. Li, and L. Fei-Fei, "Imagenet: A large-scale hierarchical image database," in *2009 IEEE conference on computer vision and pattern recognition*, pp. 248–255, Ieee, 2009.
13. A. Krizhevsky, I. Sutskever, and G. E. Hinton, "Imagenet classification with deep convolutional neural networks," *Communications of the ACM*, vol. 60, no. 6, pp. 84–90, 2017.
14. K. Simonyan and A. Zisserman, "Very deep convolutional networks for large-scale image recognition," *arXiv preprint* arXiv:1409.1556, 2014.
15. C. Szegedy, W. Liu, Y. Jia, P. Sermanet, S. Reed, D. Anguelov, D. Erhan, V. Vanhoucke, and A. Rabinovich, "Going deeper with convolutions," in *Proceedings of the IEEE conference on computer vision and pattern recognition*, pp. 1–9, 2015.
16. K. He, X. Zhang, S. Ren, and J. Sun, "Deep residual learning for image recognition," in *Proceedings of the IEEE conference on computer vision and pattern recognition*, pp. 770–778, 2016.
17. S. Xie, R. Girshick, P. Dollár, Z. Tu, and K. He, "Aggregated residual transformations for deep neural networks," in *Proceedings of the IEEE conference on computer vision and pattern recognition*, pp. 1492–1500, 2017.
18. C. Szegedy, V. Vanhoucke, S. Ioffe, J. Shlens, and Z. Wojna, "Rethinking the inception architecture for computer vision," in *Proceedings of the IEEE conference on computer vision and pattern recognition*, pp. 2818–2826, 2016.
19. C. Szegedy, S. Ioffe, V. Vanhoucke, and A. A. Alemi, "Inception-v4, inception-resnet and the impact of residual connections on learning," in *Proceedings of the Thirty-First AAAI Conference on Artificial Intelligence*, pp. 4278–4284, 2017.

20. G. Huang, Z. Liu, L. Van Der Maaten, and K. Q. Weinberger, "Densely connected convolutional networks," in *Proceedings of the IEEE conference on computer vision and pattern recognition*, pp. 4700–4708, 2017.
21. F. Chollet, "Xception: Deep learning with depthwise separable convolutions," in *Proceedings of the IEEE conference on computer vision and pattern recognition*, pp. 1251–1258, 2017.
22. D. Gangwani, Q. Liang, S. Wang, and X. Zhu, "An empirical study of deep learning frameworks for melanoma cancer detection using transfer learning and data augmentation," in *2021 IEEE International Conference on Big Knowledge (ICBK)*, pp. 38–45, IEEE, 2021.
23. H. M. Balaha and A. E.-S. Hassan, "Skin cancer diagnosis based on deep transfer learning and sparrow search algorithm," *Neural Computing and Applications*, pp. 1–39, 2022.
24. V. Miglani and M. Bhatia, "Skin lesion classification: A transfer learning approach using efficientnets," in *Advanced Machine Learning Technologies and Applications: Proceedings of AMLTA 2020*, pp. 315–324, Springer, 2020.
25. D. N. Le, H. X. Le, L. T. Ngo, and H. T. Ngo, "Transfer learning with class-weighted and focal loss function for automatic skin cancer classification," *arXiv preprint* arXiv:2009.05977, 2020.
26. M. A. Khan, T. Akram, Y.-D. Zhang, and M. Sharif, "Attributes based skin lesion detection and recognition: A mask rcnn and transfer learning-based deep learning framework," *Pattern Recognition Letters*, vol. 143, pp. 58–66, 2021.
27. D. Moldovan, "Transfer learning based method for two-step skin cancer images classification," in *2019 E-Health and Bioengineering Conference (EHB)*, pp. 1–4, IEEE, 2019.
28. V. Anand, S. Gupta, D. Koundal, S. R. Nayak, J. Nayak, and S. Vimal, "Multi-class skin disease classification using transfer learning model," *International Journal on Artificial Intelligence Tools*, vol. 31, no. 02, p. 2250029, 2022.
29. K. Thurnhofer-Hemsi and E. Domínguez, "A convolutional neural network framework for accurate skin cancer detection," *Neural Processing Letters*, vol. 53, no. 5, pp. 3073–3093, 2021.
30. Z. Rahman and A. M. Ami, "A transfer learning based approach for skin lesion classification from imbalanced data," in *2020 11th international conference on electrical and computer engineering (ICECE)*, pp. 65–68, IEEE, 2020.
31. M. A. R. Ratul, M. H. Mozaffari, E. Parimbelli, and W. Lee, "Atrous convolution with transfer learning for skin lesions classification," *BioRxiv*, p. 746388, 2019.
32. Y. Gu, Z. Ge, C. P. Bonnington, and J. Zhou, "Progressive transfer learning and adversarial domain adaptation for cross-domain skin disease classification," *IEEE journal of biomedical and health informatics*, vol. 24, no. 5, pp. 1379–1393, 2019.
33. A. Vaswani, N. Shazeer, N. Parmar, J. Uszkoreit, L. Jones, A. N. Gomez, Ł. Kaiser, and I. Polosukhin, "Attention is all you need," *Advances in neural information processing systems*, vol. 30, 2017.
34. C. Xin, Z. Liu, K. Zhao, L. Miao, Y. Ma, X. Zhu, Q. Zhou, S. Wang, L. Li, F. Yang, *et al.*, "An improved transformer network for skin cancer classification," *Computers in Biology and Medicine*, vol. 149, p. 105939, 2022.
35. S. Aladhadh, M. Alsanea, M. Aloraini, T. Khan, S. Habib, and M. Islam, "An effective skin cancer classification mechanism via medical vision transformer," *Sensors*, vol. 22, no. 11, p. 4008, 2022.
36. Z. Zhao, "Skin cancer classification based on convolutional neural networks and vision transformers," in *Journal of Physics: Conference Series*, p. 012037, IOP Publishing, 2022.
37. M. M. K. Sarker, C. F. Moreno-García, J. Ren, and E. Elyan, "Transslc: Skin lesion classification in dermatoscopic images using transformers," in *Medical Image Understanding and Analysis: 26th Annual Conference, MIUA 2022, Cambridge, UK, July 27–29, 2022, Proceedings*, pp. 651–660, Springer, 2022.
38. K. Nakai, Y.-W. Chen, and X.-H. Han, "Enhanced deep bottleneck transformer model for skin lesion classification," *Biomedical Signal Processing and Control*, vol. 78, p. 103997, 2022.
39. S. Ayas, "Multiclass skin lesion classification in dermoscopic images using swin transformer model," *Neural Computing and Applications*, pp. 1–10, 2022.

40. J. Chen, J. Chen, Z. Zhou, B. Li, A. Yuille, and Y. Lu, "Mt-transunet: Mediating multi-task tokens in transformers for skin lesion segmentation and classification," *arXiv preprint* arXiv:2112.01767, 2021.
41. X. He, E.-L. Tan, H. Bi, X. Zhang, S. Zhao, and B. Lei, "Fully transformer network for skin lesion analysis," *Medical Image Analysis*, vol. 77, p. 102357, 2022.
42. P. Tschandl, C. Rosendahl, and H. Kittler, "The ham10000 dataset, a large collection of multi-source dermatoscopic images of common pigmented skin lesions," *Scientific data*, vol. 5, no. 1, pp. 1–9, 2018.
43. O. Russakovsky, J. Deng, H. Su, J. Krause, S. Satheesh, S. Ma, Z. Huang, A. Karpathy, A. Khosla, M. Bernstein, *et al.*, "Imagenet large scale visual recognition challenge," *International journal of computer vision*, vol. 115, pp. 211–252, 2015.
44. M. Tan and Q. Le, "Efficientnet: Rethinking model scaling for convolutional neural networks," in *International conference on machine learning*, pp. 6105–6114, PMLR, 2019.
45. A. Dosovitskiy, L. Beyer, A. Kolesnikov, D. Weissenborn, X. Zhai, T. Unterthiner, M. Dehghani, M. Minderer, G. Heigold, S. Gelly, *et al.*, "An image is worth 16x16 words: Transformers for image recognition at scale," *arXiv preprint* arXiv:2010.11929, 2020.

A New CNN-Based Deep Learning Model Approach for Skin Cancer Detection and Classification

Halit Çetiner and Sedat Metlek

Abstract Depending on some environmental or genetic factors, skin abrasions, and tumors may occur. Basal cell carcinoma (BCC) and Actinic Keratosis (Akiec) are the most common of these tumors. Although BCC and Akiec species can be found anywhere on the skin, they are usually seen in areas exposed to direct sunlight, such as the head and neck. Although the risk of metastasis in BCCs is low, if not diagnosed and treated, they can grow aggressively and even cause loss of tissue. When diagnosing BCCs, they can often be confused with a similar species, Akiecs. In order to solve the stated problem, a new decision support system has been proposed based on convolution-based deep learning methods. The proposed system was developed in three steps. In the first step, the input images were evaluated in different color spaces in order to determine in which color space the lesion regions were more prominent. In the second step, Geodesic Active Contour (GAC), Chan and Vese (C-V), Selective Binary and Gaussian Filtering Regularized Level Set (SBGFRLS), Online Region Active Contour (ORACM) methods were used to segment the ROI regions from the images. The best results in the first two steps were obtained with the C-V segmentation method in the HSV color space. In the last step, the obtained images were classified with the CNN-based MatConvNet-1.0-beta15 architecture. As a result of classification, accuracy, and F1 score were obtained as 0.859–0.863, respectively, with MatConvNet-1.0-beta15 architecture. At this stage, a deep learning model that can compete with CNN-based models has also been proposed. The accuracy and F1 score of the proposed model were obtained as 0.914–0.913, respectively. The success rates obtained in the study with the proposed model are promising in terms of its application in different lesion types.

H. Çetiner (✉)
Isparta University of Applied Sciences, Isparta, Turkey
e-mail: halitcetiner@isparta.edu.tr

S. Metlek
Burdur Mehmet Akif Ersoy University, Burdur, Turkey
e-mail: sedatmetlek@mehmetakif.edu.tr

H. Ali et al. (eds.), *Advances in Deep Generative Models for Medical Artificial Intelligence*, Studies in Computational Intelligence 1124,
https://doi.org/10.1007/978-3-031-46341-9_7

1 Introduction

Some of the deadliest skin cancers known are Basal Cell Carcinoma (BCC) and Actinic Keratoses (Akiec) skin lesion types. It is also one of the most difficult types of cancer to detect. However, if it is diagnosed and treated early, almost 100% recovery can be achieved. Cancer can spread rapidly if not diagnosed early. This situation makes the treatment process very difficult and sometimes it may be too late for treatment, although it is not desired. BCC and Akiec are more common among the population than other skin cancers. However, if not diagnosed early, it can be much more dangerous than other types of skin cancer. More than 75% of deaths due to skin cancer are caused by BCC and Akiec [38].

According to data from the World Health Organization, approximately 2 million people have BCC and Akiec skin cancer every year [38]. In 2021, the number of new BCC and Akiec cases diagnosed in the United States is estimated to increase by around 5.8% [40]. Akiec and Intraepithelial Carcinoma (Bowen) are common non-invasive variants of squamous cell carcinoma that can be treated locally without surgical intervention. However, there is a consensus that if these lesions are left untreated, they can develop into invasive squamous cells that are usually non-pigmented. Usually, when exposed to UV light, Akiec in the skin triggers Bowen's disease due to infections. For this reason, it is important to receive the necessary medical treatment, especially against UV light. In the absence of early diagnosis and treatment, lesions can turn into malignant tumors.

Early diagnosis is of great importance in BCC. It is a common variant of epithelial skin cancer that grows very rapidly, especially when confused with other skin diseases such as Akiec and when the treatment process is started late. Therefore, it must be diagnosed correctly for correct treatment. Medical interventions such as biopsy may be required for correct diagnosis [20, 39]. However, it cannot always be diagnosed at the first biopsy. At the same time, intervention with biopsy may cause discomfort to the patient. For all these reasons, the importance of non-invasive diagnosis is one more step forward. Considering the population growth and disease diversity, the importance of developing auxiliary decision support systems in diagnosing patients with non-invasive methods becomes even more important. Due to the increase in skin cancer cases, there have been some studies in the literature that can help dermatologists diagnose [34, 38, 40]. This study, it was aimed to develop an active contour and deep learning-based auxiliary decision support system without the need for special diagnostic devices and biopsy. Contribution of the study to the literature;

1. Unlike many other studies in the literature, the images used in the study were subjected to 4 different segmentation methods in 10 different color spaces. The aim here is to first determine the ROI region and then classify it instead of extracting the feature from the whole image and performing the classification process. Thus, both the process cost is reduced and the negative effects caused by environmental factors during image capture are minimized. Among the color spaces tested in

the study, it was determined that the color space in which the lesion regions are best displayed is the HSV color space.
2. Active contour-based segmentation algorithms have been tested to determine the relevant area on the used data set. In the study, GAC, C-V, SBGFRLS, and ORACM segmentation algorithms were used to determine the ROI region consisting only of lesions. It was detected that the best and fastest result obtained in the study was determined by C-V active contour method.
3. With Active Contour, only the relevant area (ROI) is detected and used in the deep learning algorithm, thus reducing the transaction cost. As a result, the training phase is completed in less time.
4. In the study, unlike many studies in the literature, BCC and Akiecs, which are a type of skin lesions, are identified and classified. ROI and class information were presented to expert healthcare personnel, allowing the person concerned to evaluate the results of the system together with their own observations.
5. In the study, MatConvNetBeta1.15 architecture in the literature was used for classification [13, 44, 45] and a new CNN-based deep learning model was proposed. In the model proposed in the study, the highest accuracy and F1 score were obtained with the C-V segmentation method in the HSV color space.

The decision support system developed consists of three steps. In the first step, different color spaces were tested and it was determined in which color space the relevant area was more prominent. Using different segmentation methods, skin lesions were detected on the images used in the second step. In the third step, ROI regions were classified using machine learning algorithms. In the rest of the study, firstly, literature studies on the subject are presented. Afterward, the data set and the methods used were explained. Subsequently, experimental applications related to these methods were shared and finally, the results obtained from the study were conveyed.

2 Related Works

Types of skin lesions are usually in irregular forms [12]. However, the forms that exist on the skin are constantly changing. These forms from time to time can turn into other types of lesions without showing any symptoms. If the lesions are not intervened, inflammation, ulceration, itching, or bleeding can be seen. Therefore, the lesion area should be examined by a specialist dermatologist and the change in the lesion area should be followed up continuously. It is anticipated that the decision support system to be developed will be a helpful tool for dermatologists in tracking the lesion area. There are machine learning-based classification algorithms developed for different lesions in the literature [4, 46, 48, 50]. Some of these are presented below, along with the methods they use below.

Pomponiu et al. [35] experimentally studied 399 images. In their work, they first pre-processed the images they obtained. Afterward, they obtained features from the preprocessed images with the AlexNet architecture used. Using the KNN classification algorithm in the obtained features, they reached an accuracy rate of 93.64%. Codella et al. [10] studied 2624 images from the ISIC database in their studies. In the application they developed, they classified images with 93.10% accuracy using AlexNet CNN architecture and Support Vector. Rahim et al. [36] developed a deep convolution neural network-based model for computer-aided detection of polyps in colonoscopy images. The model they developed also achieved an F1 score of 88.30%. Zhang et al. [52] proposed a computer-aided system for tumor detection in chest ultrasound images. They also used deep learning architectures in the system they proposed. They classified ultrasound images with a sensitivity of 0.88 using YOLOV4 architecture. Different from other studies in the literature, Gazioğlu and Kamaşak [3] examined the effect of blurry, noisy, or low-contrast images on classification success using ResNet50, DenseNet121, VGG16, and AlexNet architectures.

Mendes and Silva [27] aimed to classify Melanoma and BCC using the ResNet-152 CNN architecture in their study. For this purpose, it obtained AUC values of 0.96 for Melanoma and 0.91 for BCC. Kwasigroch et al. [23] compared performance results using ResNet, VGG19, and hybrid VGG19 architectures to classify skin lesions. In their study, they obtained 75.5, 81.2, and 80.7 accuracy rates for ResNet, VGG19, and hybrid VGG19 algorithms, respectively. Kawahara et al. [18] studied a total of 1300 volumes of images in 10 different classes. They classified the features on the images, which they obtained with a CNN-based algorithm, using a linear classifier. They achieved an accuracy rate of 81.8% in their work. Jafari et al. [17], studied one of the most aggressive types of cancer, melanoma. It has determined local and global lesion regions on the skin with the algorithm it has used to detect the correct lesion areas. Li et al. [24], propose a lesion segmentation algorithm based on deep neural networks. Ichim et al. [16], are based on extracting features such as perimeter, area, diameter, fractal size, lacunarity, pixel sum of directional slopes, and local binary patterns to define the lesion. Each feature classifier they obtained was rated.

Generally in the literature, experimental results are tested on a data set accessible to everyone [22, 25, 42]. As can be seen in the literature research, the common point of the studies is based on the logic of obtaining features with convolution-based algorithms over the entire image. Since CNN-based algorithms work on the entire image, computational costs are high. In the study, unlike CNN-based applications in the literature, it was used only in the relevant lesion area, not on the whole image. Segmentation algorithms were used to determine the relevant lesion regions on the image, and the success of different segmentation algorithms was also examined.

3 Material and Method

In order to detect skin diseases using machine learning methods, the system to be designed must be trained first. At this point, the importance of the data set to be used and the importance of the images in different classes in the data set stand out one step further. For this purpose, HAM10000 ("Human Against Machine with 10,000

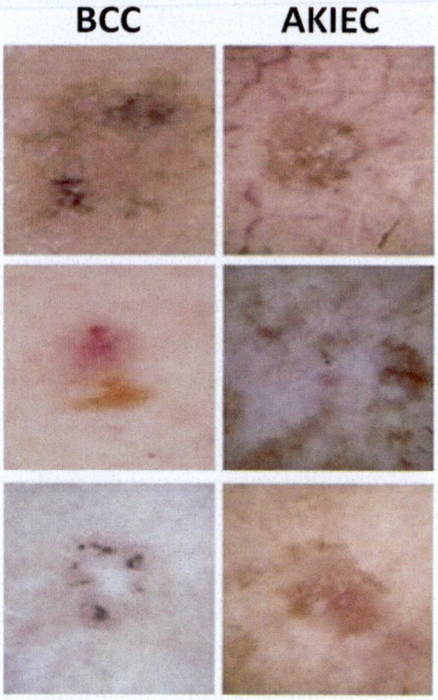

Fig. 1 Two different classes of lesions

training images") data set, which contains many images and different classes at the same time, was used. The data set used in the study was obtained from 2 different Dermatology departments in Austria over a period of 30 years [43]. There are a total of 10,015 lesion images in the data set using 7 different lesion classes.

Some of the images from the preferred data set are shown in Fig. 1. Each labeled image in the specified classes is 450 × 600 in size. The skin cancer classes basal cell carcinoma (BCC), actinic keratoses, and intraepithelial carcinoma / Bowen's disease (Akiec) in the HAM1000 dataset are shown in Fig. 1. There are 514, 327 images from BCC and Akiec skin cancer types, respectively.

Due to the difference in the number of images belonging to both classes, 320 of the 514 BCC images that can best express BCCs were selected by the specialist physicians. The same procedure was applied to 327 Akiec images 320 Akiec images were selected and an experimental study was carried out on a total of 640 images in the study.

In the study, it is an important issue to be able to accurately identify the lesion areas. Therefore, in practice in the literature; Geodesic Active Contour (Geodesic Active Contour, GAC), Chan and Vese (CV), Selected Binary Gaussian Filtering (Segmentation of medical images using Selective Binary and Gaussian Filtering Regularized Level Set, SBGFRLS), and Online Region Active Contour Model (ORACM) models were used as segmentation algorithms. In this section, firstly, brief information about the segmentation models used in the study is presented.

3.1 Segmentation

3.1.1 Geodesic Active Contour (GAC) Method

ORACM is a method developed to overcome two shortcomings in the geodesic active contour (Geodesic Active Contour, GAC) model. One of these shortcomings is that it distorts the active contour model using only the level iterative current gradient and runs slowly.

The second issue that is considered a deficiency is that the images used as the input parameter require the α parameter. The α parameter in question here is called the balloon force and is used to control the dimensions of the contour curves obtained from the image. In the GAC approach, these two problems, which are considered deficiencies in the literature, are solved. In addition, the GAC method creates a structure that represents the set of points where the values of the dual-level function are equal. In Eq. 1, the GAC model for any I image is presented [7];

$$\frac{\vartheta\phi}{\vartheta t}=g\,|\nabla\phi|\left(div\left(\frac{\nabla\phi}{|\nabla\phi|}\right)+\alpha\right)+\nabla g.\nabla\phi \tag{1}$$

$\vartheta\phi$ in Eq. 1 denotes the change in the Lipschitz function expressed by ϕ. ϑg is the amount of change in the function g that decreases in the I image and is used as a positive edge detection function, and α is the balloon force. The α coefficient is used to reduce or enlarge the contours. Calculation of $\vartheta\phi$ and ϑg in each iteration in GAC model causes high calculation cost. This situation is presented in Eqs. 2–5 [7].

$$\left.\begin{array}{l}\phi_x=\phi*G_x,\ G_x=I\,(x+1,y)-I\,(x-1,y)\\ \phi_y=\phi*G_y,\ G_y=I\,(x,\,y+1)-I\,(x,\,y-1)\end{array}\right\}\ First\ derivatives \tag{2}$$

$$\left.\begin{array}{l}\phi_{xx}=\phi*G_{xx},\ G_{xx}=I\,(x+1,y)+I\,(x-1,y)-2*I(x,\,y)\\ \phi_{yy}=\phi*G_{yy},\ G_{yy}=I\,(x,\,y+1)+I\,(x,\,y-1)-2*I(x,\,y)\\ \phi_{xy}=\phi*G_{xy},\ G_{xy}=I\,(x+1,y)+I\,(x-1,y)-2*I(x,\,y)\end{array}\right\}\ Second\ derivatives \tag{3}$$

$$\nabla g=\sqrt{\phi_x^2+\phi_y^2}\ \Big\}\ Gradient \tag{4}$$

$$\nabla\phi=\frac{\phi_{xx}.\phi_{yy}-\phi_{xy}^2}{(1+\phi_x^2+\phi_y^2)}\ \Bigg\}\ Curvature \tag{5}$$

In noisy entrances, the results can be adversely affected by the slope due to local minimum and maximum points.

3.1.2 Chan and Vese Model (C-V Method)

For the C-V model, the level adjustment formula used in the I image and the φ domain is presented in Eq. 6. ϕ in Eq. 6 denotes the level adjustment parameter, and C represents the active curve in the image [7].

$$\begin{aligned} C &= \{x \in \varphi : (\phi) = 0\} \\ inside\ (C) &= \{x \in \varphi : (\phi) > 0\} \\ outside(C) &= \{x \in \varphi : (\phi) < 0\} \end{aligned} \tag{6}$$

Equation 7 is used to update the level adjustment parameter to zero in the C-V Method. In Eq. 7, μ are fixed parameters to control the smoothness of the level adjustment, υ iteration speed, and γ_1 and γ_2 of the inner and outer frame of the contour. ∇ is the slope operator.

$$\frac{\vartheta\phi}{\vartheta t} = \delta(\phi)\left[\mu\nabla\left(\frac{\nabla\phi}{|\nabla\phi|}\right) - \upsilon - \gamma_1(I-c_1)^2 + \gamma_2(I-c_2)^2\right] \tag{7}$$

The content of c_1 and c_2 values are presented in Eqs. 8 and 9. The terms H(ϕ) and $\delta(\phi)$ used in these equations express heaviside and dirac functions, respectively [47].

$$C_1(\phi) = \frac{\int^{I}(x).H(\phi)dx}{\int^{H}(\phi)\,dx} \tag{8}$$

$$C_2(\phi) = \frac{\int^{I}(x).(1-H(\phi))dx}{\int^{H}(1-H(\phi))dx} \tag{9}$$

The C-V model aims to segment the desired object with the appropriate starting contour. However, only the global segmentation feature is used in this model. Therefore, when all objects are wanted to be extracted, they cannot do this without adjusting the starting points in the image.

3.1.3 Selective Binary and Gaussian Filtering Regularized Level Set (SBGFRLS)

SBGFRLS is an Active Contour Model (ACM) based segmentation model where the starting points are defined by the user and then these points are continuously updated by the regional marked printing function (SBF). The SBF function used in the SBGFRLS model is presented in Eq. 10 [51].

$$\mathrm{spf}\,(\mathrm{I}\,(\mathrm{x},\mathrm{y})) = \frac{\mathrm{I}\,(\mathrm{x},\mathrm{y}) - \frac{c_1+c_2}{2}}{\max\left(\left|I\,(x,y) - \frac{c_1+c_2}{2}\right|\right)} \tag{10}$$

3.1.4 Online Region Active Contour Model (ORACM)

ORACM is generally a region-based ACM method. Similar to ACM, user-defined initiation criteria are used in the ORACM method. In this model, the thresholding process produces rigid boundaries and many small particles. These small particles are removed by applying morphological processes. Afterwards, the active contour used in ORACM is constantly updated. The most important advantage of ORACM compared to ACM is that it can perform segmentation by using less time and parameters. The function used in ORACM different from other ACM is presented in Eq. 11 [41].

$$\frac{\vartheta \phi}{\vartheta t} = H\left(spf\left(I\left(x\right)\right)\right).\phi\left(x\right) \tag{11}$$

The H(.) expression used in Eq. 9 is also used in Eq. 11, but the spf() expression is the same as in Eq. 10. The expression $\phi(x)$ is given in Eq. 6 in detail. The α parameter, which is used to adjust the input images and presented in Eq. 1, is not used in this method. In addition to this, the parameter, which is presented in Eq. 1 and has a high cost, $\nabla\phi$ has been removed.

3.2 Classification

Two different platforms were used in the classification phase. The first of these is the MATLAB platform, which uses the MatConvNet architecture. Secondly, it is the python platform where the tensorflow and keras libraries where the proposed model is developed. All segmentation carried out up to this stage has been carried out on each platform itself.

3.2.1 MatConvNet

After Krishevsky et al. [45], Deep Convolution Neural Network and ImageNet classification study, CNNs became a preferred method in computer vision applications instead of traditional image applications in the literature. For this reason, libraries on the subject have been developed on many different platforms. MatCovNet is a special library designed to develop CNN-based architectures for use in the Matlab environment. There are many different versions used in the literature.

There are convolution blocks of different content and sizes in this library. In addition, there are fully connection and pooling blocks as well as activation blocks. In the literature, there are application-specific architectures in which researchers are created with these blocks [28]. In the study, unlike these, MatConvNet-1.0-beta 15 version, which is one of the generally developed architectures in MatCovNet, was used. There are five basic convolution layers in the architecture used. ReLU(activation) and pooling processes were carried out alternately between convolution layers.

In the architecture used, there are seven activations, fully connection, dropout and classification layers in addition to convolution layers.

A filter in the form of $H(s_1, s_2)$ is used in each pooling layer. In the study, the largest value (max pooling) matrix of $H(2, 2)$ was used. The layer number is expressed as d in Eq. 12 [2].

$$y_{i,j,d} = \max_{1 \leq i' \leq s_1,\ 1 \leq j' \leq s_2} x_{i+i'-1,\ j+j'-1,d} \tag{12}$$

According to Eq. 12, the y output matrix is obtained from the x input matrix. The output matrix (y) obtained here is the input matrix (x) of the next matrix. The activation result of the $x_{i,j,d}$ matrix coming to the ReLU layer is calculated according to Eq. 13 [2].

$$y_{i,j,d} = max\left\{0,\ x_{i,j,d}\right\} \tag{13}$$

At the end of the process, there is data information for skin lesion class estimation at the 20th layer. In the implemented application, there are a total of $1 \times 1 \times 1000 \times 43{,}469$ feature information, including 1000 features for each data in the 20th layer.

The classification process was provided by sending the attributes and class information data obtained as a result of the deep learning algorithm to SVM, which is a linear classifier. The class information generated is between 0 and 1. The highest of these values gives the information of the class to which the image belongs. At this stage, the k-fold value was tested as 5 in order to reliably evaluate the data entered into the SVM.

While the general graphic of the architecture used in the study is presented in detail in Fig. 2, the sizes and numbers of the filters used in the architecture are presented in detail in Table 1.

3.2.2 Proposed Model

In parallel with the development of technology, data increase is observed in many areas [8, 21, 29, 31, 32]. Depending on the increasing amount of data, it has become an important issue to extract meaningful information from these data. Especially, the importance of the data to be used in many machine learning methods has increased even more [30]. Because feature extraction and feature detection directly affect the success rate.

For this reason, feature selection in newly developed machine learning algorithms is performed in an integrated manner with the model. In the study, it is aimed to develop a DNN model based on the convolutional neural network model that can automatically extract features.

For this purpose, a CNN-based model that automatically classifies skin lesions was designed by taking the basic layers presented in Fig. 3 as an example. The general flow diagram of the model designed as a result of experimental studies is presented

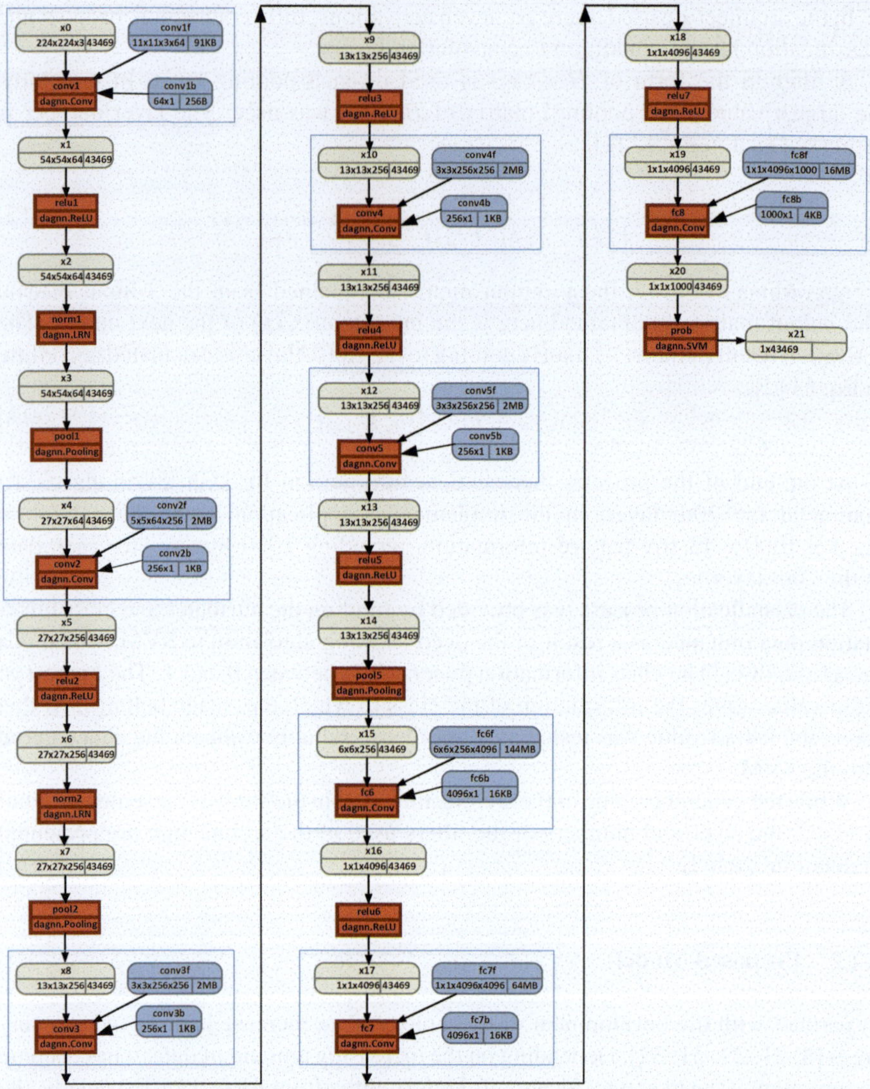

Fig. 2 Architecture of MatConvNet-1.0-beta 15 [26]

in Fig. 4. In addition, the pseudocode Algorithm 1 and Algorithm 2 of the study are also shared below.

The data used as input in the first layer of the proposed model consists of $224 \times 224 \times 3$ images. There are six blocks in the continuation of the input layer. In the first block, there are convolution, activation, max pooling, and dropout layers. The python codes of the created structure are briefly given below.

Table 1 Convolution layers used in MatConvNet-1.0-beta15 architecture

No	Filter size	Number	Layer
1	11×11	64	Conv1f
2	5 × 5	64 × 256	Conv2f
3	3 × 3	256 × 256	Conv3f
4	3 × 3	256 × 256	Conv4f
5	3 × 3	256 × 256	Conv4f

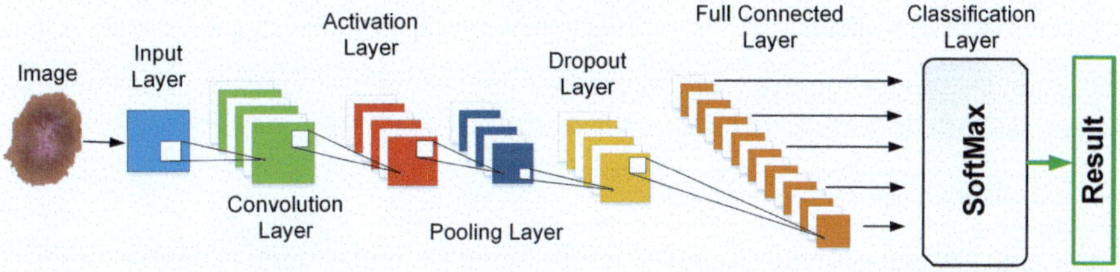

Fig. 3 A deep neural network layers

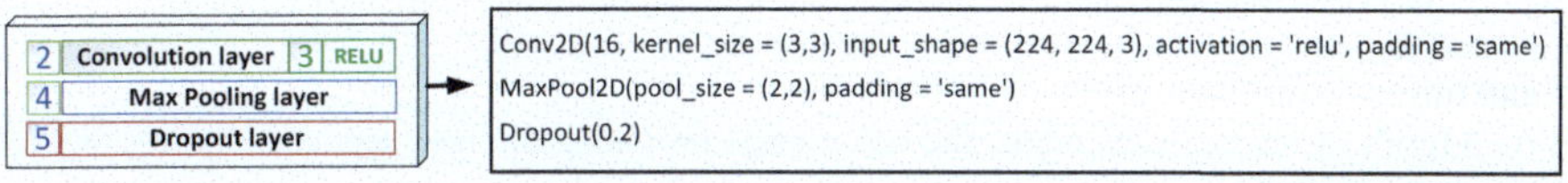

Fig. 4 Internal structure detail of Block 1

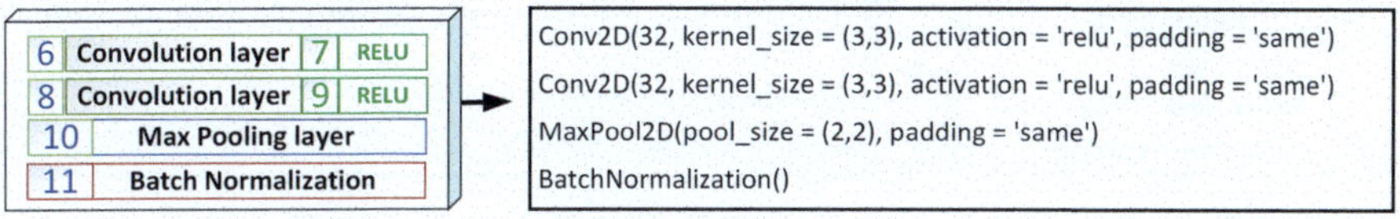

Fig. 5 Internal structure detail of Blocks 2, 3 and 4

In the second block, two consecutive convolutions and activations were performed. Afterward, max pooling and batch normalization were performed in the same block. In the third and fourth blocks, the operations made in the second block were repeated. The internal structure of the created block is presented in Fig. 5.

In the fifth block, dropout layer, dense layer, and batch normalization processes were performed. The internal structure of this block is also presented in Fig. 6.

In the last block, there are flatten, dense, dense and fully connected layers, respectively. The Flatten layer transforms the features from other layers into one dimension. Dense layers contain 100 hidden neurons each. With these layers, the classification performance is increased by reinforcing the features. The internal structure of the last block is presented in Fig. 7.

In the last layer of the block, a fully connected layer with softmax activation function is defined for BCC and Akiec classes. According to this layer output, the

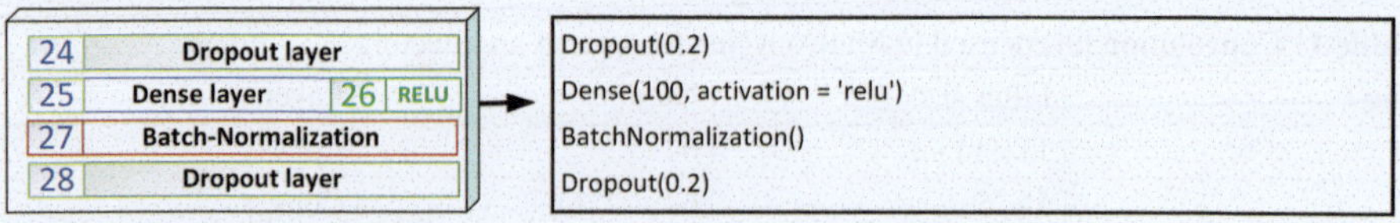

Fig. 6 Internal structure detail of Blocks 5

Algorithm 1 Detection of color spaces and ROI region

1: Input: Read labeled data from dataset
x_i=(x_a,x_b:3) : $i \in$ (1, ..,640), x_a=224dp, x_b=224dp
2: Four different segmentation models and 10 different color spaces were used in the study. At this stage, the contents of the functions used are defined
segmentation=[GAC, CV, SBGFRLS, ORACM]
colorspace=[RGB, YCbCr, HSV, HSI, CIELab, CIELuv, CMY, YIQ, YUV, CIEXYZ]
3: **for** $sg = 1, 2, \ldots, 4$ **do**
//for each different segmentation model
4: **for** $cs = 1, 2, \ldots, 10$ **do**
//for each different color space model
x_{RES_i}=$segmentation_{sg}(colorspace_{cs}(x_i))$
5: ShowResult(x_{RES_i})
6: **end for**
7: **end for**
8: As a result of the analyzes made, the color space providing the best segmentation result was determined (Fig.11).

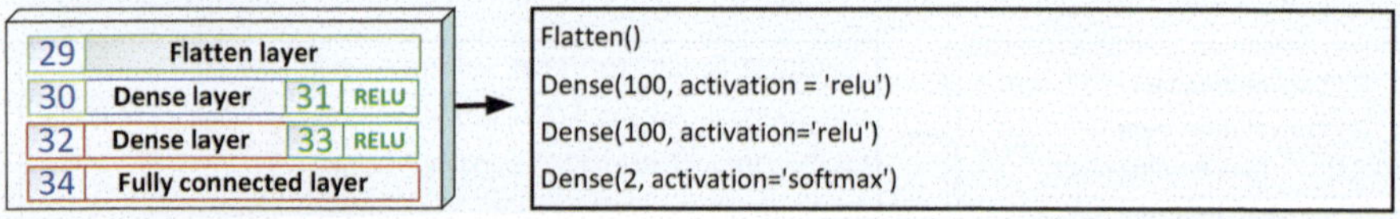

Fig. 7 Internal structure detail of Blocks 6

estimation result of the classes is obtained. The created structure consists of a total of 35 layers with the specified order and features. While the proposed model is presented in Fig. 8, the limitations of the model are also shared in Table 2.

4 Experimental Studies

Experimental studies carried out within the scope of this study were carried out on a computer with NVIDIA RTX 3060 GPU graphics card with a 3.2 GHz processor. Experimental studies were carried out in two different platform environments. MatConvNet-1.0-beta 15 has been tested on a platform with Matlab 2021b version on Windows 10 operating system. Tensorflow 2.5.0 [1] and Keras [19] artificial intel-

Algorithm 2 Training and testing processes for classification

Input: Read image in detected color space (HSV)
x_{RES_i}=(x_a,x_b:3) : $i \in (1, ..,640)$, x_a=224dp, x_b=224dp
Divide into two groups as training and testing according to Cross-Validation 5 value.
$TrainX_{RES_i}$=(x_a,x_b:3) : $i \in (1, ..,512)$
$TestX_{RES_i}$=(x_a,x_b:3) : $i \in (1, ..,128)$
Identify four different segmentation models
segmentation=[GAC, CV, SBGFRLS, ORACM]
Identify two different classification models and parameters
ClassificationModel=[MatCovNet,Proposed Models]
Identify of Evaluation Metrics
EvaluationMetrics=[Accuracy, Recall, Sensitivity, F1Score]
Train classification models in each segmentation model
for $sg = 1, 2, \ldots, 4$ **do**
//for each different segmentation model
    for $cl = 1,2$ **do**
//for each different classification model
$Model_{(sg,cl)}$=$Train(ClassificationModel_{cl}(segmantation_{sg}(TrainX_{RES_i})))$
    end for
end for
for $sg = 1, 2, \ldots, 4$ **do**
//for each different segmentation model
    for $cl = 1,2$ **do**
//for each different classification model
$Results_{(sg,cl)}$=$Test(Model_{(sg,cl)}(TestX_{RES_i}))$
        for $ev = 1,4$ **do** $EvaResults_{(ev,sg,cl)}$=; $EvaluationMetrics(Results(sg, cl))$
        end for
    end for
end for
As a result of the analyzes made, the color space providing the best segmentation result was determined (Fig.11).

ligence libraries were used in the design and implementation of the proposed model. Python 3.9.7 version platform was used in the creation of the proposed model by utilizing the specified libraries. In both platforms, the data is divided into two groups training and testing according to the cross-validation 5 value.

4.1 Evaluation Metrics

Confusion matrices are used to measure the overall success of the system in the study. The accuracy, recall, sensitivity, and F1 score values obtained from the confusion matrix shows at what rate the classifiers predicted. Calculations of accuracy, recall, sensitivity, and F1 score values of both models used in the developed algorithm are shown in Equations (14)–(19), respectively.

$$Accuracy\ rate = \frac{TP + TN}{(TN + FP + TP + FN)} \tag{14}$$

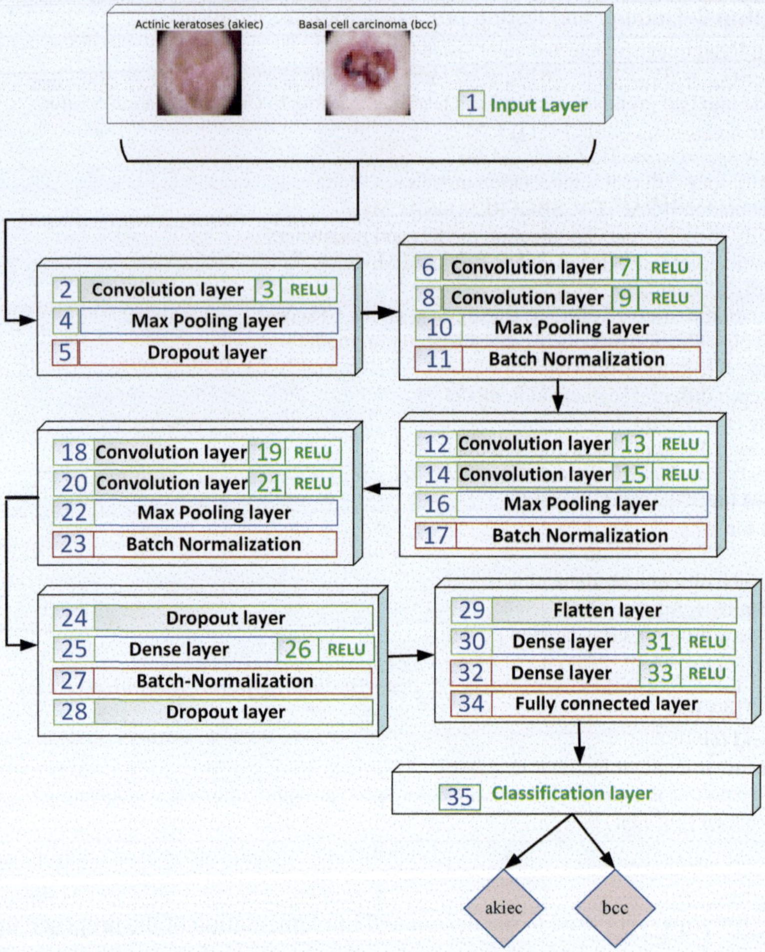

Fig. 8 Proposed model

$$Recall\ for\ Positive = \frac{TP}{(TP + FN)} \tag{15}$$

$$Recall\ for\ Negative = \frac{TN}{(TN + FP)} \tag{16}$$

$$Sensitivity\ to\ Positive = \frac{TP}{(TP + FP)} \tag{17}$$

Table 2 Some limitation parameters of the proposed model and the best parameter values determined

Parameters	Limitation ranges	Best value
Input image size	–	224 × 224 × 3
Initialization weight	Random, 1	Random
Learning rate	0.01–0.00090	0.00150
Batch size	2–512	32
Activation function	ReLU, Tanh	ReLU
Optimizer	RMSProp, SGD, Adamax, Nadam, AdaGrad, Adam	Adam
Loss function	Categorical Cross, Sparse Categorical Cross	Sparse Categorical Cross
Number of epochs	50–100	100
Output size	–	1 × 2

$$Sensitivity\ to\ Negative = \frac{TN}{(TN + FN)} \tag{18}$$

$$F1\ Score = 2x \frac{Precision\ X\ Recall}{Precision\ +\ Recall} \tag{19}$$

Between equations (14) and (19);

1. TP (True Positive): The algorithm outputs Akiec, in real case it should be Akiec,
2. FP (False Positive): The algorithm outputs Akiec, it should be BCC in the real case,
3. FN (False Negative): The algorithm outputs BCC, in real case it should be Akiec,
4. TN (True Negative): The algorithm outputs BCC, in real case it should be BCC, expresses.

The accuracy ratio shown in Eq. 14 is expressed as the ratio of the number of correct predictions to the total number of predictions. The Recall mentioned in Eqs. 15 and 16 shows how successfully Positive or Negative states are predicted. The sensitivity expression in Eqs. 17 and 18 is the ratio of those correctly predicted for Positive or Negative cases to the total predicted. F1 Score in Eq. 19 is the measurement of the accuracy of the tested data. It is the harmonic mean of the sensitivity and recall metrics. By using the harmonic mean instead of the normal mean, extreme cases are ignored.

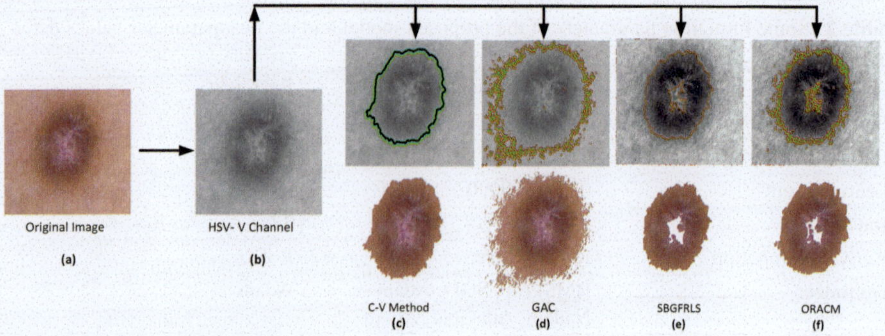

Fig. 9 Results of the segmentation methods tested

Table 3 Tested color spaces

No	Filter size	Number	Layer
1	RGB	6	YUV
2	HSV	7	YIQ
3	HSI	8	CIE lab
4	CMY	9	CIE XYZ
5	YCbCR	10	CIE LUV

4.2 Experimental Segmentation

In the study, 640 images belonging to BCC and Akiec species in the HAM10000 data set were first subjected to the segmentation process. During the segmentation stage, C-V Method, GAC, SBGFRLS, ORACM methods were used. Figure 9 shows the values obtained from 4 different segmentation methods for a single image.

The images obtained during the segmentation stage were reduced to $224 \times 224 \times 3$ RGB dimensions. The color spaces presented in Table 3 were tested in order to detect the regions of different colors on the obtained images. As a result of the experimental study, the best results were found in the HSV color space. The results detected in the HSV color space are presented in Fig. 10. When the color spaces given in Table 3 are applied to the segmentation result obtained by the C-V method shown in Fig. 9c, the results in Figure 10 are obtained.

4.3 Evaluation Results

In the study, 2 different models were designed according to 4 segmentation models for the MatConvNet 15 architecture and proposed model, and the classification successes obtained are presented in Table 4.

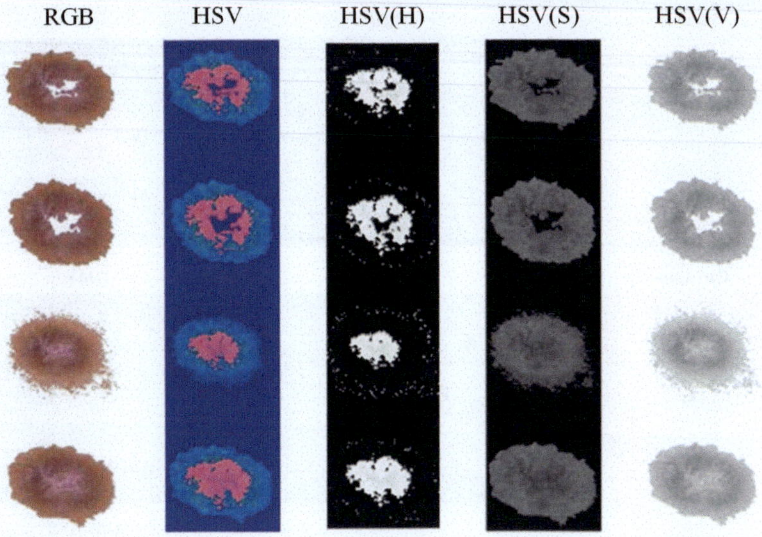

Fig. 10 Results of the segmentation methods tested

Table 4 Tested color spaces

	GAC		C-V		SBGFRLS		ORACM	
	MatConv Net 15	Proposed model	MatConv Net 15	Proposed Model	MatConv Net 15	Proposed model	MatConv Net 15	Proposed model
Accuracy rate	0.789	0.828	**0.859**	**0.914**	0.835	0.820	0.804	0.851
Recall for positive	0.793	0.838	0.838	0.920	0.830	0.836	0.800	0.846
Recall for negative	0.784	0.818	0.883	0.907	0.841	0.806	0.809	0.857
Sensitivity to positive	0.781	0.812	0.890	0.906	0.843	0.796	0.812	0.859
Sensitivity to negative	0.796	0.843	0.828	0.921	0.828	0.843	0.796	0.843
F1 score for positive	0.787	0.825	**0.863**	**0.913**	0.837	0.816	0.806	0.852
F1 score for negative	0.790	0.830	0.854	0.914	0.834	0.824	0.803	0.850

Bold show highest values for C-V segmentation

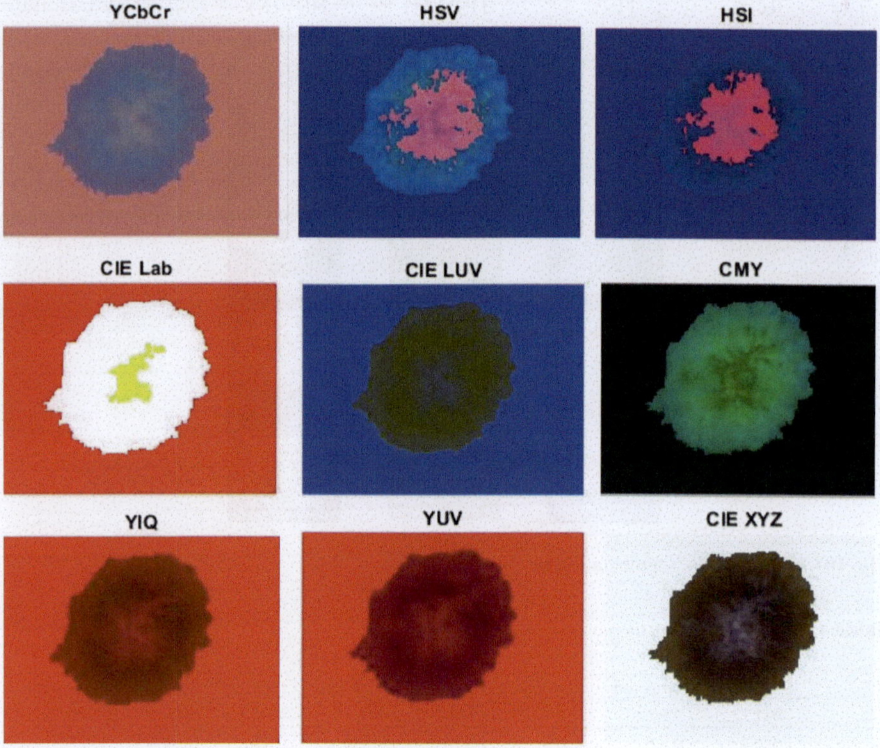

Fig. 11 Results of the segmentation methods tested

As seen in Table 4, the highest accuracy rate was obtained with C-V segmentation, respectively, 0.859 and 0.863, with the MatConvNet 15 model. The lowest accuracy ratio and F1 Score were obtained by GAC segmentation as 0.789 and 0.787, respectively. With the proposed model, the highest accuracy rate and F1 score were obtained with C-V segmentation as 0.914 and 0.913, respectively. The lowest accuracy ratio and F1 Score were obtained with SBGFRLS segmentation as 0.820 and 0.816, respectively (Fig. 11).

Comparison results with other studies in the literature using the same data set are presented in Table 5. As can be understood from here, the proposed model provides higher performance results than many studies using the same data set in the literature.

The training parameters and computational complexity of the CNNs blocks used in the proposed model are presented in Table 6 in detail. The values in Table 6 show that the results of the training parameters are reasonable. Much lower computational complexity was also obtained in the testing of the proposed model.

Table 5 Comparison results on the same datasets

Model	Accuracy
Yao's et al., single model deep learning [49]	86.40
Shen's data classification augmentation [37]	85.30
Charan's et al., two path CNN model [9]	88.60
Ameri's, AlexNet [6]	84.00
Huang's et al., efficientNets and DenseNet [14]	85.80
Huo's, CNN [15]	75.00
Karar's et al., efficientNets [5]	87.91
Garg's et al. CNN [11]	90.51
Nugroho's et al., CNN [33]	78.00
Proposed model	91.40

Table 6 Training parameters and computational complexity of CNNs

	Filters	Kernels	Activation	Pooling	Parameters (M)	Training time (s)	Testing time (s)
CNN Block-1	16	(3,3)	ReLU	(2,2)	448	0.54	0.0009
CNN Block-2	32	(3,3)	ReLU	(2,2)	4640	5.64	0.01
	64	(3,3)	ReLU	(2,2)	93770	11.39	0.02
CNN Block-3	64	(3,3)	ReLU	(2,2)	18,502	22.50	0.04
	64	(3,3)	ReLU	(2,2)	37,184	45.23	0.08
CNN Block-4	128	(3,3)	ReLU	(2,2)	73,856	89.84	0.16
	128	(3,3)	ReLU	(2,2)	148,096	180.15	0.32

5 Conclusion and Discussion

In the study, images obtained from the data set named HAM10000 were used. Images containing 320 Akiec and 320 BCC lesion classes from the data set used were selected by health professionals who are experts in the field. These data were split into two groups as training and test sets according to the cross-validation value of 5. Contrary to the studies in the literature in which convolution is performed on the whole image, this study primarily focused on finding the ROI region. For this, 10 different color spaces have been tested and it has been determined that the color space in which the ROI region is most prominent is the HSV color space. In order to segment the ROI region over the image, 4 different segmentation models, namely GAC, C-V, SBGFRLS, and ORACM, were tested. It was determined that the best result among the tested models was obtained with the C-V method as shown in Fig. 9c.

The main purpose of this part of the study is to do less convolution processing by focusing only on the determined ROI region instead of performing convolution on the entire image in the classification algorithm. Thus, both the processing cost is reduced and the negative effects caused by environmental factors during the image obtained are minimized. Convolution-based MatConvNet-1.0-beta15 architecture, one of the existing pre-trained machine learning methods, was used to classify the determined ROI region. Later, a new model was proposed based on the convolution model used in this model.

In the classification process in which the C-V segmentation method was used together with the MatConvNet-1.0-beta15 model and the HSV color space, the highest accuracy and F1 score were obtained as 0.859 and 0.863, respectively. Similarly, with the proposed model, images in HSV color space, and the C-V segmentation method, the highest accuracy and F1 score were obtained as 0.914 and 0.913, respectively. Detailed results of the segmentation models and classification algorithms used in the study are presented in Table 4. It has been determined that the proposed model on the ROI regions obtained by the C-V segmentation model in the HSV color space, as can be seen in Table 4, has higher success than the pre-trained MatConvNet-1.0-beta15 architecture. It was an expected result at the beginning of the study that focusing only on the ROI region in the study would directly reduce the training and testing time. However, with the proposed model, in addition to this result, the classification success has been increased. Along with this, it turned out that the HSV color space is very important in the determination of the ROI region. Therefore, it is recommended to focus on the HSV color space first in similar skin cancer studies. In the next future times, it should be planned to carry out studies in the HSV color space with advanced deep learning methods in different skin cancer studies.

In the study, distinctive feature maps were created by using appropriate filters and window sizes in convolution layers. After this stage, in order to increase the effect of distinctive features on classification performance, the features were reinforced with dense layers. The success values obtained as a result of the study also confirm this process. A deep learning model that can compete with the performances of pre-trained high-dimensional architectures such as MatConNet has been created within the scope of the study. Based on the proposed architecture, it can be developed for different problems in the future.

References

1. Martín Abadi, Paul Barham, Jianmin Chen, Zhifeng Chen, Andy Davis, Jeffrey Dean, Matthieu Devin, Sanjay Ghemawat, Geoffrey Irving, and Michael Isard. TensorFlow: a system for Large-Scale machine learning. In *12th USENIX symposium on operating systems design and implementation (OSDI 16)*, pages 265–283, 2016.
2. Brahim Ait Skourt, Abdelhamid El Hassani, and Aicha Majda. Mixed-pooling-dropout for convolutional neural network regularization. *Journal of King Saud University - Computer and Information Sciences*, 34(8, Part A):4756–4762, 2022.

3. Bilge Süheyla Akkoca-Gazioğlu and Mustafa Kamasak. Effects of objects and image quality on melanoma classification using Deep Neural Networks. 2020.
4. Fayadh Alenezi, Ammar Armghan, and Kemal Polat. Wavelet transform based deep residual neural network and ReLU based Extreme Learning Machine for skin lesion classification. *Expert Systems with Applications*, 213:119064, 2023.
5. Karar Ali, Zaffar Ahmed Shaikh, Abdullah Ayub Khan, and Asif Ali Laghari. Multiclass skin cancer classification using EfficientNets - a first step towards preventing skin cancer. *Neuroscience Informatics*, 2(4):100034, 2022.
6. A Ameri. A Deep Learning Approach to Skin Cancer Detection in Dermoscopy Images. *Journal of Biomedical Physics and Engineering*, 10(6):801–806, 2020.
7. Vicent Caselles, Ron Kimmel, and Guillermo Sapiro. Geodesic active contours. *International journal of computer vision*, 22(1):61–79, 1997.
8. Halit Çetiner. Multi-Label Text Analysis with GRU and CNN Based Hybrid Deep Learning Model. Technical report, 2022.
9. Dusa Sai Charan, Hemanth Nadipineni, Subin Sahayam, and Umarani Jayaraman. Method to classify skin lesions using dermoscopic images. *arXiv preprint* arXiv:2008.09418, 2020.
10. Noel Codella, Junjie Cai, Mani Abedini, Rahil Garnavi, Alan Halpern, and John R Smith. Deep learning, sparse coding, and SVM for melanoma recognition in dermoscopy images. In *International workshop on machine learning in medical imaging*, pages 118–126. Springer, 2015.
11. Rishu Garg, Saumil Maheshwari, and Anupam Shukla. Decision Support System for Detection and Classification of Skin Cancer Using CNN BT - Innovations in Computational Intelligence and Computer Vision. pages 578–586, Singapore, 2021. Springer Singapore.
12. Qi Han, Hongyi Wang, Mingyang Hou, Tengfei Weng, Yangjun Pei, Zhong Li, Guorong Chen, Yuan Tian, and Zicheng Qiu. HWA-SegNet: Multi-channel skin lesion image segmentation network with hierarchical analysis and weight adjustment. *Computers in Biology and Medicine*, 152:106343, 2023.
13. Md Anwar Hossain and Md Mohon Ali. Recognition of handwritten digit using convolutional neural network (CNN). *Global Journal of Computer Science and Technology*, 2019.
14. Hsin-Wei Huang, Benny Wei-Yun Hsu, Chih-Hung Lee, and Vincent S Tseng. Development of a light-weight deep learning model for cloud applications and remote diagnosis of skin cancers. *The Journal of Dermatology*, 48(3):310–316, mar 2021.
15. Y Huo. Full-Stack Application of Skin Cancer Diagnosis Based on CNN Model. In *2021 IEEE International Conference on Computer Science, Electronic Information Engineering and Intelligent Control Technology (CEI)*, pages 754–758, 2021.
16. Loretta Ichim, Dan Popescu, and Oana Chenaru. Advanced processing techniques for detection and classification of skin lesions. In *2018 22nd International Conference on System Theory, Control and Computing (ICSTCC)*, pages 498–503. IEEE, 2018.
17. Mohammad H Jafari, Nader Karimi, Ebrahim Nasr-Esfahani, Shadrokh Samavi, S Mohamad R Soroushmehr, K Ward, and Kayvan Najarian. Skin lesion segmentation in clinical images using deep learning. In *2016 23rd International conference on pattern recognition (ICPR)*, pages 337–342. IEEE, 2016.
18. Jeremy Kawahara, Aicha BenTaieb, and Ghassan Hamarneh. Deep features to classify skin lesions. In *2016 IEEE 13th international symposium on biomedical imaging (ISBI)*, pages 1397–1400. IEEE, 2016.
19. Nikhil Ketkar. Introduction to keras. In *Deep learning with Python*, pages 97–111. Springer, 2017.
20. Azize Kilic, Ali Kilic, Ali E Kivanc, and Abdullah Sisik. Biopsy Techniques for Skin Disease and Skin Cancer: A New Approach. *Journal of cutaneous and aesthetic surgery*, 13(3):251–254, 2020.
21. Ecir Uğur Küçüksille and Mahmut Tokmak. Yapay Arı Kolonisi Algoritması Kullanarak Otomatik Ders Çizelgeleme. *Journal of Natural & Applied Sciences*, 15(3), 2011.

22. Devender Kumar, Sadasivan Puthusserypady, Helena Dominguez, Kamal Sharma, and Jakob E Bardram. An investigation of the contextual distribution of false positives in a deep learning-based atrial fibrillation detection algorithm. *Expert Systems with Applications*, 211:118540, 2023.
23. Arkadiusz Kwasigroch, Agnieszka Mikolajczyk, and Michal Grochowski. Deep neural networks approach to skin lesions classification - A comparative analysis. In *2017 22nd International Conference on Methods and Models in Automation and Robotics (MMAR)*, pages 1069–1074. IEEE, aug 2017.
24. Hang Li, Xinzi He, Feng Zhou, Zhen Yu, Dong Ni, Siping Chen, Tianfu Wang, and Baiying Lei. Dense Deconvolutional Network for Skin Lesion Segmentation. *IEEE Journal of Biomedical and Health Informatics*, 23(2):527–537, mar 2019.
25. Shuai Liu, Peng Gao, Yating Li, Weina Fu, and Weiping Ding. Multi-modal fusion network with complementarity and importance for emotion recognition. *Information Sciences*, 619:679–694, 2023.
26. Team MatConvNet. Architecture of MatConvNet-1.0-beta 15.
27. Danilo Barros Mendes and Nilton Correia da Silva. Skin lesions classification using convolutional neural networks in clinical images. *arXiv preprint* arXiv:1812.02316, 2018.
28. Sedat Metlek. Forecasting of Dow Jones Sukuk Index Prices Using Artificial Intelligence Systems. *Economic Computation and Economic Cybernetics Studies and Research*, 56(1/2022):107–124, mar 2022.
29. Sedat Metlek. Forecasting of Dow Jones Sukuk Index Prices Using Artificial Intelligence Systems. *Economic Computation and Economic Cybernetics Studies and Research*, 56(1/2022):107–124, mar 2022.
30. Sedat Metlek. A new proposal for the prediction of an aircraft engine fuel consumption: a novel CNN-BiLSTM deep neural network model. *Aircraft Engineering and Aerospace Technology*, 95(5):838–848, jan 2023.
31. Sedat Metlek and Halit Çetiner. *Matlab Ortamında Derin Öğrenme Uygulamaları*. iksad publishing house, Ankara, 2021.
32. Maryam M Najafabadi, Flavio Villanustre, Taghi M Khoshgoftaar, Naeem Seliya, Randall Wald, and Edin Muharemagic. Deep learning applications and challenges in big data analytics. *Journal of big data*, 2(1):1–21, 2015.
33. Ardan Adi Nugroho, Isnandar Slamet, and Sugiyanto. Skins cancer identification system of HAMl0000 skin cancer dataset using convolutional neural network. *AIP Conference Proceedings*, 2202(1):20039, dec 2019.
34. Sameena Pathan, K Gopalakrishna Prabhu, and P C Siddalingaswamy. Techniques and algorithms for computer aided diagnosis of pigmented skin lesions-A review. *Biomedical Signal Processing and Control*, 39:237–262, 2018.
35. Victor Pomponiu, Hossein Nejati, and N-M Cheung. Deepmole: Deep neural networks for skin mole lesion classification. In *2016 IEEE International Conference on Image Processing (ICIP)*, pages 2623–2627. IEEE, 2016.
36. Tariq Rahim, Syed Ali Hassan, and Soo Young Shin. A deep convolutional neural network for the detection of polyps in colonoscopy images. *Biomedical Signal Processing and Control*, 68:102654, 2021.
37. Shuwei Shen, Mengjuan Xu, Fan Zhang, Pengfei Shao, Honghong Liu, Liang Xu, Chi Zhang, Peng Liu, Zhihong Zhang, and Peng Yao. A low-cost high-performance data augmentation for deep learning-based skin lesion classification. *BME Frontiers*, 2022, 2022.
38. Doaa A Shoieb, Sherin M Youssef, and Walid M Aly. Computer-aided model for skin diagnosis using deep learning. *Journal of Image and Graphics*, 4(2):122–129, 2016.
39. Robert Skaggs and Brett Coldiron. Skin biopsy and skin cancer treatment use in the Medicare population, 1993 to 2016. *Journal of the American Academy of Dermatology*, 84(1):53–59, 2021.
40. American Cancer Society. Cancer Facts & Figures 2021. Technical report, American Cancer Society, 2021.

41. M Fatih Talu. ORACM: Online region-based active contour model. *Expert Systems with Applications*, 40(16):6233–6240, 2013.
42. Poornima Singh Thakur, Tanuja Sheorey, and Aparajita Ojha. VGG-ICNN: A Lightweight CNN model for crop disease identification. *Multimedia Tools and Applications*, 82(1):497–520, 2023.
43. Philipp Tschandl, Cliff Rosendahl, and Harald Kittler. The HAM10000 dataset, a large collection of multi-source dermatoscopic images of common pigmented skin lesions. *Scientific data*, 5(1):1–9, 2018.
44. Andrea Vedaldi and Karel Lenc. Matconvnet: Convolutional neural networks for matlab. In *Proceedings of the 23rd ACM international conference on Multimedia*, pages 689–692, 2015.
45. Andrea Vedaldi, Mathias Lux, and Marco Bertini. MatConvNet: CNNs are also for MATLAB users. *ACM SIGMultimedia Records*, 10(1):9, 2018.
46. Lituan Wang, Lei Zhang, Xin Shu, and Zhang Yi. Intra-class consistency and inter-class discrimination feature learning for automatic skin lesion classification. *Medical Image Analysis*, 85:102746, 2023.
47. Xiao-Feng Wang, De-Shuang Huang, and Huan Xu. An efficient local Chan-Vese model for image segmentation. *Pattern Recognition*, 43(3):603–618, 2010.
48. Yiguang Yang, Fengying Xie, Haopeng Zhang, Juncheng Wang, Jie Liu, Yilan Zhang, and Haidong Ding. Skin lesion classification based on two-modal images using a multi-scale fully-shared fusion network. *Computer Methods and Programs in Biomedicine*, 229:107315, 2023.
49. Peng Yao, Shuwei Shen, Mengjuan Xu, Peng Liu, Fan Zhang, Jinyu Xing, Pengfei Shao, Benjamin Kaffenberger, and Ronald X Xu. Single model deep learning on imbalanced small datasets for skin lesion classification. *IEEE transactions on medical imaging*, 41(5):1242–1254, 2021.
50. Mehwish Zafar, Javeria Amin, Muhammad Sharif, Muhammad A Anjum, Ghulam A Mallah, and Seifedine Kadry. DeepLabv3+-Based Segmentation and Best Features Selection Using Slime Mould Algorithm for Multi-Class Skin Lesion Classification, 2023.
51. Kaihua Zhang, Lei Zhang, Huihui Song, and Wengang Zhou. Active contours with selective local or global segmentation: a new formulation and level set method. *Image and Vision computing*, 28(4):668–676, 2010.
52. Yu Zhang and Qiang Yang. A survey on multi-task learning. *IEEE Transactions on Knowledge and Data Engineering*, 2021.

Machine Learning Based Miscellaneous Objects Detection with Application to Cancer Images

Zahid Mahmood, Anees Ullah, Tahir Khan, and Ali Zahir

Abstract With the technological developments in artificial intelligence, traditional machine learning methods, and recently Deep Convolutional Neural networks (DCNNs) have accomplished great success in several vision related tasks. For example, object detection, object classification or recognition, and image segmentation are effectively achieved with the aid of aforementioned technologies. To train an effective DCNN model generally needs a big amount of diverse and balanced data. However, the DCNNs are quite often constrained by several aspects, such as (i) data annotation cost, (ii) long-tailed dispersal of data or imbalanced data, and (iii) scarcity of relevant data. Moreover, these days Generative Adversarial Networks (GANs) are widely used in image generation and synthesis related tasks. Object detection, being an important but challenging problem in the field of image processing and computer vision, plays an important role for several applications. While different methods exist to detect objects that appear in an image, a detailed analysis regarding common object detection is still lacking. This chapter pertains to detect objects that appear in an image with complex backgrounds using the Adaptive Boosting Algorithm (ABA). Different from several previously published chapters or research articles that focus on detection of six different objects, such as ships, vehicles, face, or eyes on standard datasets, this chapter focuses on real life objects, which include: (i) Melanoma (actual Malignant Melanoma, Nevus Spilus, and Blue Navy), (ii) license plates, (iii) vehicles, (iv) pedestrians, (v) players, and (vi) football. The ABA is applied on 8525

Z. Mahmood (✉) · T. Khan · A. Zahir
Department of Electrical and Computer Engineering, COMSATS University Islamabad, Abbottabad Campus, Islamabad, Pakistan
e-mail: zahid0987@cuiatd.edu.pk

T. Khan
e-mail: tahirkhan10@gmail.com

A. Zahir
e-mail: alizahir@cuiatd.edu.pk

A. Ullah
Department of Electronics Engineering, University of Engineering Technology Peshawar, Abbottabad Campus, Peshawar, Pakistan
e-mail: aneesullah@uetpeshawar.edu.pk

H. Ali et al. (eds.), *Advances in Deep Generative Models for Medical Artificial Intelligence*, Studies in Computational Intelligence 1124,
https://doi.org/10.1007/978-3-031-46341-9_8

test images, which include: 251 Melanoma, 2512 license plates, 2400 vehicles, 2502 pedestrians, 590 players/sportsmen, and 270 football images. The chapter also analyses the challenges of current study during investigating real life several objects' images and proposes a promising research direction, namely supervised learning cloud-based object detection. We are optimistic that this study will be useful for the researchers, practitioners, and beginners as a quick review with better understanding about object detection.

Keywords Adaptive Boosting · Generative Adversarial Networks (GAN) · Melanoma · Object detection

1 Introduction

Object detection, which is one of the fundamental tasks in computer vision has achieved a great deal of attention in the research community in various domains. Object detection aims to locate visible objects, such as melanoma, pedestrians, vehicles, or sportsmen in an input image [1]. Typically, object detection is achieved through understanding grown through analysis of a set of labelled objects and non-objects exemplars. Significant progress has been made in the last decade in this area due to its practical use in many computer vision applications, such as video surveillance, robotics, and human computer interaction.

In continuous image frames, accurate detection of objects assists to understand the movement patterns of objects to uncover suspicious events. Real-life systems are desired to accurately detect objects in various conditions, for example in static background scenes, non-uniform illuminations, abrupt object motion, change in color contrast, or rise in image noise level [2].

Many times, the task of object detection becomes hard due to inevitable variations in target appearance, such as lighting, pose, occlusion, or low-resolution. Recently, several object detection methods have been proposed, most of which analyse objects on standard datasets in controlled environments. Different from many of the published literature, this chapter simultaneously explores six different objects under diverse conditions. Particularly, this chapter investigates object detection in the context of (i) Malignant Melanoma (MM), (ii) license plates, (iii) vehicles, (iv) pedestrians, (v) players in the field, and (vi) football. In addition, we report experiments on real life images that have substantial variations from image appearance up to abruptly varying and complex backgrounds. We are hopeful that this study will be helpful for researchers to modify this method as per their needs. For readers' better understanding, below we categorise the investigated objects along with their recent developments.

Malignant Melanoma: As per the World Health Organization (WHO) report, skin cancer represents one-third of all types of cancers diagnosed in the world [3]. A matter of concern is that this disorder has climbed globally significantly in past 10

years at a constant rate. In the aforementioned disorder, the Malignant Melanoma (MM) has been observed as the fifth most common type of cancer that is affecting humans rapidly all over the world [3]. Moreover, an alarming fact is that the increase of Melanoma is on the order of 10–12/0.1 Millions in Europe, 18–20/0.1 Millions in the USA, and 30–40/0.1 Millions in Australia [3]. In its matured stage, the Melanoma becomes incurable and the treatments, such as chemotherapy or skin operation barely benefit the patients. Unfortunately, no low-priced instrument for melanoma screening exists throughout the world, where the public can get a free advice without visiting an office of a dermatologist. The aforementioned point highlights the need to timely detect this fatal disease [4–9]. Standard approach opted by medical staff to detect melanoma is Total Body Skin Examination (TBSE). The TBSE approach analyzes each of the Pigmented Skin Lesions (PSL) independently to identify possible melanoma. Besides being extremely tiresome and arduous for patients having abnormal mole pattern [10] or enormous nevi, for example, greater than 80, the aforementioned procedure suffers from observer's subjectivity as well as difficulties to track the lesion. For instance, without previous photographs, it is hard to conclude accurately whether a PSL having unclear skin marks is: (a) a lesion that existed but grew after the last check-up, (b) a lesion that existed and not changed but remained unobserved, and (c) an a newly grown lesion. Aforementioned or similar evidence regarding the previous states of the lesions are significantly important and encourage the prediction of malignancy by utilizing reliable marks of the melanoma, such as variations in lesion's shape, color, and size [11]. To identify varying moles all through the TBSE method usually a baseline is needed for the doctors to start. In [12], authors discussed an automated early melanoma diagnosis using sequential dermoscopic images. In their method, they initially, align sequential dermoscopic images of skin lesions. Later, they develop a spatio-temporal network to investigate the dermoscopic alterations from aligned lesion samples and its relevant difference images. The aforementioned listed approaches are very nice efforts to address the melanoma localization.

License Plates: License Plate Detection (LPD) is an emerging technology that is used nowadays to automatically locate vehicles' plates. The LPD is mostly employed for diverse purposes, such as to search stolen vehicles, to monitor road traffic, airport gates, speed, and automatic parking-lots access control. Several methods ranging from baseline algorithms, for instance Corner Template Matching and Hough Transform (HT) to sophisticated mechanisms, such as Vector Quantization (VQ), Neural Networks (NN), Support Vector Machine (SVM), or Likely-hood Ratio (LLR) have been developed to detect plates based on the features of plate characteristics [13, 14]. Mostly the LPD is achieved through machine learning techniques under various environment conditions [15].

Vehicles: Vehicles detection technology is normally employed in various applications for public safety purposes. For example, vehicle detection is the foundation of the planning and control of automated and self-driving vehicles. Due to the developments of the CNNs, there has been rapid progress in object detection domain. An important mainstream in vehicle detection method is YOLO based algorithm [16], which addresses the vehicles detection under diverse environments and conditions. The YOLO based methods have proved quite efficient to detect the complex objects, such as vehicles. Recent advancements in vehicles detection can be seen in [17].

Pedestrians: The aim of pedestrian detection is to localize pedestrian instances in a given image. In recent years, pedestrian detection algorithms have achieved a consistent improvement [18]. Several techniques proposed in the literature to achieve the pedestrian detection mainly differ in the way that they model object's appearance, shape, motion, or occlusion handling [19]. In [20], pedestrians are located using K-means algorithm. More advances in pedestrian detection can be seen in [21].

Players: To detect players' in large sports arena is also a challenging task. In this situation, low-resolution of players poses the main detection threat to any algorithm. In addition, players' pose, such as running, diving, or jumping severely affects the detection accuracy of state-of-the-art object detection and recognition algorithms [22]. In [23], multiple players are detected in sports arena during play. While in [24], authors discuss player detection and labelling in a soccer match video. Aforedescribed are nice efforts that enhance the viewers' experience. However, in such a dynamic environments where objects instantly change their position and pose, the accuracy of the developed algorithms have yet to reach a satisfactory level.

Football: Football detection is a challenging research domain due to the fact that a football match involves 22 players. As a result, this game demonstrates combined behavior in a highly dynamic environment with randomly changing position of football. As we will see shortly that football/soccer can be accurately detected through machine learning technology. Aforementioned are nice efforts in the object detection domain in which researchers from all over the world address the specific object detection challenges. However, we believe that literature lacks a comprehensive chapter that could address the aforementioned objects in a single study. The main contributions of this chapter are summarized as under.

- We present an empirical study on six different objects, which are melanoma, license plates, vehicles, pedestrians, players, and football/soccer under various backgrounds and lighting conditions. For each of the aforementioned objects, we report the object detection accuracy along with its computational complexity.
- We cover large and challenging ranges of several objects under diverse situations in our experiments to explore the detection phenomenon. We believe that the detection rates reported in this chapter provides detailed insight about several objects. We are hopeful that the experimental results shown in this chapter will provide a quick research overview to research beginners and practitioners to modify or improve the object detection algorithm for their specified tasks.
- Our experimental study reports multiple objects that appear in the input image. In all of the cases, objects are located using a popular supervised learning based

Adaptive Boosting Algorithm (ABA). For each of the category, we collect large number of samples to generate our own classifiers.

Rest of this chapter is organized as follows. Section 2 briefly reviews the Adaptive Boosting Algorithm (ABA). Detailed simulation results are presented in Sect. 3 and finally Sect. 4 concludes the chapter and highlights future research directions.

2 The Adaptive Boosting Algorithm (ABA)

This section briefly describes details of the Adaptive Boosting Algorithm (ABA) used to detect six different objects. To detect objects, we apply the well-known algorithm developed through joint research collaboration of Mitsubishi Lab and Compaq Lab by P. Viola and M. Jones from 2001 to 2004 [25]. The ABA was primarily developed to automate the phenomenon of human face localization in still images/videos. Algorithm-1 shows the pseudocode of the ABA method. Following are several motivations for us to employ the ABA based approach to locate miscellaneous objects presented in this study.

- Features extraction is a crucial step to successfully locate any object. The approach introduced by [25] utilizes the concept of Integral Image Representation (IIR) that evaluates features very quickly. One of the major characteristics of the IIR is that it does not depend on image intensities.
- Our study indicates that selecting the too many features will degrade the classifier's performance, which will result in peaking phenomenon. Therefore, an important characteristics of the approach developed by [25] applies a unique feature set that are reminiscent of Haar Basis Functions (HBF). The IIR was applied to compute the HBFs very rapidly, which is feasible for real-time object detection applications.
- Our study indicates that the ABA is an effective learning technique that constructs a robust and strong classifier by selecting few features. In [25], a weak learner is constrained in such a way that each of the returned weak classifiers is dependent on merely a single feature. Moreover, the ABA successively combines complex classifiers in a cascade that enhances the detection speed.

For our implementation, during training phase, we collected a total of 32,431 images with following important details. We refer aforementioned images as positive images, which contain object of interest only.

- **Skin cancer images**: We collected a total of 3531 skin images that had the resolution of 25×25 pixels of patients who suffered from cancer.
- **License plates images**: We gathered a total of 4800 license plates images that have the resolution of 25×40 pixels.
- **Vehicle images**: For our simulations, we gathered a total of 5700 images of vehicles with image 20×40 pixels.
- **pedestrian images**: We collected 6400 images of pedestrian with resolution of 20×40 pixels.

Algorithm 1 The adaptive boosting algorithm

1: Given example images (x_1, y_1),..., (x_n, y_n) where $y_i = 0, 1$ for negative and positive examples respectively.
2: Initialize weights $w_{1,i} = 1/2m, 1/2l$ for $y_i = 0, 1$ respectively. Where m and l are the number of negatives and positives respectively
3: For $t = 1, \ldots, T$:

- Normalize the weights $w_{t,i} \leftarrow \frac{w_{t,i}}{\sum_{j=1}^{n} w_{t,j}}$
- Select the best weak classifier with respect to the weighted error
  $\epsilon_t = \min_{f,p,\theta} \sum_i w_i |h(x_i, f, p, \theta) - y_i|$
  Implementation details are available in [25]
- Define $h_t(x) = h(x, f_t, p_t, \theta_t)$ where f_t, p_t and θ_t are the minimizers of ϵ_t.
- Update the weights:
  $w_{t+1,i} = w_{t,i} \beta_t^{1-e_i}$
  where $e_i = 0$ if example x_i is classified correctly, $e_i = 1$ otherwise, and $\beta_t = \frac{\epsilon_t}{1-\epsilon_t}$.
- The final strong classifier is:
  $h(x) = \begin{cases} 1 & \sum_{t=1}^{T} \alpha_t h_t(x) \geq \frac{1}{2} \sum_{t=1}^{T} \alpha_t \\ 0 & otherwise \end{cases}$
  where $\alpha_t = log \frac{1}{\beta_t}$

- **Player images**: For our simulations, we collected 5000 images of players from various sports arena, in which player resolution was 18×36 pixels.
- **Football/soccer images**: To generate a robust football classifier, we gathered a total of 7000 images of football in image resolution of 18×18 pixels.

We also collected 15000 negative images from several Internet sources. The negative images have the resolution of 640×480 pixels. Negative images are general scene images and do not contain above mentioned object of interest. Using Algorithm-1, we trained the ABA to obtain six different classifiers. The general expression for the classifier is shown in Eq. 1.

$$h(x) = \begin{cases} 1 & \sum_{t=1}^{T} \alpha_t h_t(x) \geq \alpha_t, \\ 0 & \text{otherwise.} \end{cases} \tag{1}$$

where α_t shows the error distribution and $\alpha_t = log(1/\beta_t)$ and h_t are the weak classifiers that are obtained during each round of boosting. The h(x) denotes the final classifier, which is a linear combination of many weak classifiers. In our experimental setup, we set T=40 to obtain the final classifier for each of the aforesaid objects. Readers are referred to [25] for a detailed description of the ABA classifier generation mechanism. Next section discusses experimental setup and results obtained therein along with detailed discussions.

3 Experimental Setup and Results

We performed simulations on Dell Precision Tower 7810, Dual Intel Xeon Processor E5-2699 V3, Storage: 2×1 TB Hard Drives with 96×2 GB of RAM. The aforementioned is a high-performance machine that can execute complex machine learning algorithms. All of the simulations were performed using MATLAB.

3.1 Investigations on Melanoma

3.1.1 Melanoma Detection

We evaluated Melanoma detection in three different phases. In the phase-1, we evaluated the classifier to classify images of actual pigmented lesions. In the phase-2, we examine the system on Dermnet dataset.[1] Finally, we assessed our conclusions by interviewing experts. It is important to state here that to identify the lesion, the dermatologists typically use stored slides of lesion images. We collected 84 images of benign and malignant lesions from patients. This study includes various age groups. The lesion images are in the RGB color with at least 0.5 cm diameter. Figure 1a shows the melanoma detection results on patients that suffered from skin cancer. From Fig. 1a key points are listed as follows:

- For all the seven images shown in Fig. 1a, it is clear that classifier successfully locates the melanoma in the captured images. These results are important, as the images captured and shown therein have much low-resolution than professional equipment.
- The classifier successfully detects for non-uniform lesions as shown in the left most image on top row in Fig. 1a. Although lower small part of the lesion is missed during detection, yet it is reasonable due to the extreme irregular shape and symmetry of the lesion.
- An interesting observation during melanoma detection is successful detection of particularly small size, such as 0.5 cm as depicted in the right most image in top row of Fig. 1(a). The small rectangle besides the larger one shows the successful detection of the low-resolution lesion.
- In few cases, double detection was achieved as shown in right most bottom image in Fig. 1a. We believe that such detection will be very helpful to further analyze the severity of the lesion.
- Out of 84 patients, melanoma detection experiments were conducted on different age groups as shown in Table 1. The ABA was more successful on patients that aged above 60. We believe that our evaluations are useful for the dermatologist community and for those outside specialized centres due to automatic processing of each intermediate module.

[1] www.dermnet.com.

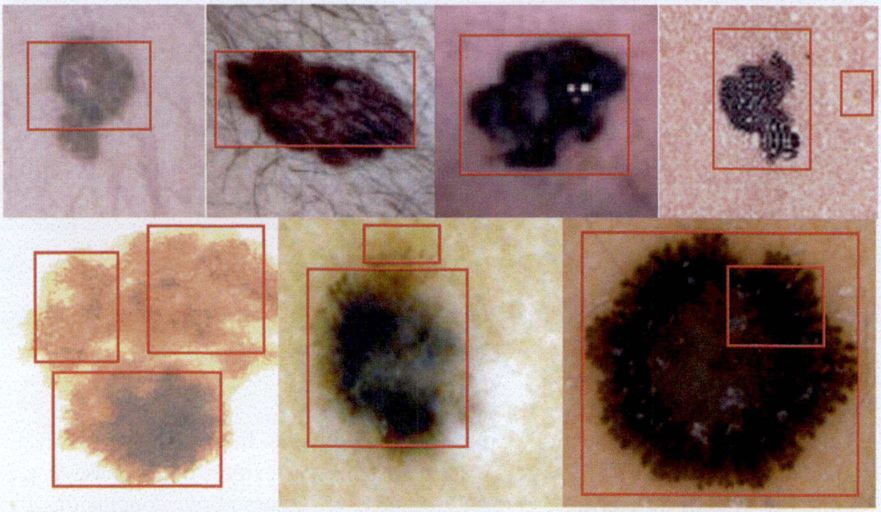

(a) Melanoma detection results on patients

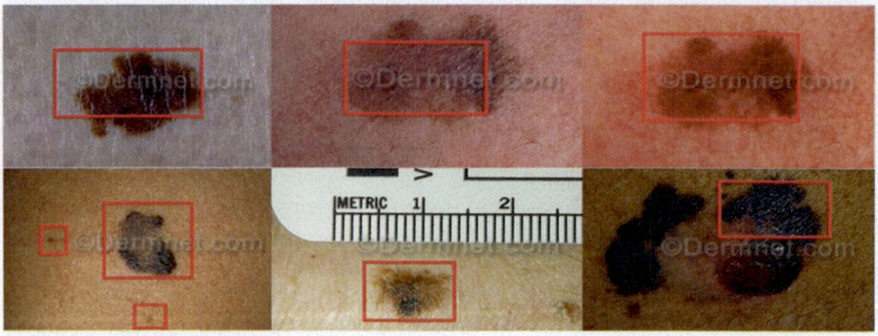

(b) Malignant melanoma detection results on the Dermnet dataset.

Fig. 1 Melanoma detection

Table 1 Melanoma detection on different age groups

Age group (years)	< 10	10–25	25–40	40–60	>60
No. of Patients	0	7	9	27	41
Detection accuracy %	Rare	3.50	4.50	16	44
Sensitivity %	Not evaluated	54	57	57.80	62.67

Although there are diverse types of skin lesions as mentioned on Derment database, such as Atypical Nevi, Becker Nevus, Halo Nevus, Nevus Spilus, Mongolian Spot, and Melanocytic Nevi. For our experiments, we chose Malignant Melanoma, Nevus Spilus, and Blue Navy to test the detection ability of our trained algorithm. The reason to choose them for experiments is their more prevalent and wild effect on the society. Figure 1b shows some malignant melanoma detection result on Dermnet dataset. Key observations in Fig. 1b are highlighted below:

- Malignant melanoma dataset on Dermnet dataset is challenging due to the fact that it contains large number of diverse images captured on different patients under non-uniform illuminations. Moreover, the disorder in these images varies in different orientations on human body. The ABA is more sensitive to detect brown and light brown skin lesion as shown in the first row in Fig. 1b.
- A dark lesion on skin is a harsh entity to be spotted in the captured images. As shown in last image in second row, only a small part is detected, while the rest is not located by the algorithm.
- Simulation results revealed that out of 19 dark lesion images, only six (6) were successfully detected. Therefore, the ABA produces a detection accuracy of 31.57% on such images. On 41 brown images that included dark brown and light brown lesion, the ABA achieved 30.13% accuracy. Aforementioned discussion summarizes that on 60 test images from Dermnet dataset, the ABA shows an average detection accuracy of 61.70%.

3.1.2 Nevis Spilus (NS) Detection

In the next phase of our study, we focused on Nevis Spilus, which is another type of skin lesion that appears in mix shapes, such as light brown, tan macule, speckled with smaller/darker macules, or papules on skin. Figure 2a shows Nevis Spilus detection results on Dermnet dataset. Key observations in Fig. 2a are highlighted below.

- Nevis Spilus on Dermnet dataset is also a challenging task due to the fact that it contains large number of lesions on the skin. The images in which lesion size was greater than 0.5 cm was located by the ABA as shown in first row of Fig. 2a. However, for the images in which extremely small and tiny lesions are present on the skin as shown in second row of Fig. 2a, very low detection accuracy was observed. In such conditions, the ABA partially detected portion of the lesion as shown in second row of Fig. 2(a). For few of such images, the ABA could not locate any lesion.
- We also observed the ABA to be very sensitive under non-uniform lighting for Nevis Spilus. For images captured under dark contrast conditions, the ABA produces very low detection accuracy. Middle image in second row of Fig. 2a is an example of this situation. Table 2 summarizes the results for Nevis Spilus.
- On 60 test images from Dermnet dataset, the ABA yields an average detection accuracy of 56.50% on Nevis Spilus images.

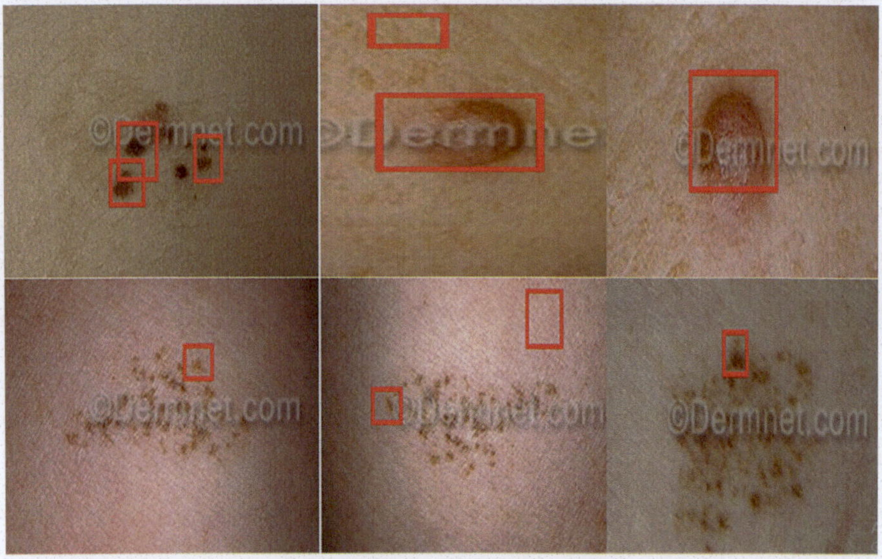

(a) Nevis Spilus detection results

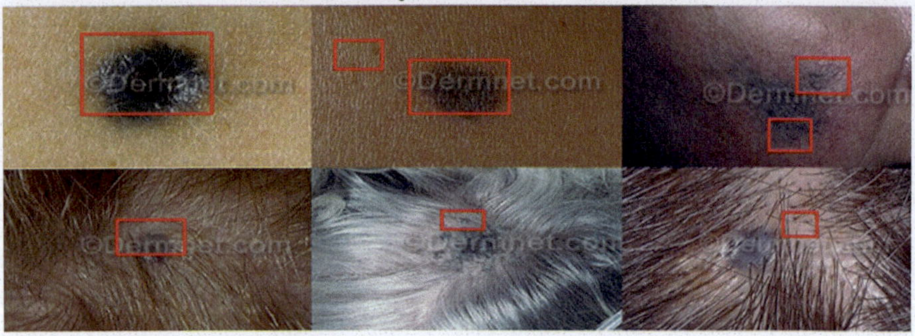

(b) Blue Nevus detection results.

Fig. 2 Nevis Spilus and Blue Nevus detection results on the Dermnet dataset

Table 2 The ABA classification accuracy on MM, NS, and BN categories

Source	Detection accuracy %	True positive %	True negative %
Melanoma on patients	68.30	82.05	55.45
Malignant Melanoma	61. 70	79.00	66.87
Nevus Spilus	56.50	81.60	64.79
Blue Navy	51.70	76.66	67.66

3.1.3 Blue Nevus (BN) Detection

In the final phase of our study, we study the detection accuracy of the ABA to detect Blue Nevus (BN) on Dermnet dataset. The Blue Nevus (BN) was supposed to be uncommon and harmless mole. The BN has usually dark blue appearance because the pigment cells, such as melanocytes accumulate deep in the epidermis. Normally, the BN view is observed as a constant steel-blue pattern. Due to aforementioned reason, the BN is also a challenging task to be located in real-time. Figure 2b shows few BN images along with detection result. From Fig. 2b, key observations are highlighted below.

- The BN that appeared on the skin, for example, nose, cheek, or neck was reasonably detected by the ABA as shown in the first row of Fig. 2b.
- For extremely irregular and large BN, the ABA partly detected the symptom as shown in the last image in first row of Fig. 2b.
- For cases, where BN appeared in congested hair, such as on top of head, under arms, or on legs, very low detection accuracy was observed. To strengthen the classifier, we integrated the MM classifier with the BN classifier. In that situation, partial detection was achieved. This case is shown in the second row of Fig. 2b.
- The BN detection is a challenging task when it appears with hair. In future, we expect to resolve this issue by introducing the image segmentation algorithm to effectively isolate hair from the BN spot. Table 2 summarizes the BN results on 47 images along with the MM and the NS categories.

3.1.4 Performance, Limitations, and Future

Performance: We presented detailed simulation results to locate the melanoma on various age groups. The ABA applied to detect melanoma is a realistic effort to locate melanoma in real-time on users' smartphone. The following items highlight the performance of the ABA.

- The ABA worked more effectively on patients' skin that aged greater than 60. We can expect that in future the ABA can be improved to reliably detect the melanoma in all age groups. This will surely help people to regularly monitor their health. Consequently, we find the ABA to be more sensitive on patients that aged greater than 60 followed by 40–60 years.
- The ABA was least effective on patients that aged 10–25 years. We keep it as our future study to investigate the skins of the growing people. It is stated here for readers' information that to investigate the skins of the patients in the age range of 10–25 years is a challenging task due to fact that an individual is in the growing stage of youth. In such age, many factors simultaneously affect the skins of the individuals.
- From Table 2, it is obvious that the ABA is also least effective to detect the Blue Nevis due to extreme irregular shape of this lesion. Similarly, the BN found on top

of head in hair is still a challenge to be reliably detected. Our effort to integrate two different classifiers to detect the BN could not produce encouraging results.

Limitations: Points below highlight the limitations of the ABA.

- Although the ABA yielded encouraging results to detect the melanoma. In most of the cases, we observed the partial detection of the ABA in various melanoma images, such as the results shown in Fig. 1a. Similarly, results shown in Fig. 2a depict the fact that still there is a considerable room to improve the accuracy of the applied ABA.
- Currently, we performed experiments under certified surgeons to conclude about the melanoma detection. Therefore, we present this study to be reasonably suitable for doctors and surgeons.
- We believe that in a short time this study can be helpful to develop a health monitoring application to be used on smartphones. However, one major hurdle to achieve the high detection accuracy is low-resolution images that are obtained through the cameras embedded in smartphones.
- Similarly, non-uniform lightings are also a big challenge to reliably detect the melanoma. The ABA performed much better on images that were captured in hospital under controlled conditions. However, images captured in sun light have very low melanoma detection.

Future: Points below highlight the future of the ABA.

- The ABA can assist the medical staff to reliably detect the melanoma. Moreover, a complete reliable melanoma identification system can be developed.
- Aforementioned discussion also points to the development of a system that can even specify the severity level of the melanoma on skin image.

3.2 License Plate Detection (LPD)

The LPD is also a challenging task because it contains characters and may contain decorations, such as sceneries, frames, and screws. To locate license plates, we selected the NCTU license plate dataset.[2] Aforesaid is a challenging dataset due to fact that the license plates here are obtained in diverse conditions. Few of such cases are indicated in Fig. 3. Moreover, to locate license plates in real-time becomes challenging due to following factors.

Location: License plates may exist in different locations on the vehicle.
Size: Plates with different sizes may exist in an image or different images.
Colors/backgrounds: Plates may have different colors/background due to different plate styles. In our simulations, we consider vehicles' own headlight effects, natural illuminations, and plate like backgrounds. Few of the license plate detection results are shown in Fig. 3 with following key observations:

[2] http://lpr.csie.nctu.edu.tw.

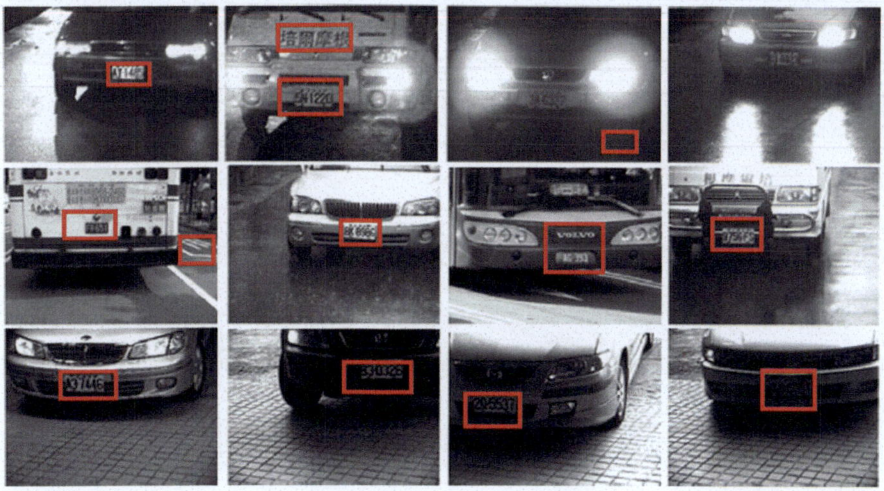

Fig. 3 The LP detection results: **top row**: vehicle headlights, **medium row:** natural illuminations, and **bottom row**: plate like background

- The ABA detects license plates under normal vehicle's headlines. For high intensity lights, the ABA fails to detect license plates as shown in 3rd and 4th image in top row in Fig. 3.
- Under natural illuminations or normal lighting conditions, the ABA accurately detects the license plates. However, in some cases, there are false detections as shown in 1st image in 2nd row in Fig. 3.
- For plate like background, such as vehicle standing on a tile that has similar appearance like plates, the ABA accurately locates the license plate as shown in 3rd row in Fig. 3.

Table 3 summarizes the results on 2512 test images. Clearly, under natural illuminations, the ABA delivers encouraging results followed by plate like background and headlights, respectively. We observe under very high beam headlights, the license plated detection was extremely low, which resulted in the least detection accuracy of the top row in Table 3. We perform experiments on license plates that had resolution of 25×35 pixels and 20×30 pixels. The results found were same and listed in Table 3. Moreover, the ABA was unable to detect any license plate less than 20×30 pixels.

Table 3 License plated detection summary

Database	Plate condition	No. of plates	Detection accuracy %
NCTU	Natural Illuminations	1450	87. 7000
	Plate like Background	262	84.5000
	Headlights	800	68.3000
Total/ Average		**2512**	**80.1600**

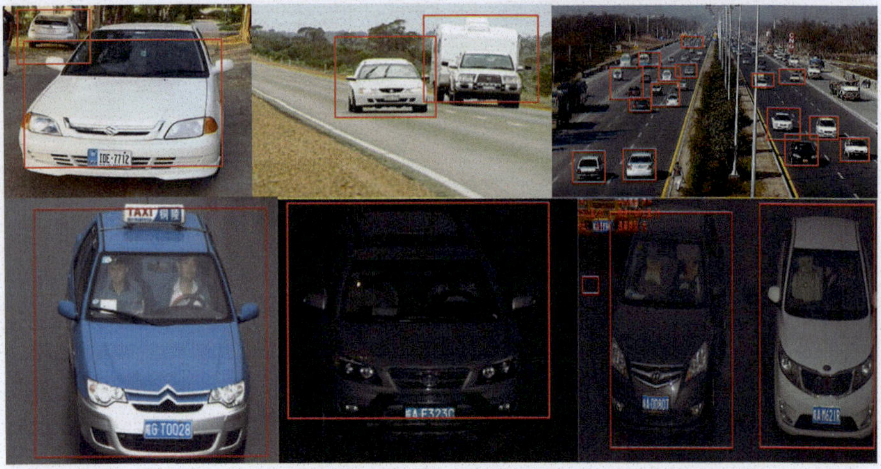

Fig. 4 Vehicle detection: **top row**: real life images and **2nd row**: PKU database

3.3 Vehicle Detection

Vehicle detection is another challenging task because a vehicle may appear in different orientations with different colors. To locate vehicles, we selected the local PKU dataset[3] along with local Pakistani traffic real life images as shown in top row in Fig. 4. As can be seen that vehicle detection is successfully achieved on images that contain numerous vehicles. In addition, the ABA successfully handles varying illuminations and vehicle pose deviations. Vehicle detection module successfully locates vehicles from PKU database in different conditions as shown in 2nd row in Fig. 4. Table 4 summarizes the ABA results on vehicle detection. From Fig. 4 and Table 4, few observations are in order:

- The ABA has 100% detection accuracy up to 11 vehicles that appear in an image. Similarly, for up to 41 vehicles that appear in an image, the ABA yields over 85% detection accuracy, which we believe is encouraging
- For different orientations, the ABA effectively detects vehicles in the images. In Fig. 4, all vehicles are detected from frontal up to straight view. In some cases, we find false negative as shown in right side of top row in Fig. 4. In particular, the ABA yields over 90% detection accuracy on the PKU dataset.
- As shown in Table 4 that our developed vehicle classifier yields 100% detection accuracy up to 11 vehicles that appear in an image. On real life images, the vehicle classifier yields 94.93% detection accuracy. The PKU database contains five distinct categories of vehicles with maximum 3 vehicles per image. Our developed

[3] https://github.com/ofeeler/LPR.git.

Table 4 Vehicles detection accuracy summary

Dataset	Vehicles per image	Detection accuracy %	Detection accuracy %
Real life images	1–11	100	94.93
	12	95	
	15	95	
	17	**88**	
	19	88	
	21	88	
	34	87.50	
	41	87.50	
	45	84.90	
PKU	Randomly chosen 800 images to test the detection accuracy. The PKU database contains vehicles in 5 different scenarios with maximum maximum 3 images in an image		94.94
Average (on 2400 test images)			94.9352

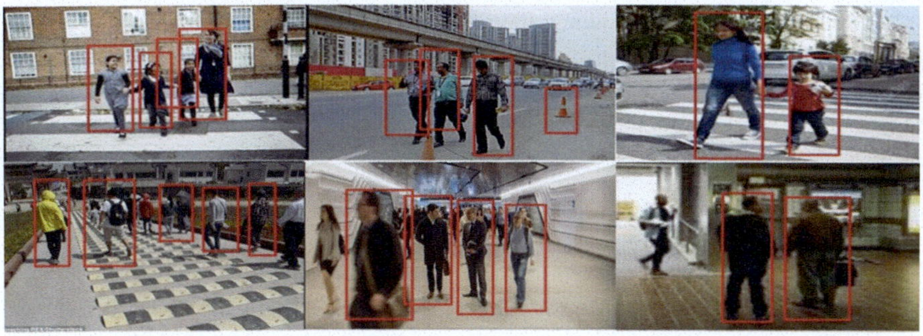

Fig. 5 Pedestrian detection

classifier yields 94.94% detection accuracy on standard PKU dataset. The overall accuracy generated by the vehicle classifier is 94.9352%, which we believe is encouraging.

3.4 Pedestrian Detection

Pedestrian detection was performed on google publicly pedestrian dataset.[4] Figure 5 shows real-life captured images with detected pedestrians. As shown in 1st image in 2nd row of Fig. 5, pedestrian detection is achieved on images that contain ten

[4] www.Google.com/pedestrian-walking.

pedestrians. These objects have also significant variations in pose, yet the pedestrian classifier handles them effectively. Table 5 summarizes the ABA results on pedestrian detection. From Fig. 5 and Table 5, few observations are in order:

- The ABA has 100% detection accuracy up to 9 pedestrians that appear in an image. Up to 50 pedestrians that appear in an image, the ABA yields over 85% detection accuracy.
- For different walking pose, the ABA effectively detects pedestrians in the images. In Fig. 5, all pedestrians are detected from frontal up to side view. In some cases, we observe undetected pedestrians as shown in 2nd row in Fig. 5.
- Experiments performed on 2502 general outdoor images, revealed over 90% accurate pedestrian detection.

3.5 Players' Detection

Since to detect players', no public database is available. Therefore, to locate players' in the input images and to enhance the aesthetic sense, we collected player images during various sports as shown in Fig. 6. As shown in Fig. 6, several players are successfully detected in images that have diverse variations in pose. Table 5 summarizes the ABA results on players' detection. From Fig. 6 and Table 5, few observations are in order:

- The ABA has 100% detection accuracy up to 9 players that appear in an image. Up to 13 players that appear in an image, the ABA yields over 95% detection accuracy.
- The ABA yields same detection accuracy up to 9 pedestrians or players that appear in the input image. On 590 players images, the ABA yields, 98.65% detection accuracy.

Experiments performed on 590 images reveal that the ABA yields 98.6555% detection accuracy. This point reveals the robustness of the ABA to detect various objects. Especially, players are in various pose during play, such as running, jumping, diving, or bending.

3.6 Football Detection

Figure 7 shows few images with detected football/soccer confined by a square bounding box. As shown in Fig. 7 that football is accurately detected in all scenarios, such as on ground and in the air. We also observe false detection during football detection as shown in 1st row of Fig. 7. On 270 football images, the ABA yields 92.47% detection accuracy. We believe that in future, the football detection will be useful for several purposes as highlighted in points below.

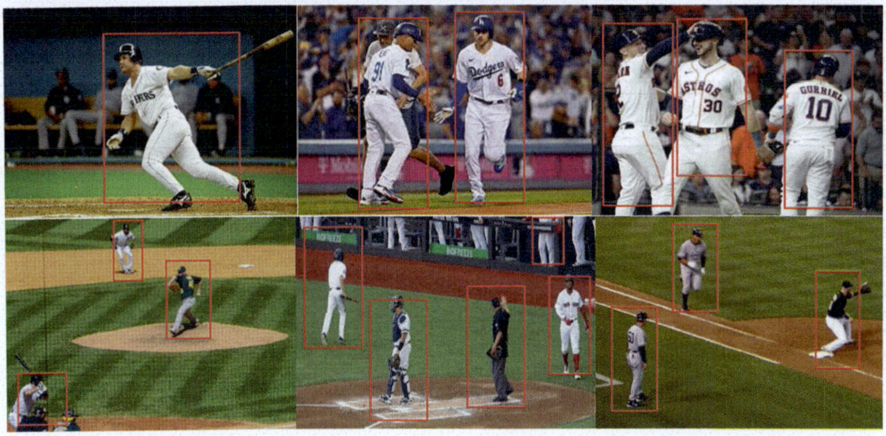

Fig. 6 Players detection

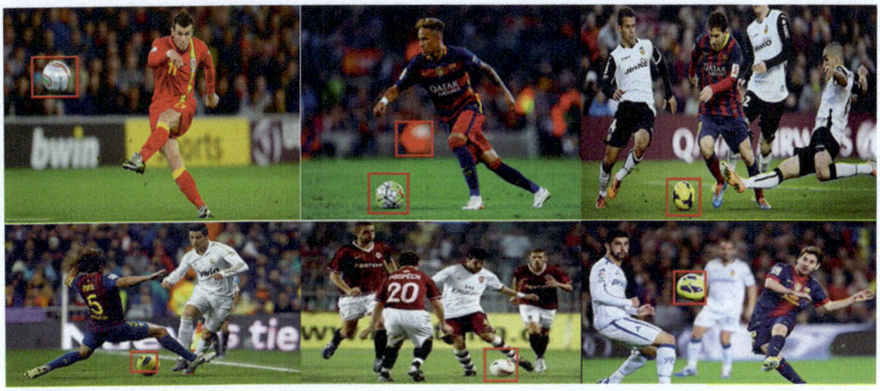

Fig. 7 Football detection

- **Coaches**: They want to know what the weaknesses and strengths of their players are. For example, during a football game, players can have high shooting power and low acceleration so that they can provide personalized training to their players.
- **Directors**: They want to know which player is best for a given position in field, which player to hire for their clubs, etc.
- **TV and Entertainment Industry**: They want to provide more interesting information about the game, such as average speed of the ball, of a player, or was it an offside or not?
- **Miscellaneous**: There are other potential users, such as newspaper editors who want a summary of the match to publish, sports analyst, and gaming industry.

The aforementioned applications are based on accurate player detection and tracking. Once the locations of the players are found, all the useful statistics can be derived.

3.7 Computational Complexity

We report the computational complexity of the ABA in terms of time consumed to yield the output image that contains the specified object. Table 5 lists the execution time of objects detection. As can be seen that the Blue Navy is computationally more expensive than rest of the objects. Similarly, Malignant Melanoma also requires nearly 2 s to be located within the image. We observe that the Melanoma detection is relatively an expensive object than the other objects that are investigated in this study. Mean detection time to detect Melanoma and its categories is found to be 2.3210 s. Table 5 also indicates that the pedestrians and football have least detection time. On the average, the ABA consumes about 1.1388 s to detect the six objects, which are reported in this chapter. Therefore, the ABA can be used in real-time applications.

Table 5 Computational complexity

Object		Execution time (s)
Melanoma	Melanoma on patients	1.8860
	Malignant Melanoma	1.9900
	Nevus Spilus	2.7112
	Blue Navy	2.6970
License Plates		0.1211
Vehicles		0.1311
Pedestrians		0.1111
Players		0.4908
Football		0.1111
Average		1.1388

3.8 Discussion

This section sheds further light on the ABA detection capability along with few state-of-the-art methods.

- The ABA was tested on 8525 different object images out of which contain 251 melanoma images including patients and Dermnet dataset. The ABA yields 59.55% detection accuracy. Many times, on conventional desktops, training phase takes several days to generate a classifier. Out of various types of melanoma, the Blue Navy was harder to detect and was more computationally expensive than rest of the objects. Achieving high accuracy in object detection and recognition is still a challenging task in computer vision due to several reasons. These include but are not limited to factors, for example large variations in the shapes of the objects, low sizes of the images, and huge computational demands of the underlying algorithms.

- Our study indicates that the GANs based method can significantly fulfill the tasks of object detection or recognition. To reliably detect challenging objects, such as in medical imaging, recently GAN method proposed [26] lessens the adverse effects of undesirable textures to enhance the implicit association between desired object and it texture.
- Moreover, the GANs based methods can be handy enough to segment the images from their desired region of interest. For instance, cancer and melanoma images could be analyzed through segmentation or mask generations [27].
- The GANs can be made intelligent enough to discriminate between the melanoma image from the non-melanoma, or the normal skin lesion from the abnormal one through various training, encoding, and decoding methods [28].

3.9 Future Research Direction

This section proposes a promising research direction, namely supervised learning-based cloud enabled object detection. Based on the presented study in this chapter, we propose a cloud-based environment to solve most of the aforementioned problems. Figure 8 shows the tentative flow of cloud-based object detection architecture. Apart from the requirement of fast analysis of image data of exponentially growing scales and sizes, there also exists a need to accurately and uniquely capture the image features without loss or destruction during analysis. All of the tasks including the training phase, features extraction, object detection, and objection recognition incur high computational complexities and are beyond the capabilities of conventional computing machines due to their limitations in terms of compute-power, storage, and memory. Therefore, the aforementioned tasks can be effectively performed on a cloud-based infrastructure due to greater capabilities in terms of tasks parallelization and storage.

3.10 Final Remarks

As evident from the results section in this chapter, we conclude that machine learning is an effective tool to assist humans by training an algorithm on appropriate data as per desired applications. Moreover, machine learning has diverse effects on society that include healthcare, industrial mass productions, education, and transportations. Furthermore, machine learning is transforming the world around us very quickly. This chapter also indicated that machine learning methods can be used to detect and track humans in multimedia streams. For object detection, in addition to the conventional

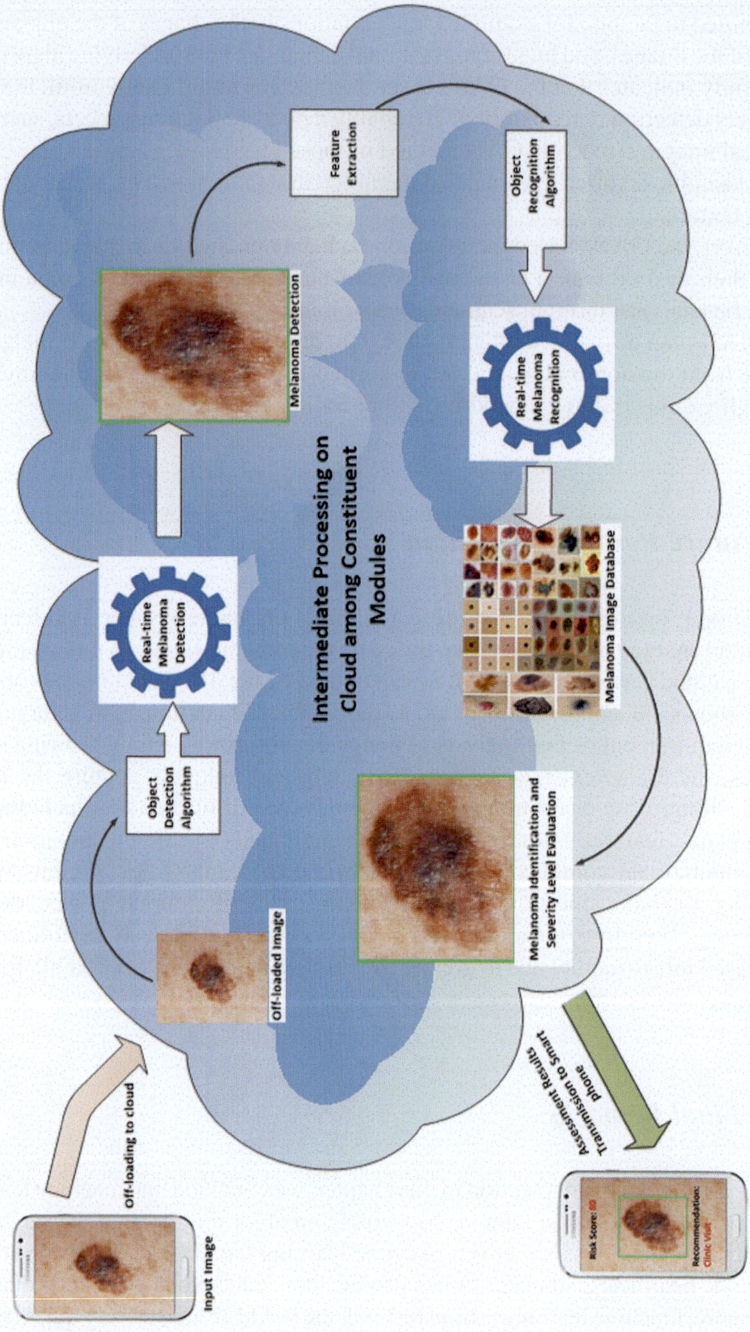

Fig. 8 Cloud-based melanoma detection architecture

machine learning, a rapidly growing paradigm is to use deep learning algorithms, for instance the RCNN, the YOLO, the SSD. In addition to MatLab, few software libraries that can be used to detect objects are Tensor Flow, ImageAI, and GluonCV. Furthermore, Bayesian networks, the CNNs, and recurrent neural networks can also be used to detect various objects [29].

4 Conclusions

This chapter pertained to detect six different objects that appear in an image with complex background using the Adaptive Boosting Algorithm (ABA). This chapter focused on real life generic objects including 251 images from Melanoma, 2512 images of license plates, 2400 images of vehicles, 2502 images of pedestrians, 590 images of players/sportsmen, and 270 images football each of which contained one or more objects. In particular, a publicly available Dermnet dataset was used to investigate the melanoma. The ABA yields high accuracy for all objects except melanoma. Besides, this chapter also analysed and discussed the challenges of object detection in current study and proposed a promising research direction, namely supervised learning cloud-based melanoma detection. Authors believe that this study will be useful for researchers, practitioners, and beginners to better investigate this research domain. In future, a parallel version of the ABA can be developed to further reduce the processing time. For all of the objects except melanoma, the ABA yields over 80% detection accuracy. Therefore, the efficiency of the ABA can further be investigated under non-uniform and bad lighting conditions to detect general out door objects. Similarly, for generic objects the ABA can be trained to handle to short term or long-term occlusions.

References

1. W. Lisheng, K. Ding, and H. Huosheng, "Automatic skin cancer detection in dermoscopy images based on ensemble lightweight deep learning network," IEEE Access, vol. 8, pp. 99633–99647, 2020.
2. Y. Long, Y. Gang, Z. Xiao, and Q. Liu, "Accurate object localization in remote sensing images based on convolutional neural networks," IEEE Transactions on Geoscience and Remote Sensing, vol. 55, no. 5, pp. 2486–2498, 2017.
3. WHO, "Ultraviolet (UV) Radiation and Skin Cancer," World Health Organization (WHO), 2020, Accessed: January 4, 2022. [Online]. Available: https://www.who.int/news-room/q-a-detail/ultraviolet-(uv)-radiation-and-skin-cancer
4. A. G. Pacheco and R. A. Krohling, "The impact of patient clinical information on automated skin cancer detection," Comput. Biol. Med., vol. 116, art. no. 103545, 2020.
5. M. E. Celebi, N. Codella, and A. Halpern, "Dermoscopy image analysis: Overview and future directions," IEEE Journal of Biomed. Health Informat., vol. 23, no. 2, pp. 474–478, 2019.
6. T. J. Brinker et al., "Deep learning outperformed 136 of 157 dermatologists in a head-to-head dermoscopic melanoma image classification task," Eur. J. Cancer, vol. 113, pp. 47–54, 2019.

7. N. Gessert, M. Nielsen, M. Shaikh, R. Werner, and A. Schlaefer, "Skin lesion classification using ensembles of multi-resolution efficient nets with meta data," MethodsX, pp. 1–8, 2020.
8. A. G. Pacheco et al., "PAD-UFES-20: A skin lesion dataset composed of patient data and clinical images collected from smartphones," Data Brief, vol. 32, pp. 1–10, 2020.
9. Y. Liu et al., "A deep learning system for differential diagnosis of skin diseases," Nature Med., vol. 26, no. 6, pp. 1–9, 2020.
10. Silva, J., et al.: 'Atypical mole syndrome and dysplastic nevi: Identification of populations at risk for developing melanoma-review article', Clinics (Sao Paulo), 2011, 66, (3), pp. 493–499.
11. B. Negin, E. Riedel, S. Oliveria, and M. Berwick, "Symptoms and signs of primary melanoma," Cancer, vol. 98, no. 2, pp. 344–348, 2003.
12. Z. Yu, J. Nguyen, T. Nguyen, J. Kelly, C. Mclean, and P. Bonnington, "Early Melanoma Diagnosis with Sequential Dermoscopic Images," IEEE Transactions on Medical Imaging, vol. 41, no. 3, 633–646, 2022.
13. Z. Mahmood, K. Khan, U. Khan, S. H. Adil, S. S. A. Ali, and M. Shahzad, "Towards Automatic License Detection," Sensors, vol. 22, no. 3, pp. 1–19, 2022.
14. K. Khan, A. Imran, H. Z. Rehman, A. Fazil, M. Zakwan, and Z. Mahmood, "Performance Enhancement Method for Multiple License Plate Recognition in Challenging Environments," EURASIP Journal on Image and Video Processing, no. 30, pp. 1–23, 2021.
15. Z. Mahmood, M. U. S. Khan, M. Jawad, S. U. Khan, and L. T. Yang "A parallel framework for object detection and recognition for secure vehicle parking," 17th International Conference on High Performance Computing and Communications (HPCC), pp. 892–895, USA, 2015.
16. N. Zarei, P. Moallem, and M. Shams, "Fast-Yolo-Rec: Incorporating Yolo-base detection and recurrent-base prediction networks for fast vehicle detection in consecutive images," IEEE Access, vol. 10, pp. 120592–120605, 2022.
17. L. Chen, S. Lin, X. Lu, D. Cao, H. Wu, C. Guo, C. Liu, and F. Wang, "Deep neural network based vehicle and pedestrian detection for autonomous driving: a survey," IEEE Transactions on Intelligent Transportation Systems, vol. 22, no. 6, pp. 3234–3246, 2021.
18. A. Abdelmutalab C. Wang, "Pedestrian detection using MB-CSP model and boosted identity aware non-maximum suppression," IEEE Transactions on Intelligent Transportation Systems, vol. 23, no. 12, pp. 24454–24463, 2022.
19. W. Hsu and P. Chen, "Pedestrian detection using stationary wavelet dilated residual super-resolution," IEEE Transactions on Instrumentation and Measurement, vol. 71, pp. 5001411 , 2022.
20. M. I. Shahzad, Y. Shah, Z. Mahmood, A. W. Malik, and S. Azmat, "K-Means based Multiple Objects Tracking with Long-term Occlusion Handling," IET Computer Vision, 2017, Vol. 11, No. 1, pp. 68–77.7.
21. J. Cao. Y. Pang, J. Xie, F. Khan, and L. Shao, "From handcrafted to deep features for pedestrian detection: a survey," IEEE Transactions on Pattern Analysis and Machine Intelligence, vol. 44, no. 9, pp. 4913–4934, 2022.
22. Z. Mahmood, N. Muhammad, N. Bibi, and T. Ali, "A Review on state-of-the-art Face Recognition Approaches," Fractals, Complex Geometry Patterns and Scaling in Nature and Society, vol. 25, no. 2, pp. 1750025-1–1750025-19, 2017.
23. Z. Mahmood, T. Ali, N. Muhammad, N. Bibi, I. Shahzad, and S. Azmat, "EAR: Enhanced Augmented Reality System for Sports Entertainment Applications," KSII Transactions on Internet and Information Systems, vol. 11, no. 12, pp. 6069–6091, 2017.
24. Liu et al., "Automatic player detection, labeling and tracking in broadcast soccer video," Pattern Recognition Letters, 103–113, 2009.
25. P. Viola, and M. Jones, "Robust real-time face detection," International Journal of Computer Vision, vol. 57, no. 2, pp. 137–154, 2004.
26. R. Zhang, W. Lu, and X. Wei, J. Zhu, H. Jiang, Z. Liu, J. Gao, X. Li, J. Yu, and R. Yu, "A progressive generative adversarial method for structurally inadequate medical image data augmentation," IEEE Journal of Biomedical and Health Informatics, vol. 26, no. 1, pp. 7–16, 2022.

27. J. Liu, C. Shen, T. Liu, N. Aguilera, and J. Tam, "Active appearance model induced generative adversarial network for controlled data augmentation," in Proc. Med. Image Comput. Comput. Assist. Interv. Proc., Part I, vol. 11764, pp. 201–208, 2019.
28. Y. Tang, S. Oh, Y. Tang, J. Xiao, and R. M. Summers, "CT-realistic data augmentation using generative adversarial network for robust lymph node segmentation," in Proc. Med. Imagin., Comput.-Aided Diagnosis, vol. 10950, art. no. 109503V, 2019.
29. S. V. Mahadevkar, B. Khemani, S. Patil, K. Kotecha, D. Vora, A. Abraham, and A. Gabralla, "A review on machine learning styles in computer vision-techniques and future directions," IEEE Access, vol. 10, pp. 107293–107329, 2022.

Advanced Deep Learning for Heart Sounds Classification

Muhammad Salman Khan, Faiq Ahmad Khan, Kaleem Nawaz Khan, Shahid Imran Rana, and Mohammed Abdulla A. A. Al-Hashemi

Abstract Globally, cardiovascular diseases (CVDs) constitute the leading cause of death. A heart murmur is a frequently encountered anomaly that can be detected during the process of auscultation, which involves listening to the sounds produced by the heart. Recent research has focused on identifying representative features and patterns from heart signals to precisely detect abnormal heart sounds. Short-time Fourier transforms (STFT) based spectrograms have gained attention as a means to learn characteristic patterns of normal and abnormal phonocardiogram (PCG) signals. In this study, we investigate the use of advanced deep-learning models, such as convolutional neural networks (CNNs), convolutional auto-encoders (CAEs), vision transformers (ViT), and transfer learning techniques for identifying abnormal patterns in spectrograms derived from PCGs. The PhysioNet/CinC and PASCAL publicly available challenge datasets are used for training and testing the deep learning models. Transfer learning was found to be a highly effective approach, achieving high accuracy and precision among all four approaches. ViT and CAEs performed equally well. The bespoke CNN model employed in this study was less complex and lighter than previous competing research, yet it outperformed them with relatively excellent classification precision and accuracy, making it an appropriate tool for using PCG data to screen for abnormal heart sounds. By employing the transfer learning technique, spectrogram detection achieved noteworthy performance with respect to the accuracy, F1 scores, sensitivity, specificity, and precision, yielding values of 95.3%, 95.55%, 95.8%, 96.5%, and 96.98% respectively.

M. S. Khan (✉)
Department of Electrical Engineering, College of Engineering, Qatar University, Doha, Qatar
e-mail: salman@qu.edu.qa

F. A. Khan
Department of Electrical Engineering, FE and CS, National University of Modern Languages, Islamabad, Pakistan

K. N. Khan
Department of Computer Science (GCCIS), Rochester Institute of Technology (RIT), Rochester, NY, USA

S. I. Rana · M. A. A. A. Al-Hashemi
Heart Hospital, Hamad Medical Corporation, Doha, Qatar

H. Ali et al. (eds.), *Advances in Deep Generative Models for Medical Artificial Intelligence*, Studies in Computational Intelligence 1124,
https://doi.org/10.1007/978-3-031-46341-9_9

Keywords Cardiovascular diseases · Convolutional neural networks · Heart sound · Transfer learning · Transformers

1 Introduction

Cardiovascular diseases (CVDs) are a significant public health concern globally due to their high prevalence, morbidity, and mortality rates. The WHO reports that CVDs are responsible for more than 17 million deaths annually, accounting for 31% of all deaths globally. This number is projected to increase to over 23 million by 2030. In Europe, CVDs are the leading cause of death with over 4 million deaths annually, while in the United States, heart disease and stroke account for nearly a third of all deaths [1, 2]. The critical step in finding CVDs is first to screen the PCGs for normal and abnormal heart sounds.

Early detection of abnormal heart sounds is critical for improving clinical outcomes, reducing the burden of the disease, and minimizing healthcare costs. Early detection allows for timely intervention, better management of risk factors, and improved quality of life. It also increases awareness of the importance of heart health and promotes better public health outcomes. The clinical scenario is further complicated as many murmurs are innocent or physiological and do not need further testing.

Efforts to improve the early detection and treatment of abnormal heart sounds have focused on developing novel diagnostic tools and methods, including advanced imaging technologies and machine learning algorithms. These technologies aim to screen heart sounds, monitor disease progression, and assess treatment efficacy, enabling personalized management of the disease. However, further research is needed to optimize these tools and to integrate them into routine clinical practice to improve early detection and treatment of abnormal heart sounds.

The diagnosis of abnormalities currently relies on the subjective interpretation of patient data by clinicians, which is known to be prone to error and inefficiency [3]. Furthermore, the advent of advanced cardiovascular examination and treatment technologies has resulted in the generation of vast amounts of complex data, presenting a challenge for cardiologists to effectively and efficiently analyze. As such, there is an urgent need to develop automated screening methods that are both effective and affordable, without compromising patient safety.

Artificial intelligence (AI) algorithms offer a promising solution to these challenges. By analyzing large datasets, including medical imaging and patient history, AI algorithms can identify patterns and markers that may indicate the presence of a heart sound abnormality with a high degree of accuracy. This not only improves the accuracy of diagnosis but also enables earlier detection of abnormality in heart signals, which is crucial for effective treatment.

Automated screening through AI also reduces the time and resources required for manual screening, resulting in more efficient and cost-effective healthcare delivery. By providing personalized recommendations and treatments, AI algorithms can further enhance patient outcomes and quality of life. In addition, the use of AI in screening can help make abnormality detection and early intervention more accessible to under-served communities, which may have limited access to specialist care. This has the potential to significantly reduce the burden of heart-related diseases, which currently represent a leading cause of death worldwide.

1.1 Heart Sounds and Auscultation

Auscultation, a widely used method for detecting cardiac murmurs, involves using a stethoscope to listen to the heartbeats. Proficiency in auscultation requires extensive training for physicians and cardiologists [5]. It is important to note that experienced cardiologists can diagnose patients with an accuracy rate of 80%, compared to medical students and primary care physicians who have an accuracy rate of 20–40% [6–8]. Cardiac murmurs can arise from structural or valvular diseases of the heart. Heart valve disease refers to conditions affecting one or more of the four heart valves, which can manifest as stenosis, a narrowing of the valve opening, or regurgitation, a backward flow of blood. The primary causes of these conditions include aging, rheumatic fever, endocarditis, hypertension, coronary artery disease, and Marfan syndrome, among others. Patients may experience symptoms such as fatigue, shortness of breath, chest pain, palpitations, and swelling, and severe cases may lead to heart failure, stroke, and other complications. Early diagnosis and treatment are critical for managing the disease and mitigating risks.

During auscultation, the stethoscope is placed on the chest, and the healthcare provider listens to the sounds produced by the heart. The heart sounds can provide crucial information about the functioning of the heart valves, which are essential in regulating blood flow through the heart.

Several heart sounds are commonly associated with valvular diseases. For instance, a "murmur" may indicate stenosis or regurgitation. A "click" is due to midsystolic stretch of chordae tendinae as anterior mitral leaflet prolapses lead to regurgitation. Other sounds such as "whooshing" or "rushing" can also indicate the presence of valvular disease. Normal and various abnormal heart sounds can be seen in Fig. 1.

The interpretation of heart sounds is a complex and specialized skill, requiring extensive training and experience. In the diagnosis of different murmurs, healthcare providers rely on the identification of specific heart sounds that are indicative of structural or valvular dysfunction. This process involves careful auscultation of the heart using a stethoscope, with the aim of detecting any abnormal sounds that may be associated with cardiac disease.

While auscultation is a valuable tool in the detection of valvular disease, it is not always sufficient for making a definitive diagnosis. In some cases, additional tests may be necessary to confirm the presence of valvular disease and determine its severity. These tests may include echocardiography or magnetic resonance imaging (MRI), which can provide detailed images of the heart and its valves, allowing for a more accurate diagnosis.

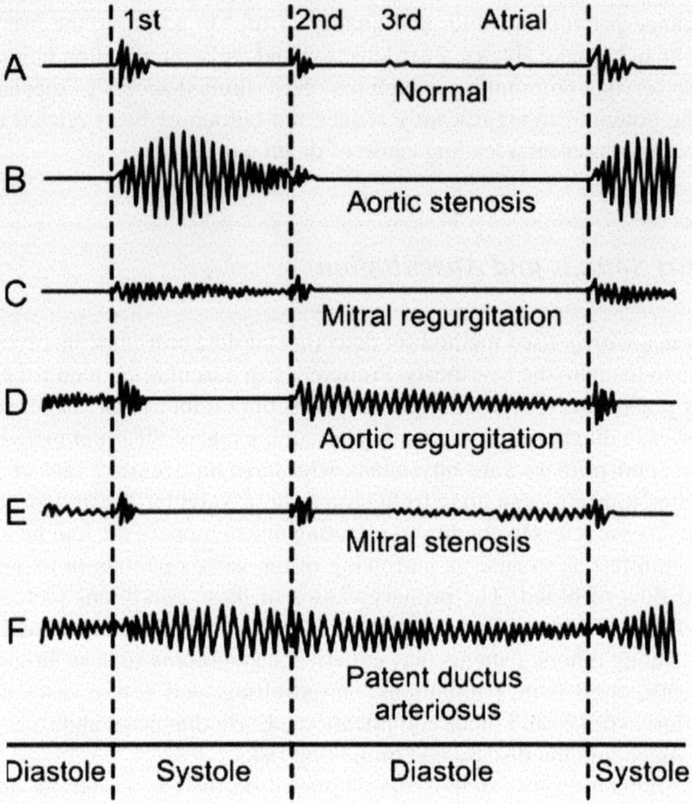

Fig. 1 Temporal analysis of heart sounds: distinguishing normal and abnormal patterns [4]

Overall, heart auscultation is an important part of the diagnostic process for valvular disease, providing healthcare providers with valuable information about the functioning of the heart valves. However, it is important to recognize its limitations and the potential need for additional testing to confirm the diagnosis and determine the appropriate treatment.

2 Datasets

2.1 PhysioNet 2016

The PhysioNet 2016 dataset [9] consists of 3153 heart sound recordings from both healthy subjects and patients with confirmed cardiac diagnoses. The heart sounds were recorded from various locations near the human heart and were divided into three categories: normal, abnormal, and unsure. Normal recordings were from healthy subjects while abnormal recordings were from patients with heart valve defects or coronary artery disease. The recordings of heart sounds have been made in an uncontrolled environment, which means that there may be various noise sources that affect the quality of the recordings, such as stethoscope motion, talking, intestinal sounds, and breathing. Due to this, few of the recorded sounds may be hard or nearly impossible to accurately classify into the normal or abnormal class. Such recordings are labeled as unsure. Both normal and abnormal recordings were contributed by both children and adults and lasted anywhere from a few seconds to over 100 s. The recordings were re-sampled to 2000 Hz and provided in .wav format, with only one PCG lead. The data was divided into five databases, with each record beginning with a letter followed by a random number. The division of the training set and test set were carefully carried out to make sure that they remain mutually exclusive, with the test set being kept private for the purpose of scoring. A total of 300 recordings from the test set were utilized as a validation dataset before performing the evaluation on the test set. The dataset is unbalanced. The stats for the PhysioNet dataset are illustrated in Table 1.

2.2 *PASCAL 2011*

The PASCAL 2011 heart sounds dataset [10] comprises audio files of variable durations, ranging from 1 to 30 s. The primary information of interest in heart sounds resides in the low-frequency components, leading to the common application of low-pass filters at 195 Hz and subsequent utilization of Fast Fourier transforms for analysis. The dataset encompasses potential sources of noise, including background noise, incidental noise from breathing, or inadvertent contact of the microphone with clothing or skin.

Table 1 PhysioNet challenge/2016 dataset specifications

Sub sets	Number of patients	Number of recordings	Proportion of recordings (%)			Length of recordings (s)		
			Abnormal	Normal	Unsure	Min	Median	Max
Set a	121	409	67.5	28.4	4.2	9.3	35.6	36.5
Set b	106	490	14.9	60.2	24.9	5.3	8	8
Set c	31	31	64.5	22.6	12.9	9.6	44.4	122.0
Set d	38	55	47.3	47.3	5.5	6.6	12.3	48.5
Set e	356	2054	7.1	86.7	6.2	8.1	21.1	101.7
Set f	112	114	27.2	68.4	4.4	29.4	31.7	59.6
Total/%	764	3153	18.1%	73.0%	8.8%	5.3 (Min)	20.8 (Median)	122.0 (Max)

Table 2 PASCAL dataset specifications

Dataset	Number of files	Total size (wav) (MB)	Total size (aif) (MB)
Dataset A	176	85.7	79.0
Training normal	31	14.0	13.2
Training murmur	34	17.3	16.4
Training extrahs	19	6.9	6.5
Training artifact	40	22.5	20.9
Unlabelled test	52	24.6	23.0
Dataset B	656	30.2	29.1
Training normal	320	13.8	13.0
Training murmur	95	5.3	5.1
Training extrasystole	46	1.9	2.1
B unlabelled test	195	9.2	8.7

Within this dataset, the "Normal" category encompasses recordings of healthy heart sounds, exhibiting heart rates ranging from 40 to 140 beats per minute. The "Murmur" category captures heart sounds characterized by distinct "whooshing, roaring, rumbling, or turbulent fluid" noises occurring either between "lub" and "dub" or between "dub" and "lub".

Dataset A comprises the "Extra Heart Sound" category, which includes additional heart sounds indicative of underlying diseases, as well as the "Artifact" category, encompassing sounds such as feedback, speech, music, and miscellaneous noise. Dataset B focuses on the "Extrasystole" category, involving recordings of irregular or skipped heartbeats, often indicative of cardiovascular conditions. Detailed statistics pertaining to this dataset can be found in Table 2.

3 Pre-processing of Heart Sounds

Pre-processing in the context of heart sounds or PCGs refers to a set of operations performed on raw cardiac signals, with the goal of enhancing the quality of the signals and removing noise and artifactual components. The purpose of pre-processing is to prepare the signals for further analysis, such as feature extraction and classification, and to ensure that the results obtained are accurate and reliable.

The pre-processing steps may include various operations such as signal filtering, artifact removal, normalization, and resampling [11–13]. Filtering to eliminate high-frequency noise and enhance low-frequency signals. Removal of unwanted noise components from the signal that may exist in higher frequency ranges, and the retention of the essential low-frequency components of the signal. This is done to improve the accuracy and reliability of the analysis or processing of the signal, as the low-frequency components may carry important information related to the intended analysis or application such as PCG analysis. During the process of recording heart sound signals using an electronic stethoscope, referred to as PCG, it is important to acknowledge the potential occurrence of artifacts originating from diverse sources. These artifacts encompass instrument noise, noise resulting from bodily sounds, disturbances arising from subject motion and movement of stethoscope diaphragms, as well as other types of interference that can compromise the overall quality of the recorded PCG signal. Instances of artifacts in PCG signals can emerge due to factors such as improper stethoscope placement, subject movement, coughing, or external influences. Artifacts in PCG signals can occur due to inappropriate placement of the stethoscope, body movement of the subject, coughing, or other external factors. For example, if the stethoscope is not properly positioned on the chest, it may pick up extraneous sounds from surrounding sources, leading to artifacts in the recorded PCG signal. Similarly, the body movement of the subject during the recording, such as breathing or shifting, can introduce motion artifacts in the PCG signal [14]. In addition, electrical artifacts can also be induced in the PCG signal. For instance, if the electronic stethoscope or its components are not properly grounded or shielded, it may pick up electrical interference from the environment or other electronic devices, resulting in electrical artifacts in the PCG signal [15]. These artifacts are typically random in time, have a high amplitude, and can last for a short duration. They can adversely affect the accuracy and reliability of PCG signal analysis, particularly in real-time point-of-care diagnosis scenarios. Therefore, artifact removal techniques are crucial for mitigating the impact of these artifacts and obtaining clean PCG signals for accurate analysis [16, 17].

To perform better, deep neural networks need a significant amount of training examples. Deep neural network models, including CNN, need fixed length input [18]. This method fixes the variable length problem while also expanding the datasets' training examples. In order to accommodate the fixed input sizes required by convolutional neural networks (CNNs) and most deep learning models, all recordings are divided into 8 s segments. The appropriate window size depends on the chosen method, and previous studies have used varying window sizes, such as 1 s [18–20], 1.5 s [21], 2 s [22], 2.5 s [23, 24], 3 s [22], 6 s [25], and 8 s [26, 27]. A recent study [27], stated that a minimum window of 8 s is needed to detect ECG arrhythmia. Motivated by this we kept the 8 s in this way the model will also be able to detect ECG arrhythmia. Since deep learning models cannot process variable-sized chunks of data [18], cardiac signals that are shorter than 8 s are discarded from the dataset. The two PASCAL sub-datasets are combined into a single dataset. Longer recordings are divided into two or three signals as needed. Since the majority of the recordings in Dataset A are under 8 s, the produced PASCAL dataset contains more than 95% of the recordings from Dataset B. The PCG signals are categorized as 0 to indicate normal signals and 1 to indicate abnormal signals. All recordings are divided into identical-sized chunks because fixed-length input is one of CNN's prerequisites, as was previously explained.

In summary, pre-processing is a critical step in the analysis of heart sounds or PCGs and plays an important role in ensuring the accuracy and reliability of the results obtained. The choice of pre-processing techniques and their parameters should be carefully considered, and the results should be validated through appropriate validation methods, such as cross-validation or bootstrapping.

4 Features Extraction

In the context of PCG or heart sound analysis, feature extraction is a crucial step that involves the identification and extraction of specific attributes or features from the heart sounds that are indicative of the heart's condition. These features can offer significant insights into the heart's functions, including its rhythm, rate, and any potential abnormalities.

PCG or heart sound features can be classified into various domains based on their nature, including time, frequency, and time-frequency. Time domain features, which are closely related to the temporal aspects of the heart sound signal, typically encompass metrics such as heart rate, duration, and inter-beat interval. These features are useful in providing information about the heart's rhythm and rate.

In contrast, frequency-domain features pertain to the spectral characteristics of the signal and can offer insights into the energy distribution across various frequencies within the heart sound signal. Spectral peaks or valleys in the frequency domain can indicate the presence of heart murmurs or other abnormalities. Commonly used frequency domain features include power spectral density and power spectral entropy, which can provide insights into the heart's sound spectrum. The time-frequency domain features are typically used to capture information about the variations in the frequency content over time, such as wavelet transform-based features. Power Spectral Density (PSD) Formula:

$$PSD(f) = \frac{|X(f)|^2}{T}$$

where
$PSD(f)$ is the Power Spectral Density at frequency f
$X(f)$ is the Fourier transform of the signal $x(t)$
T is the total duration of the signal.

Power Spectral Entropy (PSE) Formula:

$$PSE = -\sum_{i=1}^{N} p_i \log_2(p_i)$$

where
PSE is the Power Spectral Entropy
p_i is the probability of the signal's power at frequency bin i
N is the total number of frequency bins.

Time-frequency domain features are a class of features that integrate both time and frequency domain characteristics of PCGs or heart sounds. These features are useful in capturing the evolution of heart sounds over time and identifying any temporal changes in the frequency content, which can provide important diagnostic information [28–31]. Wavelet transforms and short-time Fourier transforms are two commonly used methods for extracting time-frequency domain features from heart sounds, as reported in previous studies [32, 33].

Table 3 summarizes the advantages and disadvantages of wavelet and Short-Time Fourier Transform (STFT) methods for extracting time-frequency domain features from heart sounds. This table highlights that the STFT method is simpler and more easily automated, but may not be as effective in capturing transient or non-stationary features. The wavelet transform method, on the other hand, can better capture non-stationary features, but is more complex and may require more manual intervention.

Table 3 STFT versus wavelet

Feature	Wavelet transform	Short-time Fourier transform (STFT)
Number of parameters	Moderate to high: requires setting parameters such as wavelet type, scale, and threshold method	Moderate: requires setting parameters such as window size, window type, and overlap percentage
Ease of use	Moderate: implementation may require more complex computations and specialized libraries	Relatively easy: commonly used and widely available in signal processing libraries
Automation	Limited automation: may require manual parameter tuning for optimal results	Limited automation: parameters need to be manually selected, may not adapt well to changing signal characteristics
Advantages	• Excellent time-frequency localization, allowing for fine-grained analysis of signal features	• Simpler implementation with widely available libraries
	• Effective for analyzing signals with non-stationary or transient characteristics	• Suitable for analyzing stationary signals with constant frequency components
	• Can capture both high and low-frequency features	• Computationally efficient
Disadvantages	• Requires careful parameter tuning for optimal results	• Limited time-frequency localization, may result in blurred representations of signal features
	• May be sensitive to noise and signal variations	• Less effective for analyzing signals with non-stationary or transient characteristics
	• May have limited performance in capturing high-frequency features	• May miss low-frequency features

4.1 Heart Sounds Spectrograms

Phonocardiography involves the use of Fourier analysis to decompose heart sounds into their constituent frequency components, resulting in a spectrogram that provides a visual representation of the distribution of frequency components within the sounds over time. The spectrogram serves as a means of analyzing and interpreting various aspects of heart sounds. Figures 2a and 2b illustrate example time-domain waveforms and spectrograms depicting normal and abnormal heart sounds. In the normal sound, only s1 and s2 sounds are present, whereas, the abnormal heart sound exhibits an early systolic murmur in addition to the s1 and s2 sounds. In the clinical setting, the spectrogram of heart sounds plays a crucial role in the assessment of heart function and the identification of abnormal sounds, such as murmurs or clicks. This information is pivotal in the diagnosis and management of a range of cardiovascular conditions, including congenital heart disease, heart valve disorders, and other cardiac abnormalities. To extract clinically relevant information from the spectrogram, it is essential to consider various technical factors that may affect the quality of the recorded data, including the signal-to-noise ratio, as well as both the frequency and temporal domains of the heart sounds. As such, careful consideration of these factors is crucial in achieving accurate and reliable analysis and interpretation of the heart sound spectrogram.

5 Classification

The realm of heart sound classification has garnered substantial research attention, encompassing the exploration of both traditional machine learning techniques and deep learning approaches. Traditional machine learning methods in heart sound classification entail the extraction of features from recordings, which are subsequently employed as inputs to a classifier. Prominent techniques encompass random forests, decision trees, k-nearest neighbors, and support vector machines. Although effective [32, 34, 35], these methods can encounter limitations in terms of input data quality, quantity, and feature selection.

In contrast, deep learning approaches leverage neural networks to automatically learn features directly from raw data. This paradigm has yielded improved performance in heart sound classification, as neural networks possess the capability to capture intricate patterns and relationships within the data. Common deep learning models employed in heart sound classification include CNNs, recurrent neural networks (RNNs), and hybrid models that combine both architectures. These models have demonstrated promising outcomes in detecting heart abnormalities and facilitating the diagnosis of cardiovascular diseases [36]. However, it is important to note that deep learning models often necessitate larger amounts of data and computational resources for training and validation purposes.

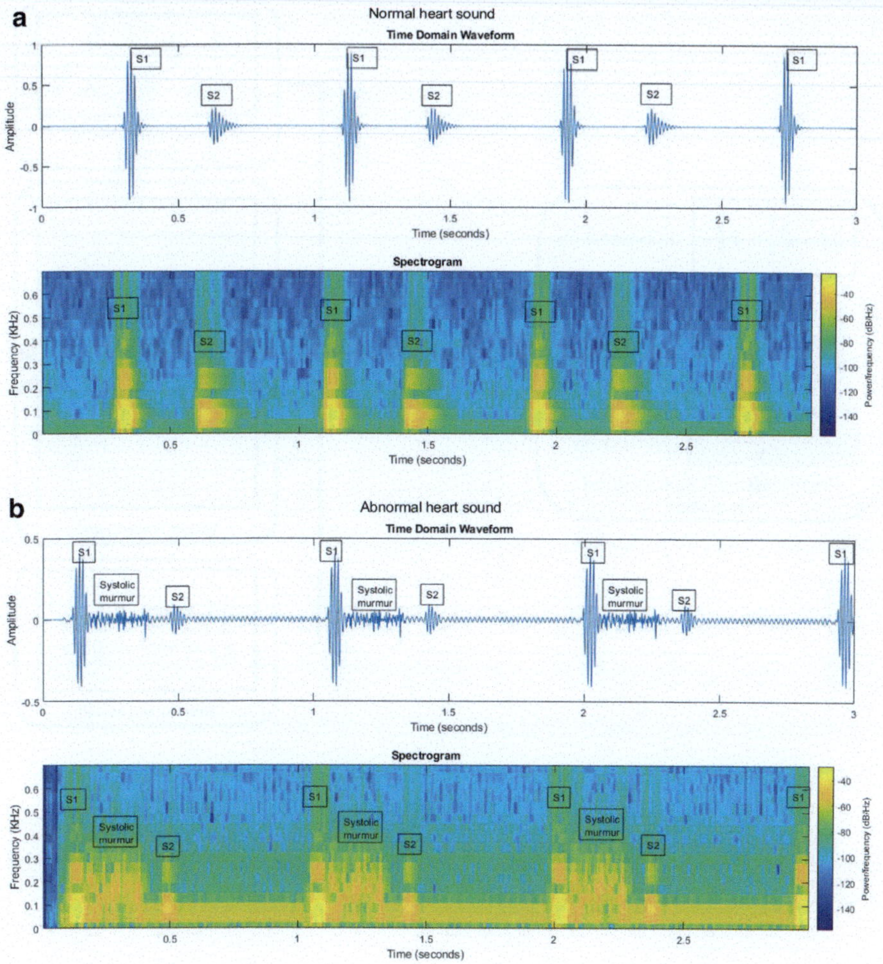

Fig. 2 **a** Normal heart sound time-domain waveform and spectrogram, **b** Abnormal heart sound time-domain waveform and spectrogram

In recent years, deep learning approaches have gained substantial traction in the field of heart sound classification. These approaches, exemplified by CNNs and RNNs, exhibit the capability to autonomously extract pertinent features from input data, thereby addressing certain limitations associated with traditional machine learning techniques. Various studies [37–39] have delved into the application of deep learning in heart sound classification, revealing that deep learning models often achieve remarkable accuracy rates across multiple scenarios.

Within this chapter, we will conduct four distinct experiments employing different classification techniques. A comprehensive depiction of the experiments and their

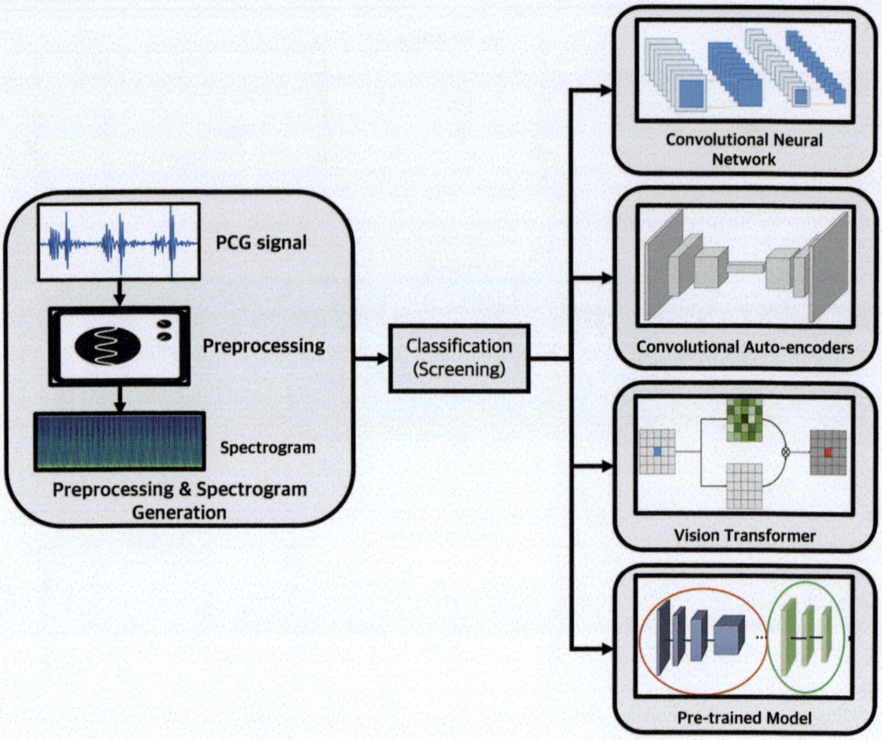

Fig. 3 Overview of the methodology

respective methodologies is presented in Fig. 3. Each experiment will be elucidated separately in subsequent sections.

5.1 Convolutional Neural Network

Convolutional Neural Networks (CNN) have shown great success in accurately detecting the spatial and temporal dependencies of images using relevant filters. CNNs are commonly used for classifying 1D signals and 2D images and utilize convolutional layers in addition to fully connected layers. One notable benefit of employing a Convolutional Neural Network (ConvNet) is its inherent advantage of demanding reduced preprocessing when contrasted with alternative machine learning models. Additionally, the network can automatically learn important features directly from the raw data, thus reducing the burden of selecting features for better classification.

In a recent study, Khan et al. [27] performed seven experiments to develop a lightweight custom CNN architecture for accurately detecting abnormalities in PCGs.

Initially, the study implemented the training, validation, and testing of published CNN architectures [21, 23, 40]. The architectures were then fine-tuned by adjusting the number and size of filters and adding or removing pooling layers [25]. The best architecture producing the highest detection rate was selected from a set of seven alternatives. The architecture details for each experiment are described in depth and listed in Fig. 4.

Once the networks were furnished with the complete training data, the training process spanned over 110 epochs, employing binary cross-entropy as the loss function and Adam optimizer with a learning rate of 0.001. Among the seven distinct variations of Convolutional Neural Networks (CNNs), the model demonstrating the highest detection rate, encompassing accuracy, specificity, and sensitivity, was chosen. The architecture details for the best-performing CNN models are given in Fig. 4. In this chapter, the CNN model used by Khan et al. [27] was employed to learn representative features for PCGs classification.

5.2 *Auto-encoders*

Auto-encoders are novel and emerging techniques in the field of deep learning that shows great potential for feature extraction and data compression. They are neural networks that aim to reconstruct their input data by encoding it into a lower-dimensional representation, which can then be decoded back to the original data. Auto-encoders consist of two pivotal components: the encoder and the decoder. Collaboratively, these components function to compress the input data and subsequently reconstruct it. In the learning process of an auto-encoder, the primary objective is to minimize the disparity between the input and the reconstructed output. This is

Experiment No.	Architectures of different investigated CNN models
1	Convolutional layers: 3 [(128 × 3 × 3)+maxpool(3 × 3)], [(256 × 3 × 3)+maxpool(3 × 3)], [(512 × 3 × 3)+maxpool(3 × 3)]
2	Convolutional layers: 3 [(128 × 3 × 3)+maxpool(3 × 3)], [(512 × 3 × 3)+maxpool(3 × 3)], [(128 × 3 × 3)+maxpool(3 × 3)]
3	Convolutional layers: 3 [(128 × 3 × 3)+maxpool(2 × 2)], [(256 × 3 × 3)+maxpool(2 × 2)], [(128 × 3 × 3)+maxpool(2 × 2)]
4	Convolutional layers: 4 [(128 × 3 × 3)+maxpool(2 × 2)], [(256 × 3 × 3)+maxpool(2 × 2)], (128 × 3 × 3), (64 × 3 × 3)
5	Convolutional layers: 5 [(96 × 11 × 11)+maxpool(3 × 3)], (256 × 5 × 5), (384 × 3 × 3), (384 × 3 × 3), [(256 × 3 × 3)+max-pool(3 × 3)]
6	Convolutional layers: 5 [(96 × 11 × 11)+maxpool(3 × 3)], [(256 × 5 × 5)+maxpool(3 × 3)], (384 × 3 × 3), (384 × 3 × 3), [(256 × 3 × 3)+maxpool(3 × 3)]
7	Convolutional layers: 6 [(16 × 3 × 3)+maxpool(3 × 3)], [(32 × 2 × 2)+maxpool(3 × 3)], (64 × 2 × 2), (128 × 2 × 2), [(256 × 2 × 2)+maxpool(3 × 3)], (256 × 2 × 2)

Fig. 4 Architectural variants of CNN for experimentation

typically achieved through the optimization of a loss function, often utilizing mean squared error. Figure 5a–c illustrate the original heart sound, encoded feature, and decoded spectrogram respectively.

Convolutional Auto-encoders (CAEs) are a specific type of auto-encoder that is well-suited for processing signals and images, such as heart sounds. The architecture of a CAEs is shown in Fig. 6. Unlike regular auto-encoders, CAEs use convolutional layers in both the encoder and decoder parts of the network. This enables them to effectively learn and capture local spatial patterns in the input data, which is particularly relevant for analyzing heart sounds that contain local patterns and variations. As such, CAEs have emerged as a promising approach for feature extraction and classification of heart sounds.

Several studies have investigated the efficacy of auto-encoders and CAEs for heart sound analysis, as evidenced by research papers such as [41–45]. In a recent study [46], the authors evaluated the effectiveness of using signal energy for direct classification of heart sounds. The resampled energy method was utilized to obtain the instantaneous energies of heart sounds, which were subsequently used for classification through a stacked auto-encoder network. The performance of the proposed method was assessed on the PASCAL B-training dataset and compared with previous studies on the same dataset. The results demonstrated that the proposed method performed similarly to segmented classification and showed the feasibility of utilizing instant energy of heart sounds and stacked auto-encoder networks for diagnosing heart diseases.

In a separate study [47], a semi-supervised methodology was introduced to identify abnormal heart sounds by utilizing a convolutional Variational auto-encoder (VAE). This method capitalizes on the VAE's ability to acquire knowledge about the spectrogram characteristics of normal heart sounds and their associated probability distribution. To detect abnormalities, the KL divergence between the encoded distribution and a known prior distribution is computed as an anomaly score. The efficacy of this proposed approach was evaluated on diverse datasets comprising open access and in-house recordings of PCG signals. These datasets encompassed a

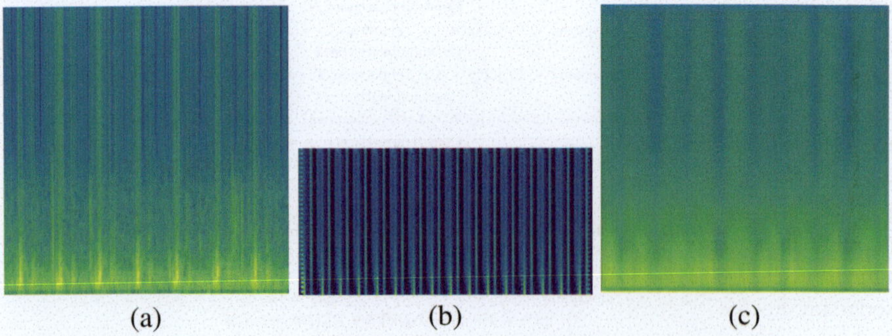

Fig. 5 **a** Original heart sound spectrogram, **b** encoded feature, **c** decoded spectrogram

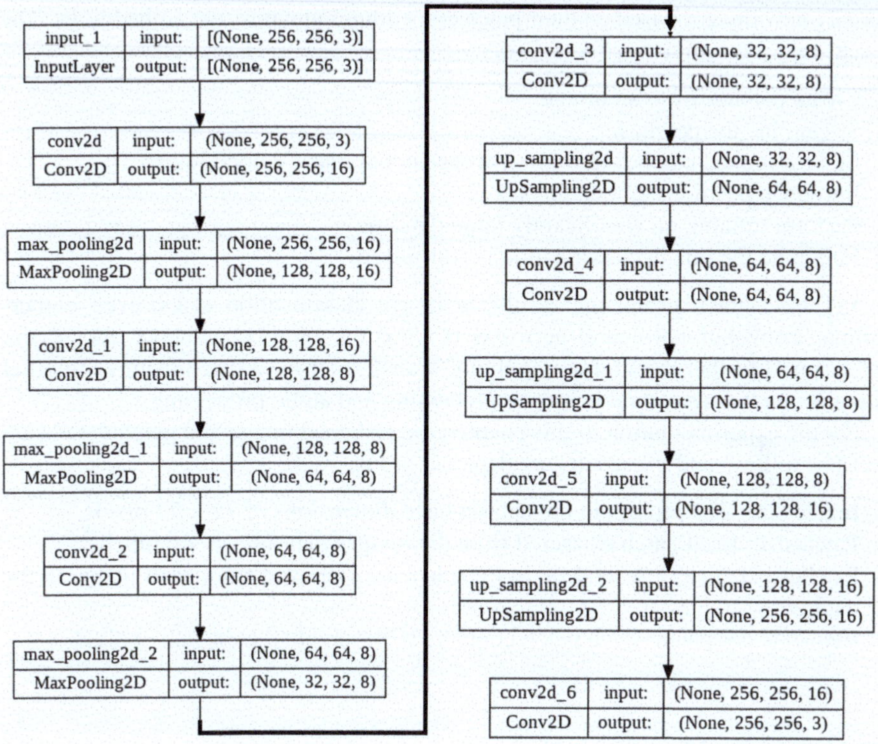

Fig. 6 Architecture of CAE

range of heart sound conditions, including normal recordings, abnormalities related to cardiovascular diseases, cardiac murmurs, and extra heart sounds.

5.3 *Vision Transformers*

The first step of the ViT methodology involves dividing an image into a set of fixed-size patches. Each patch is then linearly embedded into a low-dimensional space to produce a sequence of patch embeddings. In the second step, position embeddings are added to the patch embeddings to capture spatial information within the image. The third step involves feeding the resulting sequence of embeddings into a Transformer encoder, which processes the sequence in parallel, allowing for efficient computation. In the fourth step, a learnable "classification token" is added to the sequence, which is used to predict the image's label. The fifth step involves passing the encoded sequence through a multi-layer perceptron (MLP) to generate the final classification output. In the sixth step, the model is trained using a standard supervised learning objective, such as cross-entropy loss. Finally, in the seventh step, the trained model is used to classify new images based on their patch embeddings and position embeddings. The seven steps are summarized as follows;

1. Create patches from an image.
2. Streamline the patches.
3. Make flattened patches into lower-dimensional linear embeddings.
4. Introduce positions embeddings.
5. Perform training on significantly large datasets.
6. Fine-tune the image classification performance.

ViT has shown promising results in image classification tasks, even outperforming convolutional neural networks (CNNs) on some benchmarks. Its success has inspired further research on applying Transformer-based architectures to other domains, including natural language processing and audio processing.

For the experimentation in this chapter, the reshaped image and patch details are given as follows and the results are depicted in Fig. 7a, b.

1. Image size: The images in the dataset have dimensions of 72×72 pixels.
2. Patch size: Each patch extracted from the images measures 6×6 pixels.
3. Patches per image: A total of 144 patches are extracted from each image in the dataset.
4. Elements per patch: Each patch contains 108 individual elements or pixels.

5.4 *Transfer-Learning Using Pre-trained Models*

Transfer learning is a machine learning technique that aims to enhance the performance of a related task by utilizing the knowledge obtained from a previously learned task. In the realm of heart sound analysis, transfer learning can be employed

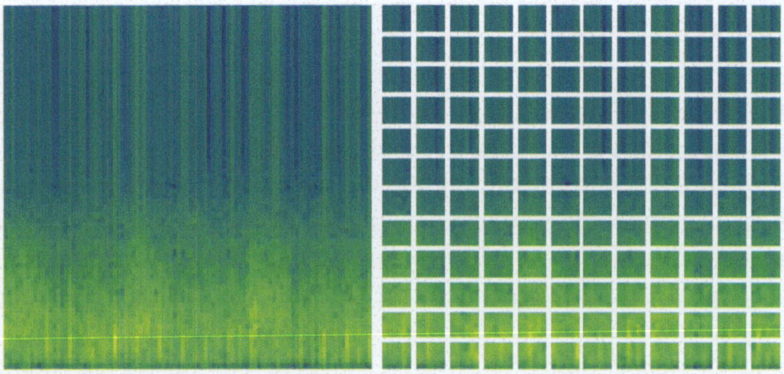

(a) (b)

Fig. 7 **a** Image size (72×72), **b** patches per image

to enhance the accuracy of heart sound classification models. This is achieved by utilizing a pre-trained model, which has been trained on a massive dataset, as a starting point for the heart sound classification task. This pre-trained model can then be fine-tuned with a smaller dataset that is specific to the task.

Transfer learning offers a pivotal advantage in leveraging the acquired knowledge from a pre-trained model, leading to reduced training time and computational resources needed for training a model from scratch. Furthermore, it effectively tackles the challenge of limited training data, a common issue encountered in heart sound analysis.

Different techniques can be used to perform transfer learning in heart sound analysis, including fine-tuning a pre-trained convolutional neural network (CNN) or utilizing a pre-trained auto-encoder as a feature extractor. These techniques have been demonstrated to enhance the performance of heart sound classification models and have been validated in various studies and experiments [27, 48]. In this chapter, we have used VGG16 + LSTM as a pre-trained model and evaluated it against the test set. The architecture of VGG16 + LSTM is depicted in Fig. 8.

6 Performance Metrics

In the domain of machine learning and deep learning, the evaluation of model effectiveness and accuracy is of paramount significance. To achieve this, a variety of performance metrics are employed, with the confusion matrix being a widely adopted metric. The confusion matrix is a tabular representation that succinctly summarizes the performance of a binary classification model by juxtaposing the predicted and actual values. By analyzing the values contained within the confusion matrix, diverse performance metrics can be derived, including True Positive (TP), True Negative (TN), False Positive (FP), and False Negative (FN). TP quantifies the instances in which the model correctly predicted the positive class and the actual class was indeed positive. TN, on the other hand, represents the count of true negative cases, wherein the model accurately predicted the negative class and the actual class was truly negative. FP encompasses the instances where the model incorrectly predicted the positive class, while the actual class was negative. Conversely, FN captures the number of instances in which the model predicted the negative class, but the actual class was positive. These values serve as the foundation for computing various performance metrics, with accuracy being one such metric. Accuracy is defined as the ratio of correctly classified instances to the total number of instances present within the dataset. The formula for accuracy is as follows:

$$Accuracy = \frac{TP + TN}{TP + TN + FP + FN} \tag{1}$$

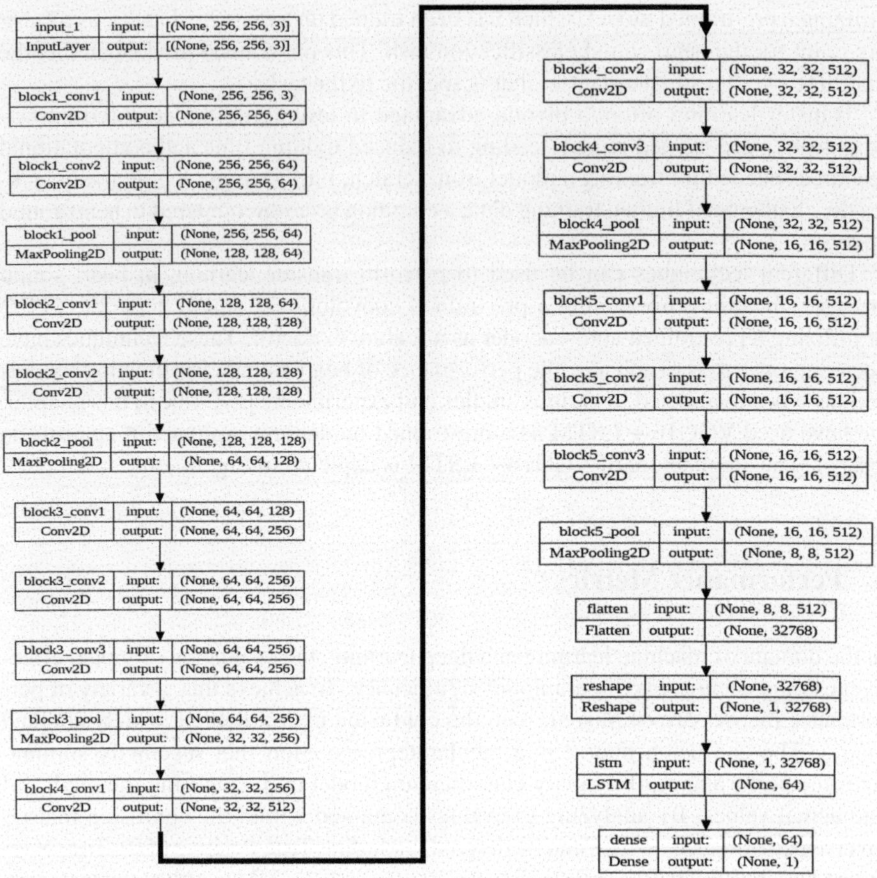

Fig. 8 Transfer learning (VGG16 + LSTM)

Precision is a key performance metric that quantifies the ratio of correctly identified positive predictions to the total number of positive predictions generated by the model. It is computed using the following mathematical expression:

$$Precision = \frac{TP}{TP + FP} \tag{2}$$

Recall, also referred to as sensitivity or true positive rate, is a pivotal metric assessing the efficacy of a model in accurately detecting positive instances from the entire set of actual positive instances present in the dataset. The calculation of the recall score is determined by the following mathematical formulation:

$$Recall = \frac{TP}{TP + FN} \tag{3}$$

The F1 Score, a comprehensive performance metric, encapsulates the harmonious fusion of both precision and recall. By taking the harmonic mean of precision and recall, it effectively balances the evaluation of a model's precision and its ability to capture all relevant positive instances. The calculation of the F1 Score involves the utilization of the following mathematical expression:

$$F1 = 2 \cdot \frac{Precision \cdot Recall}{Precision + Recall} \tag{4}$$

Specificity (True Negative Rate):

$$Specificity = \frac{TN}{TN + FP} \tag{5}$$

In heart sound analysis, these metrics are used to evaluate the performance of models in detecting and diagnosing heart diseases from heart sounds. They provide a means of comparing the performance of different models and determining the most suitable model for a given task.

7 Results

In this study, the authors experimented with four different approaches, including Convolutional Neural Network (CNN), Auto-encoders, Vision Transformer (ViT), and Transfer Learning, to classify PCGs. The input data used for all approaches were spectrograms of heart sounds obtained from the PCG signals of an 8-second window that were processed using STFT analysis. The experimentation was carried out on two publicly accessible datasets, namely PhysioNet and PASCAL, with different iterations of training and fine-tuning applied to the architectures.

To compare the performance of the four approaches, several metrics were computed and presented in Table 4. The pre-trained model achieved the highest accuracy, precision, recall, and F1-score, with scores of 95.3%, 95.8%, 96.5%, 96.98%, and 95.55%, respectively. The confusion matrices for CAEs on the PASCAL and PhysioNet datasets were presented in Fig. 9a, b, respectively, to provide a visual representation of the performance of the classification models. Finally, the training and validation loss behavior of ViT on both datasets were illustrated in Fig. 10a, b. The results of this study indicate that pre-trained models and Vision Transformers can effectively classify PCGs signals, outperforming other approaches such as CNN and convolutional auto-encoders.

8 Conclusions

This chapter presents a thorough investigation of four distinct classification techniques for classifying PCGs. All four techniques use spectrogram representations of the heart sounds to learn meaningful features. The PCG signals are analyzed using STFT, generating spectrograms of the heart sounds. The experimentation is carried out with different configurations of the architectures and datasets. The publicly available and widely used datasets, PhysioNet and PASCAL, were utilized for the experimentation. The architectures are refined through numerous training and

Table 4 Results

Techniques	Dataset	Accuracy (%)	Precision (%)	Recall (%)	F1-score (%)
Convolutional neural network	PhysioNet	95.75	97.52	96.3	96.93
	PASCAL	75.25	76.73	74.20	75.42
Convolutional autoencoder	PhysioNet	85.89	86.78	87.94	87.36
	PASCAL	77.27	82.35	87.5	84.84
Vision transformer	PhysioNet	91.01	89.78	88.94	89.36
	PASCAL	76.27	76.35	76.5	76.84
Pre-trained models	PhysioNet	95.3	95.8	96.98	95.55
	PASCAL	95.05	97.02	96.13	96.23

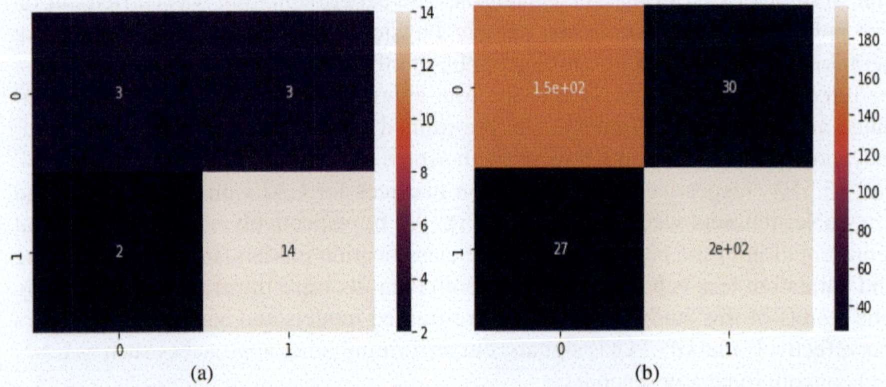

Fig. 9 **a** CAE-based architecture confusion matrix on PASCAL dataset, **b** CAE-based architecture confusion matrix on PhysioNet dataset

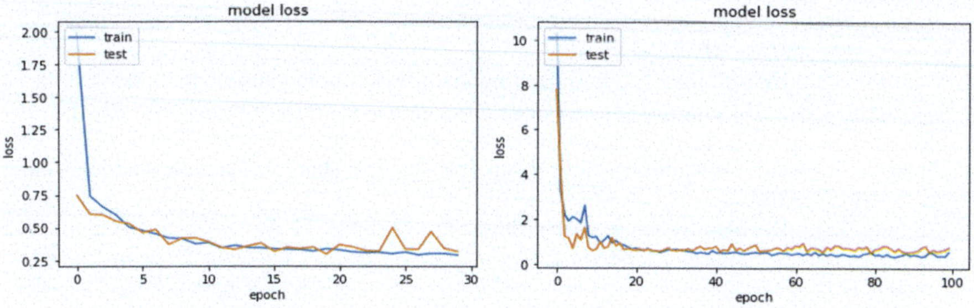

(a) (b)

Fig. 10 Vision transformer: **a** training-versus-validation loss (PhysioNet), **b** training-versus-validation loss (PASCAL)

fine-tuning iterations. The pre-trained models demonstrate superior performance in classifying PCG signals, outperforming all other classification approaches. Additionally, the Vision Transformer models also exhibit competitive performance compared to CNN and convolutional auto-encoders.

These models can aid in the identification, prognosis, and management of heart-related murmurs, resulting in more precise and effective patient care. These models, for instance, can assist in detecting irregularities in heart sounds that would not be discernible to the human ear, enabling early murmurs diagnosis and therapy. It has been established that the results of the models for detecting heart abnormalities are acceptable to medical professionals. In fact, a lot of health professionals have said they would like to use these models as a tool to help with patient care. AI/ML-based models have the potential to have a big impact on heart sound screening-related research. They can offer quicker and more precise objective diagnosis and assist with patient outcome prediction. Additionally, by effective screening at the primary care level and lowering the need for pricey diagnostic tests, these models can aid in lowering healthcare costs. Overall, models powered by AI/ML have the power to change the heart signals processing sector and enhance patient outcomes. These models are anticipated to become a more crucial tool for doctors and medical professionals in diagnosing and treating abnormal heart signals as they continue to be refined and validated via additional research.

References

1. Timmis, A. *et al.* European Society of Cardiology: cardiovascular disease statistics 2019. *European heart journal* **41,** 12–85 (2020).
2. Timmis, A. *et al.* European Society of Cardiology: cardiovascular disease statistics 2021. *European Heart Journal* **43,** 716–799 (2022).
3. Perera, I. S., Muthalif, F. A., Selvarathnam, M., Liyanaarachchi, M. R. & Nanayakkara, N. D. *Automated diagnosis of cardiac abnormalities using heart sounds* in *2013 IEEE Point-of-Care*

Healthcare Technologies (PHT) (2013), 252–255.
4. Pedrosa, J. *Heart Sound Analysis for Cardiac Pathology Identification: Detection and Characterization of Heart Murmurs* in (2013).
5. Roy, D. *et al.* Helping family physicians improve their cardiac auscultation skills with an interactive CD-ROM. *Journal of Continuing Education in the Health Professions* **22,** 152–159 (2002).
6. Etchells, E., Bell, C. & Robb, K. Does this patient have an abnormal systolic murmur? *Jama* **277,** 564–571 (1997).
7. Strunic, S. L., Rios-Gutierrez, F., Alba-Flores, R., Nordehn, G. & Bums, S. *Detection and classification of cardiac murmurs using segmentation techniques and artificial neural networks* in *2007 IEEE Symposium on Computational Intelligence and Data Mining* (2007), 397–404.
8. Ejaz, K. *et al. A heart murmur detection system using spectrograms and artificial neural networks* in *Circuits, Signals, and Systems* (2004), 374–379.
9. Liu, C. *et al.* An open access database for the evaluation of heart sound algorithms. *Physiological measurement* **37,** 2181 (2016).
10. Bentley, P., Nordehn, G., Coimbra, M., Mannor, S. & Getz, R. Classifying heart sounds challenge. *Retrieved from Classifying Heart Sounds Challenge:* https://peterjbentley.com/heartchallenge (2011).
11. Khan, F. A., Abid, A. & Khan, M. S. Automatic heart sound classification from segmented/unsegmented phonocardiogram signals using time and frequency features. *Physiological measurement* **41,** 055006 (2020).
12. Mei, N. *et al.* Classification of heart sounds based on quality assessment and wavelet scattering transform. *Computers in Biology and Medicine* **137,** 104814 (2021).
13. Xiao, B., Xu, Y., Bi, X., Zhang, J. & Ma, X. Heart sounds classification using a novel 1-D convolutional neural network with extremely low parameter consumption. *Neurocomputing* **392,** 153–159 (2020).
14. Pandia, K., Ravindran, S., Cole, R., Kovacs, G. & Giovangrandi, L. *Motion artifact cancellation to obtain heart sounds from a single chest-worn accelerometer* in *2010 IEEE International Conference on Acoustics, Speech and Signal Processing* (2010), 590–593.
15. Kumar, A. K. & Saha, G. Interpretation of heart sound signal through automated artifact-free segmentation. *Heart Res Open J* **2,** 25–34 (2015).
16. Kumar, A. K. & Saha, G. Improved computerized cardiac auscultation by discarding artifact contaminated PCG signal sub-sequence. *Biomedical Signal Processing and Control* **41,** 48–62 (2018).
17. Sharma, S. & Dhar, J. *Deep Learning Approach for Analysis of Artifacts in Heart Sound* in *Proceedings of the International Conference on Advances in Electronics, Electrical & Computational Intelligence (ICAEEC)* (2019).
18. Cherif, L. H., Mostafi, M. & Debbal, S. Digital filters in Heart Sound Analysis. *International Journal of Clinical Medicine Research* **1,** 97–108 (2014).
19. Zhang, W. & Han, J. *Towards heart sound classification without segmentation using convolutional neural network* in *2017 Computing in Cardiology (CinC)* (2017), 1–4.
20. Chakir, F., Jilbab, A., Nacir, C. & Hammouch, A. Phonocardiogram signals processing approach for PASCAL classifying heart sounds challenge. *Signal, Image and Video Processing* **12,** 1149–1155 (2018).
21. Dominguez-Morales, J. P., Jimenez-Fernandez, A. F., Dominguez-Morales, M. J. & Jimenez-Moreno, G. Deep neural networks for the recognition and classification of heart murmurs using neuromorphic auditory sensors. *IEEE transactions on biomedical circuits and systems* **12,** 24–34 (2017).
22. Bozkurt, B., Germanakis, I. & Stylianou, Y. A study of time-frequency features for CNN-based automatic heart sound classification for pathology detection. *Computers in biology and medicine* **100,** 132–143 (2018).
23. Potes, C., Parvaneh, S., Rahman, A. & Conroy, B. *Ensemble of feature-based and deep learning-based classifiers for detection of abnormal heart sounds* in *2016 Computing in Cardiology Conference (CinC)* (2016), 621–624.

24. Rubin, J. *et al.* Recognizing abnormal heart sounds using deep learning. *arXiv preprint* arXiv:1707.04642 (2017).
25. Krishnan, P. T., Balasubramanian, P. & Umapathy, S. Automated heart sound classification system from unsegmented phonocardiogram (PCG) using deep neural network. *Physical and Engineering Sciences in Medicine,* 1–11 (2020).
26. Cheng, P. & Dong, X. Life-threatening ventricular arrhythmia detection with personalized features. *IEEE access* **5,** 14195–14203 (2017).
27. Khan, K. N. *et al.* Deep learning based classification of unsegmented phonocardiogram spectrograms leveraging transfer learning. *Physiological measurement* **42,** 095003 (2021).
28. Nogueira, D. M., Ferreira, C. A. & Jorge, A. M. *Classifying heart sounds using images of MFCC and temporal features* in *Progress in Artificial Intelligence: 18th EPIA Conference on Artificial Intelligence, EPIA 2017, Porto, Portugal, September 5-8, 2017, Proceedings 18* (2017), 186–203.
29. Nogueira, D. M., Ferreira, C. A., Gomes, E. F. & Jorge, A. M. Classifying heart sounds using images of motifs, MFCC and temporal features. *Journal of medical systems* **43,** 1–13 (2019).
30. Wood, J. C., Buda, A. J. & Barry, D. T. Time-frequency transforms: a new approach to first heart sound frequency dynamics. *IEEE Transactions on Biomedical Engineering* **39,** 730–740 (1992).
31. Wood, J. C. & Barry, D. T. Time-frequency analysis of the first heart sound. *IEEE Engineering in Medicine and Biology Magazine* **14,** 144–151 (1995).
32. Dastagir, J., Khan, F. A., Khan, M. S. & Khan, K. N. *Computer-aided phonocardiogram classification using multidomain time and frequency features* in *2021 International Conference on Artificial Intelligence (ICAI)* (2021), 50–55.
33. Sejdić, E., Djurović, I. & Jiang, J. Time-frequency feature representation using energy concentration: An overview of recent advances. *Digital signal processing* **19,** 153–183 (2009).
34. Abduh, Z., Nehary, E. A., Wahed, M. A. & Kadah, Y. M. Classification of heart sounds using fractional fourier transform based mel-frequency spectral coefficients and traditional classifiers. *Biomedical Signal Processing and Control* **57,** 101788 (2020).
35. Yildirim, M. Automatic classification and diagnosis of heart valve diseases using heart sounds with MFCC and proposed deep model. *Concurrency and Computation: Practice and Experience* **34,** e7232 (2022).
36. Liu, J. *et al.* Deep learning-based computer-aided heart sound analysis in children with left-to-right shunt congenital heart disease. *International journal of cardiology* **348,** 58–64 (2022).
37. Ren, Z. *et al. Learning image-based representations for heart sound classification* in *Proceedings of the 2018 international conference on digital health* (2018), 143–147.
38. Ahmad, B., Khan, F. A., Khan, K. N. & Khan, M. S. *Automatic classification of heart sounds using long short-term memory* in *2021 15th International Conference on Open Source Systems and Technologies (ICOSST)* (2021), 1–6.
39. Deng, M. *et al.* Heart sound classification based on improved MFCC features and convolutional recurrent neural networks. *Neural Networks* **130,** 22–32 (2020).
40. Malik, S. I., Akram, M. U. & Siddiqi, I. Localization and classification of heartbeats using robust adaptive algorithm. *Biomedical Signal Processing and Control* **49,** 57–77 (2019).
41. Li, S. & Tian, K. Unsupervised phonocardiogram analysis with distribution density based variational auto-encoders. *Frontiers in Medicine* **8,** 655084 (2021).
42. Deperlioglu, O., Kose, U., Gupta, D., Khanna, A. & Sangaiah, A. K. Diagnosis of heart diseases by a secure internet of health things system based on autoencoder deep neural network. *Computer Communications* **162,** 31–50 (2020).
43. Mishra, M., Menon, H. & Mukherjee, A. Characterization of S_1 and S_2 heart sounds using stacked autoencoder and convolutional neural network. *IEEE Transactions on Instrumentation and Measurement* **68,** 3211–3220 (2018).
44. Abduh, Z., Nehary, E. A., Wahed, M. A. & Kadah, Y. M. Classification of heart sounds using fractional Fourier transform based mel-frequency spectral coefficients and stacked autoencoder deep neural network. *Journal of Medical Imaging and Health Informatics* **9,** 1–8 (2019).

45. Li, S., Tian, K. & Wang, R. *Unsupervised heart abnormality detection based on phonocardiogram analysis with beta variational auto-encoders* in *ICASSP 2021–2021 IEEE International Conference on Acoustics, Speech and Signal Processing (ICASSP)* (2021), 8353–8357.
46. Deperlioglu, O. Heart sound classification with signal instant energy and stacked autoencoder network. *Biomedical Signal Processing and Control* **64,** 102211 (2021).
47. Banerjee, R. & Ghose, A. *A semi-supervised approach for identifying abnormal heart sounds using variational autoencoder* in *ICASSP 2020–2020 IEEE International Conference on Acoustics, Speech and Signal Processing (ICASSP)* (2020), 1249–1253.
48. Ismail, S., Ismail, B., Siddiqi, I. & Akram, U. PCG classification through spectrogram using transfer learning. *Biomedical Signal Processing and Control* **79,** 104075 (2023).

The manufacturer's authorised representative in the EU is Springer Nature Customer Service Centre GmbH, Europaplatz 3, 69115 Heidelberg, Germany. If you have any concerns regarding our products, please contact ProductSafety@springernature.com

Printed and bound by CPI Group (UK) Ltd, Croydon, CR0 4YY
01/10/2026
02225855-0004